Disclaimer: This textbook is not intended to provide, and disclaims any suggestion that it does provide, medical advice of any nature. The information made available through this textbook should not be used in place of seeking professional opinions by licensed practitioners. Only licensed medical professionals may offer medical advice, diagnosis and recommendations for treatment of medical conditions. You assume full responsibility for appropriate use of the information available through this textbook.

Published by RAEducation.com LLC Publications, Gainesville, FL USA
Produced by Kristine Lyle, Printers Workshop, Kalona, IA

ISBN-10: 1-948083-13-2
ISBN-13: 978-1-948083-13-3

Johan. P. Reyneke
B.Ch.D, M.Ch.D, FCMFOS (SA), Ph.D.

Extraordinary Professor, Division of Maxillofacial and Oral Surgery,
University of the Western Cape, South Africa

Clinical Professor, Department of Oral and Maxillofacial Surgery,
University of Oklahoma, Oklahoma City, USA

Visiting Professor, Department of Oral and Maxillofacial Surgery,
College of Dentistry, University of Florida, Gainesville, FL, USA

Visiting Professor, Division of Oral and Maxillofacial Surgery,
Universidad Autonoma de Nueva Leon, Monterrey, Mexico

Private Practice, Centre for Orthognathic Surgery,
Mediclinic, Cape Town, South Africa

Dedication

To Ingrid, my wife, my best friend,
my sole mate....my giant.

The Art and Science of the
Sliding Genioplasty

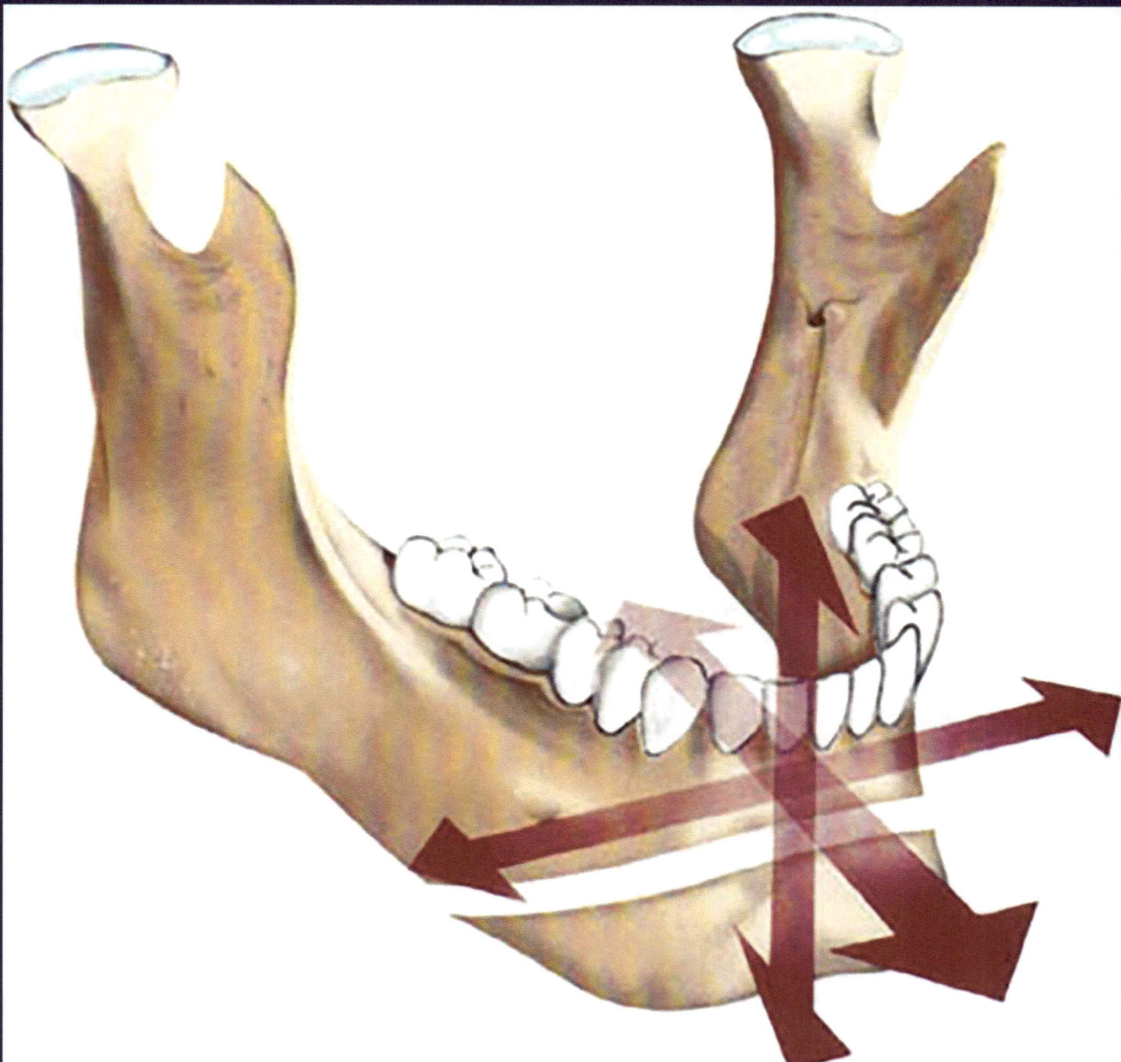

Preface

More than two thousand years ago, Cicero (106-43 BC) recognized the importance of the human face when he wrote: "Everything is in the face..." in *De Oratore, Volume III (50 BC)*. The face of an individual not only reveals his or her identity and origin, but also a person's emotions, such as happiness, sadness, fear, anger and friendliness. The chin, forms an integral part of the total facial esthetics and is often subconsciously associated with character or personality. A retruded or weak-shaped chin is generally regarded as a sign of femininity, timidity, indecision and shy behavior while a strong, square chin is often associated with aggressiveness, decisiveness, masculinity and bold behavior.

The chin is a key element of total facial harmony, however, it has no clearly defined function. Historically, the need for a strong biting action gradually became redundant with the discovery of fire - about 700,000 years ago. Tenderized food removed the need for a large strong jaw and it seems that the chin of modern man is simply a remnant of our specie's once larger jaw.

The main aims of orthognathic surgical treatment of dentofacial deformities are the correction of occlusal and oral functions, the establishment of a patent airway and to ensure well balanced and harmonious facial appearance. In our quest to achieve our treatment goals, genioplasty procedures are mostly performed as part of the orthognathic surgical correction. It is, therefore, a basic requirement for any physician wishing to practice orthognathic surgery to be well versed in the identification of any genial morphology that detracts from facial harmony and to develop an acuity in the surgical techniques required for its correction.

The orthognathic surgeon should have "the eye of an artist and the mind of a scientist." The science of the critical assessment of skeletal and soft tissue anomalies can be obtained by measurements and comparisons to the accepted norms using available data. The art, however, is a skill that should be acquired and refined by constant examination of faces. In the words of Armand Trousseau, a seventeenth century French surgeon, to his students: "Knowledge suffocates the scientist, whereas it gives the artist fresh inspiration. Therefore, learn as much as you can... but your learning must be the basis of your art and not an end to itself. A little less science and a little more art, Messieurs!"

The contemporary orthognathic surgeon recognizes the fact that the human chin should be seen as a three dimensional anatomical structure. Correction of chin deformities should therefore not only be considered in the horizontal, but also in the vertical and transverse dimensions. Harmony and balance of the chin from stomion inferius to menton, including the submental area and labio-mental fold should be a prime objective, however, the harmonious relationship of the chin in relation to overall facial esthetics is mandatory.

This text describes the clinical assessment of the hard and soft tissues of the chin and diagnosis of abnormalities. The importance of the three dimensional correction of chin deformities, and its relationship to the esthetic correction of total dentofacial deformities are emphasized, discussed and demonstrated. The radiographic evaluation and treatment planning through surgical visual objectives, the surgical techniques for genioplasty, treatment outcomes and complications are also discussed and demonstrated.

I thank Dr. Andre Boezaart for his encouragement, enthusiasm and assistance with this project. My admiration for him personally and his passion as an educator will never cease. I thank the many colleagues and post-graduate students for the pleasure I had sharing the wonders of orthognathic surgery with me.

~Johan P. Reyneke

Contents

Introduction

Over the past 2 million years, the face of the genus Homo developed a distinctive form, with our craniums expanding to accommodate an enlarging brain over the last 500,000 years. Although the chin is a prominent feature of the face, it has no clearly defined function. With the discovery of and ability to control fire about 1 million years ago, initially for heat and later for tenderizing and cooking food, the need for a strong biting action gradually became unnecessary and removed the need for a large, strong jaw. It seems, therefore, that the chin is simply a remnant of our once larger jaw.

Modern humans, Homo sapiens, evolved in Africa, most likely about 200,000 years ago. Anatomically, modern humans have features that distinguish them from various earlier humans and other apes. Our noses and jaws are in a more vertical alignment, giving us our distinctive human profile that is shared by no other animal. Our teeth and jaws became smaller and moved backward. Our skull now has a high-domed cranium and a high, smooth forehead, with no bony brow ridges. Our dental arches shifted backward, leaving a band of jawbone behind that results in the human chin (Fig 1.1).[1–5]

Faces have enchanted mankind for a very long time and even as far back as 55 BC, Cicero (106-43 BC) wrote, 'Everything is in the face...' in *De Oratore, Volume II.*[6] Psychological studies have shown that even as babies, we are drawn to faces; nine minutes after being born, when we can barely focus our eyes, we prefer to gaze at faces than at any other object.[7] Our faces form an intimate part of our lives, and each face can be considered as "custom made." All developmentally normal faces have two

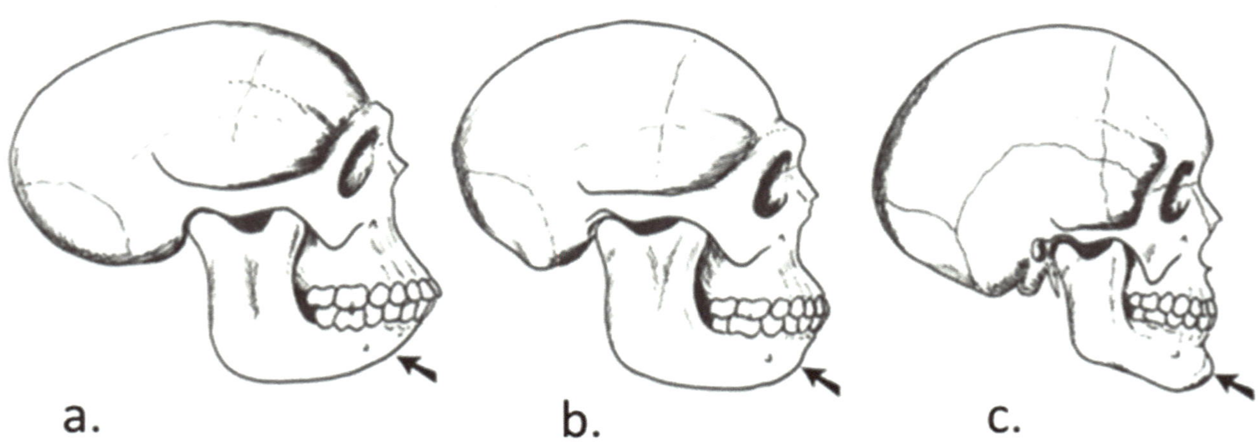

Figure 1.1 *The facial skeletons and sculls of homo erectus (a), archaic sapiens (b) and modern sapiens (c) illustrating the poorly developed chin of homo erectus compared to homo sapiens. The severe bimaxillary dental protrusion is lost and the profile has become straighter. The chin, albeit non-functional, has stayed in a forward position.*

eyes, a nose, two cheeks, a mouth, two ears, and a chin, and yet we all manage to somehow look extraordinarily different. The general ethnic differences in our facial features have evolved in response to inbreeding, subtle genetic mutations, isolation, and environmental challenges in different parts of the globe. The characteristics that are considered esthetically pleasing vary according to culture, ethnic type, and even historic period. There is also evidence that the general characteristics associated with facial beauty have changed very little throughout the history of Western European culture. However, the current preference in terms of facial beauty still differs between the various continents, for instance, in Africa, Asia, Greenland, etc.

The chin forms an integral part of the total facial esthetic, and any deformity in it will disturb the balance and harmony between the various facial components.

In an article in the STAR newspaper (June 30, 2001), David Grimes wrote, "I have come to the conclusion that my woeful situation has nothing to do with my reckless spending habits, innate laziness or the fact that I have worked at the same place for 25 years without a promotion. The fault lies entirely with my chin. Or, more specifically, my lack of chin. Chin challenged types like myself are doomed for a lifetime of overdue bills and used cars, whereas the chin-abled can look forward to his- and her-yachts, gold-plated commodes and conversations about the estate tax or at least so it would seem from an article I read recently in The New York Post."

Although this article was no doubt written tongue in cheek, we often use the words "weak" and "strong" to describe the chin, which is subconsciously associated with character or personality.[6,7] A retruded, oval-shaped chin is generally associated with femininity, whereas a strong, square chin is associated with masculinity.

Augmentation of the chin by either a horizontal osteotomy or the onlay of alloplastic material has, in the past, often been used as an adjunct to orthognathic, craniofacial, and plastic surgery procedures to improve facial balance. The decision to advance the mandible in orthognathic surgery has little, if anything, to do with chin projection. Whenever the chin is advanced by means of a sliding genioplasty as an esthetic compromise for mandibular advancement, the price is often paid in the form of poor chin shape. Chin projection is but one aspect of chin shape and good esthetics.

Numerous modifications to the basic surgical procedure of an osseous sliding genioplasty, their applications, and expected treatment results have been described.[8–11] However, the acuity of assessment of the chin and the versatility of the surgical procedure, as well as the art of achieving the esthetic demands of our patients, have not yet been specified.

The modern oral and maxillofacial surgeon can, by prudent application of artistic sense, knowledge of the principles of facial esthetics, and accurate execution of surgical techniques, change the chin contour in all three dimensions of space to improve and enhance facial beauty.

Chapter 1 - Surgical Anatomy of the Anterior Mandible

Embryology of the Chin

The skeleton of the anterior lower part of the face is formed mostly by a single bone, the anterior part of the mandible. In addition to its functional role (attachment for facial and masticatory muscles, muscles for speech, support for the teeth, and forming part of the temporomandibular articulation), the mandible plays a major part in the esthetics of the face.

The chin comprises two-thirds of the anterior mandible and is, at birth, quite small and inconspicuous. Many parents of a newborn are naturally worried about the chinless appearance of their little child. The whole mandible, however, tends to be slow in differential growth and will usually catch up with the maxilla in the normal adult face.

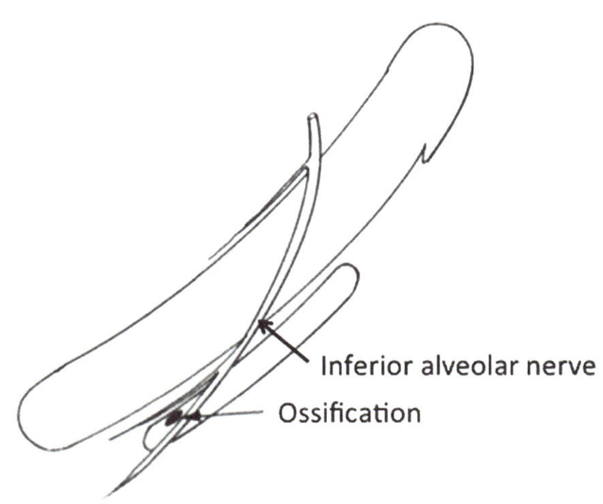

Figure 1.2 *The relationship of Meckel's cartilage to the mandibular (inferior alveolar) nerve (arrow) and the site where the first ossification starts (arrow) during the 7th intrauterine week.*

The mandible develops in relation to the first pharyngeal arch and is preceded by the cartilage of the primary cartilaginous skeleton, Meckel's cartilage. This hyaline cartilage attains full form by 6 weeks of intrauterine life and has a close relationship with the inferior alveolar (mandibular) nerve. The first ossification starts during the 7th week of intrauterine life lateral to the incisive and mental nerve *(Fig 1.2)*. As ossification continues, the bone of the two halves of the mandible come into close relationship in the middle where they are separated by fibrous tissue to form a symphysis. Bony union (synostosis) is not complete until the end of the first year of life. The mandibular symphysis in the adult patient is therefore a misnomer as it is actually a synostosis.[12]

Growth of the Mandible in the Chin Area

At birth, the mandible essentially has the structures of the adult mandible, however, the mandibular angle is obtuse and the chin is round and ill defined *(Fig 1.3)*. In the early stages of postnatal mandibular development, growth takes place by deposition and resorbtion of bone beginning at about 10 weeks around the expanding tooth germs. After about 15 weeks, the labial surface of the chin is augmented by bone deposition, while the lingual surface is resorbed *(Fig 1.4)*. This mechanism produces a forward growth movement in the incisor region.[13]

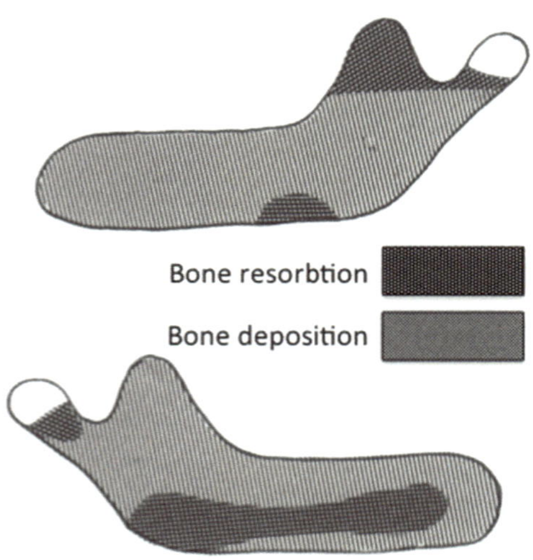

Figure 1.3 *The mandible at birth showing the areas of resorbtion and bone deposition that took place during the intrauterine development of the mandible.*

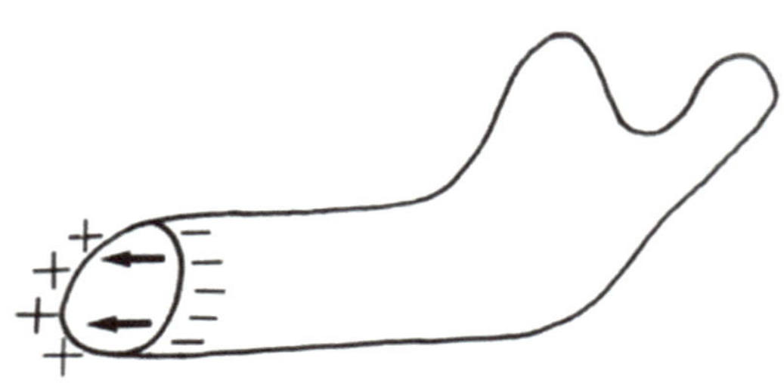

Figure 1.4 *The anterior mandible grows forward by labial bone deposition (+) and lingual resorbtion (-) starting at about 10 weeks after birth.*

Vertical growth of the alveolar process takes place stimulated by the eruption of deciduous teeth, the developing permanent teeth, and vertical growth of the mandibular ramus. During the deciduous dentition period of childhood, horizontal growth remodeling takes place in the incisor alveolar region by anterior resorbtion and lingual deposition of bone, while augmentation in the chin area takes place by anterior deposition of bone *(Fig 1.5).* The lower incisors usually undergo lingual tipping (retro-inclination) to achieve a functional relation with the upper incisors.[14]

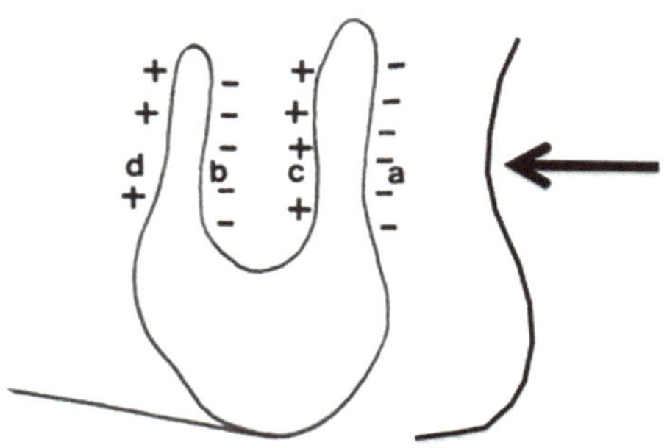

Figure 1.5 *A reversal of the growth field in the superior part of the mandible takes place and the convex surface becomes concave, eventually responsible for the depth and height of the labiomental fold (arrow). The remodeling process involves subperiosteal resorbtion on the labial side of the labial bony cortex (a) and alveolar side of the lingual cortex (b) and bone composition on the alveolar side of the labial cortex (c) and lingual side of the lingual cortex (d).*

Bone is progressively added to the external and inferior surface of the chin. This slow growth proceeds gradually throughout childhood *(Fig 1.6)* and it is from this time that the chin begins to take on a more prominent form. The mental protuberance and tubercles becomes larger and continue to grow anteriorly through bone deposition. At the same time, the alveolar bone, superior to the chin, moves posteriorly (anterior

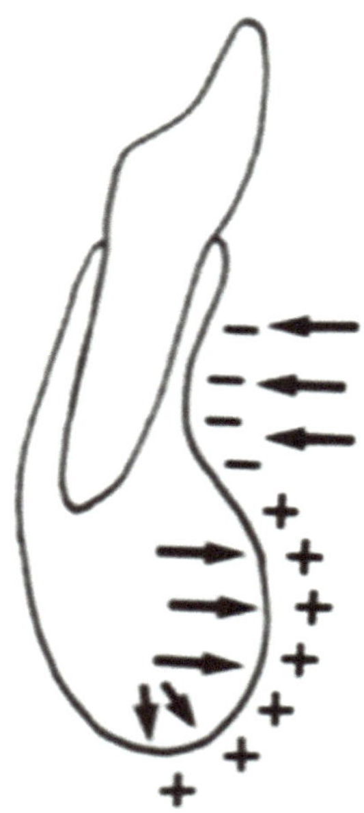

Figure 1.6 *Bone is progressively added to the chin surface including the mental protruberance (+). Deposition of bone also takes place on the inferior surface increasing the height of the chin (+arrows). Resorbtion of the anterior alveolar surface also takes place (-arrows).*

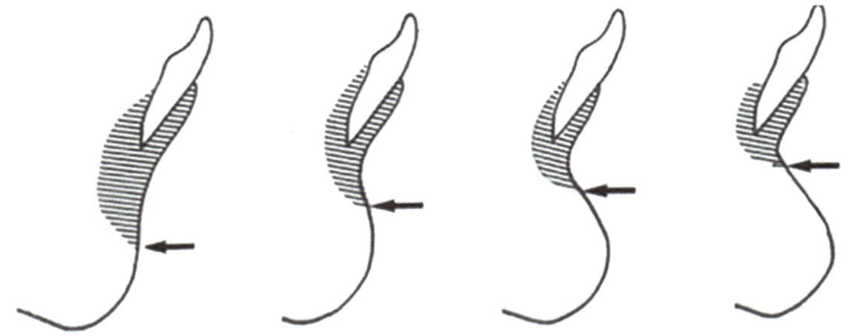

Figure 1.7 *There is a large variation of the height of the reversal line (arrows) between the anterior resorbtion of the alveolar process and deposition of bone in the chin area; it may be high or low. There is also a considerable variation in the relative amounts of bone resorbtion and deposition; which results in a corresponding variation in shape and size of the chin among individuals.*

resorbtion and bone deposition lingually) until the lower permanent incisors reach their definitive anteroposterior position.[15,16]

It is during this stage of development of the chin that the eventual shape of the chin is determined *(Figs 1.7 and 1.8).* It should, however, be kept in mind that the development of the chin forms an integral part of the development of the mandible as a whole.

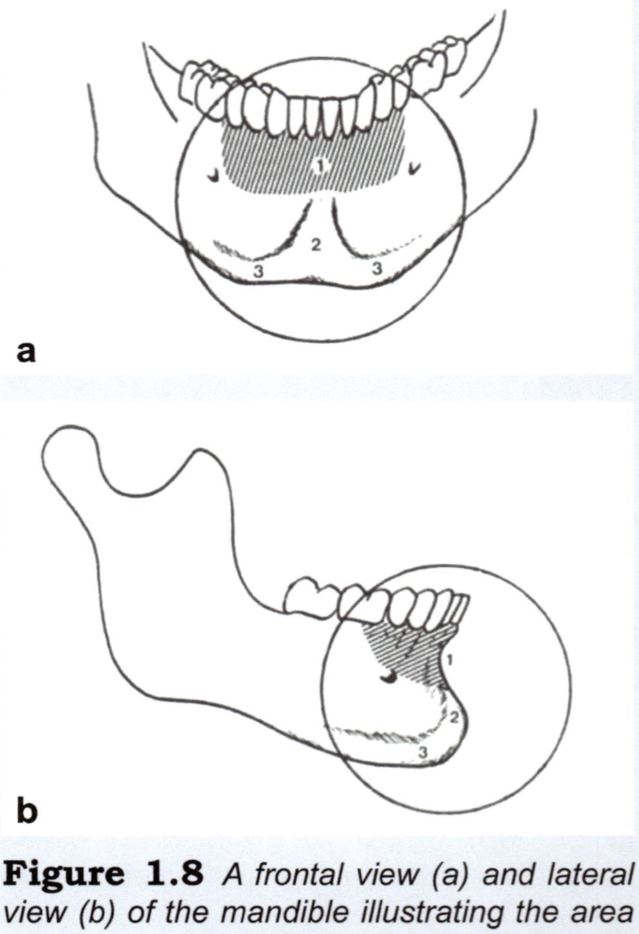

Figure 1.8 *A frontal view (a) and lateral view (b) of the mandible illustrating the area of resorbtion (1). Bone deposition on the anterior surface of the chin is responsible for the development of the mental protuberance medially (2) and the mental tubercles laterally (3). These two elements are responsible for the eventual width, size and shape of the chin.*

Increased vertical growth of the midface will lead to a clockwise rotation of the mandible, affecting the eventual anteroposterior position of the chin. The chin projection and shape may therefore be well balanced in relation to the mandible itself, however, due to the downward and backward rotation of the mandible, it may appear deficient in relation to the rest of the face *(Fig 1.9)*.

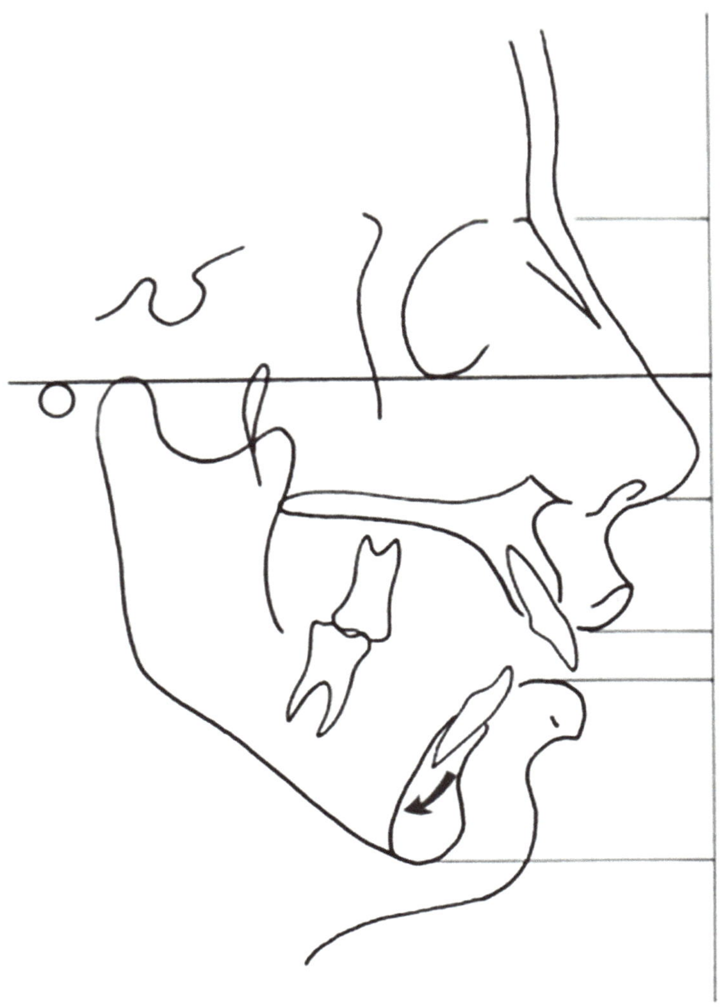

Figure 1.9 *A lateral cephalometric tracing of a patient with vertical maxillary excess and mandibular anteroposterior deficiency. The mandible has rotated clockwise, downwards and backwards (arrow). Although the chin shape and projection are balanced relative to the mandible it appears deficient in relation to the rest of the face.*

Osteology of the Anterior Mandible

The bone of the anterior mandible below the alveolar process (containing the incisor and canine teeth) forms the chin. The anterior mandible is V- or U-shaped and the mental protuberance is situated in the center of the anterior surface with a prominence on each side called the mental tubercule. The anteroposterior thickness of the mandible at the symphysis area in adults varies from 10 to 20 mm. The anteroposterior thickness may limit the amount of advancement possible with sliding augmentation genioplasty. Further posteriorly, the mental foramen is usually situated between the two bicuspid teeth halfway between the superior and inferior border of the mandible. The foramen faces backward and slightly upward and lends exit to the inferior alveolar nerve from the inferior alveolar canal *(Fig 1.10).*

On the lingual surface of the mandible, anteriorly, four mental spines also called genial tubercles (two superior and two inferior) are situated in the midline with a digastric fossa on each side, lateral and inferior to the spines. The mylohyoid line runs from posterior to anterior on the lingual surface, separating the submandibular and sublingual fossae *(Fig 1.11).*

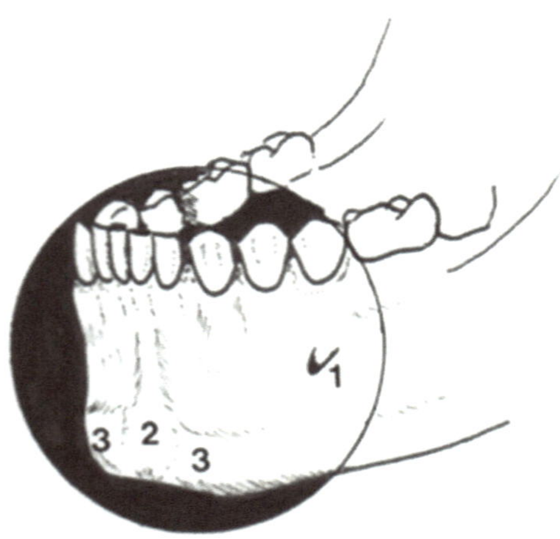

Figure 1.10 *A 45 degree lateral view of the anterior mandible illustrating the: mental foramen (1), mental protuberance in the center (2) and mental tubercles laterally (3).*

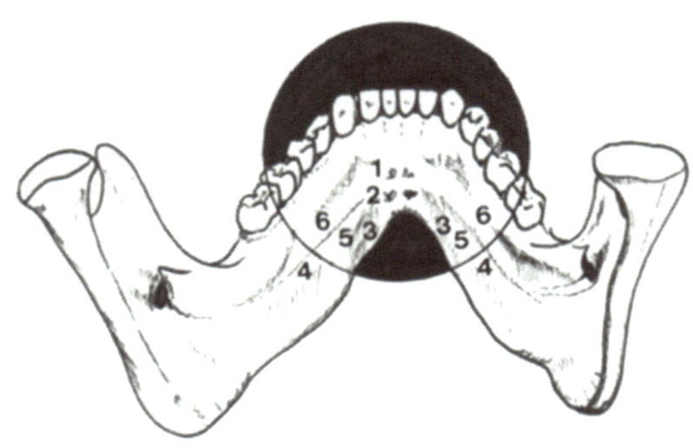

Figure 1.11 *The lingual view of the anterior mandible.*

Muscle Attachments in the Chin Area

The following muscles attach to the labial surface of the anterior mandible *(Fig 1.12)* and the orientation of the muscles in the oral and chin area appear as illustrated in Figure 1.13:

1. Mentalis
2. Depressor labii inferius
3. Depressor anguli oris
4. Platysma

When performing a genioplasty osteotomy, the mentalis muscles are the only facial expression muscles that are important from a surgical point of view. The other muscles listed in Figure 1.13 are stripped from the mandible by subperiosteal dissection and should be carefully reattached during soft tissue closure. The mentalis muscle, however, is bisected by soft tissue incision. *(See Chapter 4, Surgical Techniques.)* The mentalis muscles are paired arising from the anterior mandible from the middle of the roots of the lower incisor teeth superiorly to just inferior of the apexes of the teeth *(Fig 1.13)*. A firm septum of adipose tissue separates the two muscles. The superior fi-

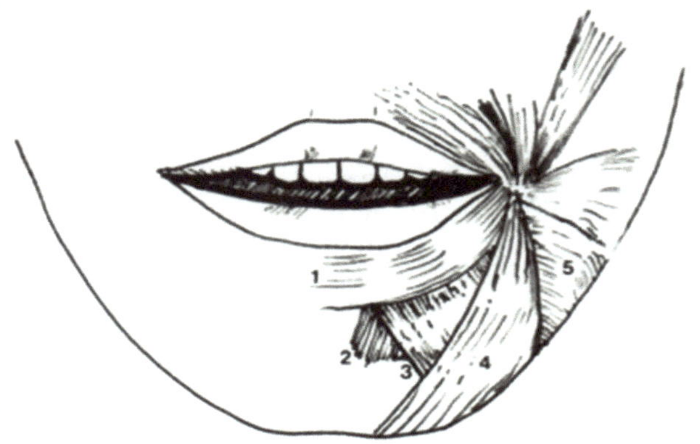

1. Orbicularis oris
2. Mentalis
3. Depressor labii inferius
4. Depressor anguli oris
5. Platysma

Figure 1.13 *The orientation of the facial muscles in the chin and peri-oral region.*

1. Mentalis muscle
2. Depressor labii,inferius
3. Depressor anguli oris
4. Platysma

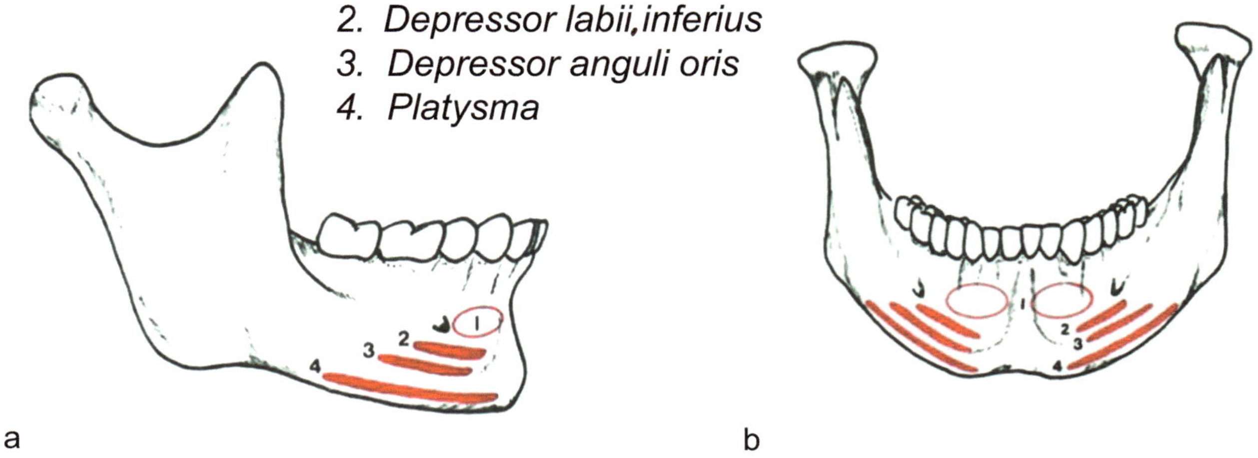

Figure 1.12 *Lateral view (a) and frontal view (b) of the mandible illustrating the muscle attachments of the anterior mandibular surface.*

bers pass almost horizontally into the skin of the upper part of the chin. The lower fibers pass vertically and obliquely to the skin of the lower part of the chin *(Fig 1.14).*

Incorrect repositioning of these muscles during suturing, after genioplasty, will lead to poor chin shape, "drooping" of the chin, and sagging of the lower lip, often exposing the lower incisor teeth. *(See Chapter 6, Complications.)* The mentalis muscle is supplied by the marginal mandibular branch of the facial nerve and is the only elevator of the lower lip and chin.

During surgery, as much of the muscle attachments as possible should be maintained:

1. to reduce postoperative bone resorbtion and
2. to increase accuracy when predicting the soft tissue result.

The following muscles *(Fig 1.15)* are attached to the lingual surface of the anterior mandible:

1. Genioglossus
2. Geniohyoideus
3. Mylohyoid
4. Digastric

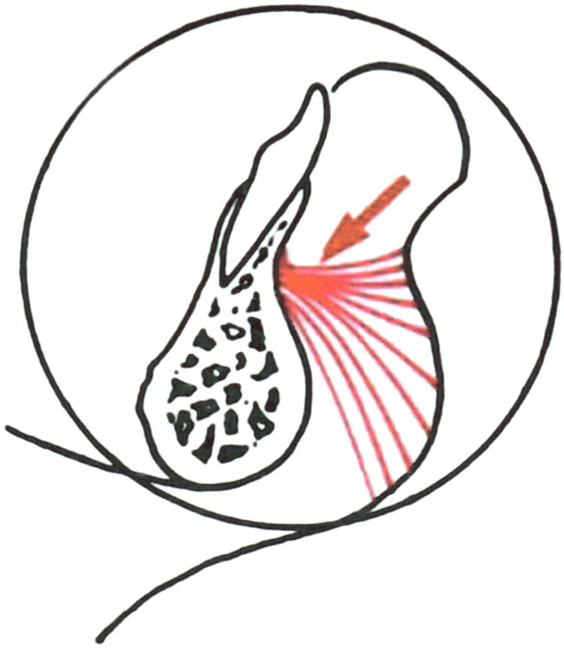

Figure 1.14 *The attachment of the mentalis muscles to the anterior mandible and the direction of the muscle fibers towards the skin are demonstrated. This muscle is bisected at an angle of 45 degrees (arrow) to the bone during the exposure of the bone when performing the genioplasty. The angulated incision facilitates easy re-approximation of the muscle during suturing.*

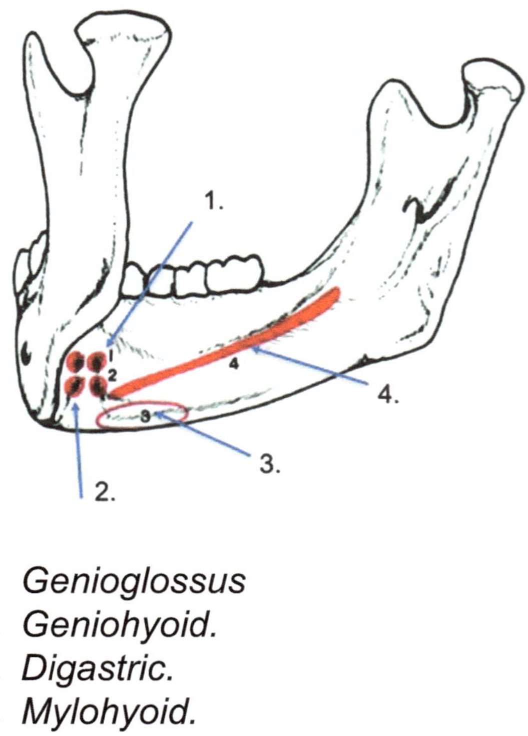

Figure 1.15 *A 45 degree posterior view of the mandible illustrating the muscle attachments on the lingual surface of the anterior part of the mandible.*

Care should be taken not to damage these soft tissue structures when performing the osteotomy through the lingual cortex. The height of the genioplasty osteotomy through the lingual cortex is indicated in Figure 1.16. *(See Chapter 4, Surgical Technique.)*

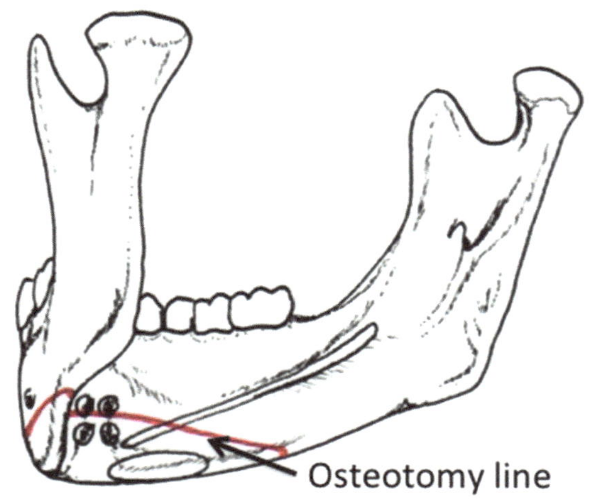

Figure 1.16 *A 45 degree posterior view of the mandible. The horizontal osteotomy line (red) demonstrates the involvement of the muscle attachments with the osteotomy on the lingual surface of the mandible.*

The Mental Nerve

The mental nerve is a cutaneous branch of the inferior alveolar nerve (originating from the mandibular third division of the trigeminal nerve [third cranial nerve]). After its exit from the mental foramen, it divides into a tuft of branches that radiate away from the foramen to supply the skin and mucous membrane of the lower lip and labial gingiva from the midline to the premolar teeth area. Some of its terminal branches run in the submucosal layer of the lip, and care should be taken not to damage the nerve by placing the soft tissue incision for the genioplasty too far labially or laterally. *(See Chapter 6, Complications.)* These branches become superficial and can usually be seen beneath the mucosa of the lower lip when it is everted.

The mental nerve is accompanied by an artery and vein, which are surgically insignificant.

Vascular Supply

The labial branch of the facial artery is the major vascular supplier of blood to the skin and muscles of the chin *(Fig 1.17)*.

The inferior alveolar artery is a branch of the maxillary artery and provides the primary supply of blood to the mandibular bone and teeth. It travels through the inferior alveolar canal in the mandible and divides into two branches at the level of the mental foramen. The mental artery exits from the bone with the mental nerve. The intraosseous branches continue anteriorly and supply the anterior mandible.

The submental artery originates as a branch of the facial artery and is given off as a branch just before the facial artery crosses the inferior border of the mandible. It then accompanies the mylohyoid nerve into the submandibular fossa where it supplies the anterior belly of the digastic and mylohyoid muscles, and it sends perforating branches through the floor of the mouth to the sublingual gland *(Fig 1.18)*.

The lingual artery supplies the musculature of the tongue and anteriorly it gives off the sublingual artery to supply blood to the sublingual gland *(Fig 1.17)*. Indiscriminate perforation of the lingual cortex of the mandible may occur in this area by oscillating or rotating instruments or a sharp osteotome may perforate this vessel. Arterial hemorrhage may lead to hematoma formation in the sublingual fossa, pushing the floor of the mouth and tongue upward. This will often distress patients and make normal speech difficult. However, it will seldom lead to airway obstruction and will usually resolve spontaneously. *(See Chapter 6, Complications.)*

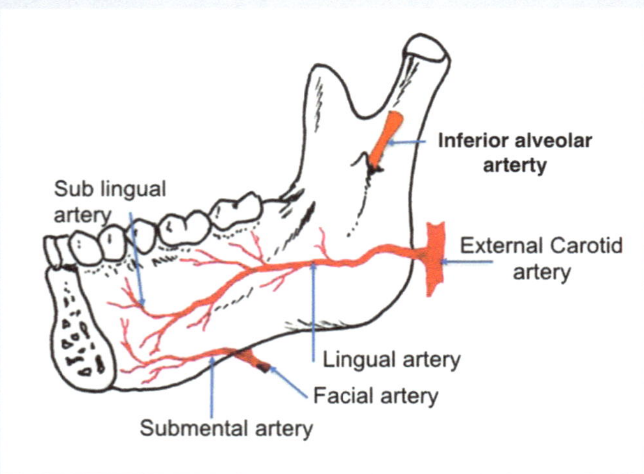

Figure 1.17 *Vascular supply to the hard and soft tissues chin. A medial view of the mandible.*

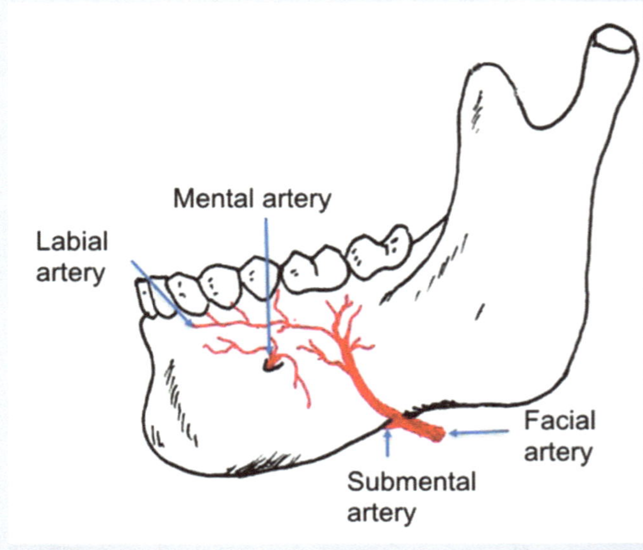

Figure 1.18 *Vascular supply of the chin. A lateral view of the mandible.*

Chapter 2 - Systematic Evaluation of Chin Deformities

Sliding genioplasty procedures are most often performed as part of the orthognathic surgical correction of dentofacial deformities. The clinical and cephalometric assessment of the chin should therefore form part of the total orthognathic evaluation of the patient. For the purpose of this evaluation, it will be assumed that all facial structures other than the chin are functional and aesthetically pleasing or will be surgically and orthodontically positioned to produce facial harmony and esthetic balance. Final assessment and surgical planning of chin esthetics are performed once the visual correction of maxillary and mandibular planning has been completed. This text will concentrate only on the evaluation of the chin, its relation to other facial structures in a normal position, and the esthetic changes that can be effected by means of surgery.

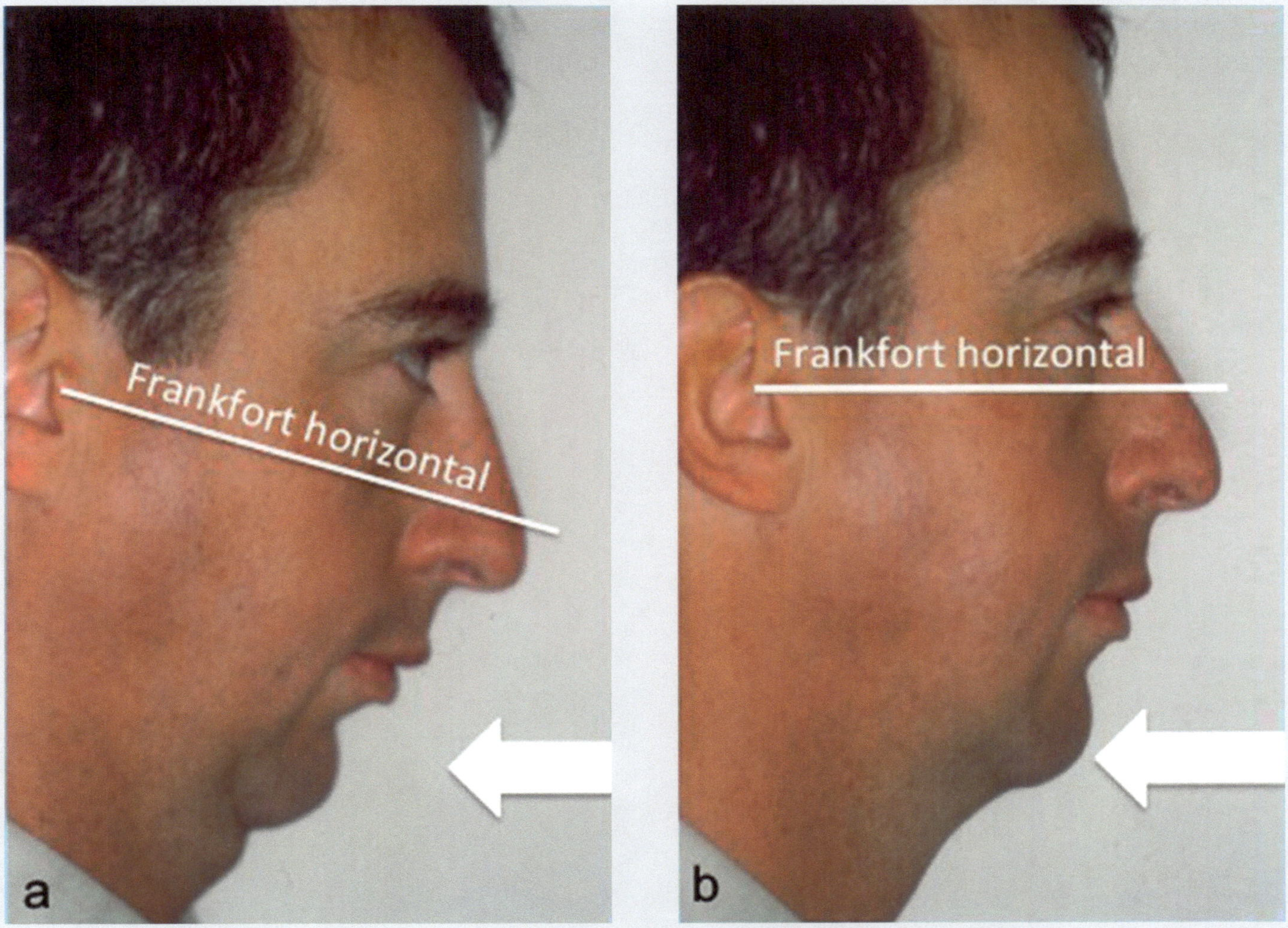

Figure 2.1 *The profound influence that head posture has on chin projection (arrows), chin-submental angle and chin-neck length is well demonstrated by comparing the profile view of this patient with head tipped down (a) and the head in natural posture (b).*

Clinical Evaluation

Anatomically, the chin is considered to be the soft tissue area below the labiomental fold. The lower lip and labiomental fold, however, form an integral part of chin esthetics. When examining the chin, the clinician should, therefore, consider all the structures that form the lower third of the face, from subnasale to soft tissue menton. It is difficult to isolate all the individual parts because the examiner should evaluate the size, shape, and position of each structure in relation to one another. In addition, the submental and neck area, as well as the nasal projection, should be included in the evaluation. Emphasis should be placed on the frontal esthetic evaluation of the chin because patients view themselves from the front and are often least aware of their profiles.

Patients should be examined in a natural head posture, with the teeth in occlusion and the lips relaxed. Figure 2.1 illustrates the profound effect a change in head posture has on the chin projection, chin–neck length, and chin–neck angle, while Figure 2.2 demonstrates the dramatic change in chin morphology with the lips in repose and when they are forced together.

A proper diagnosis can only be made and skeletal and soft tissue changes planned when the patient is examined with the head in a natural posture and the lips relaxed.

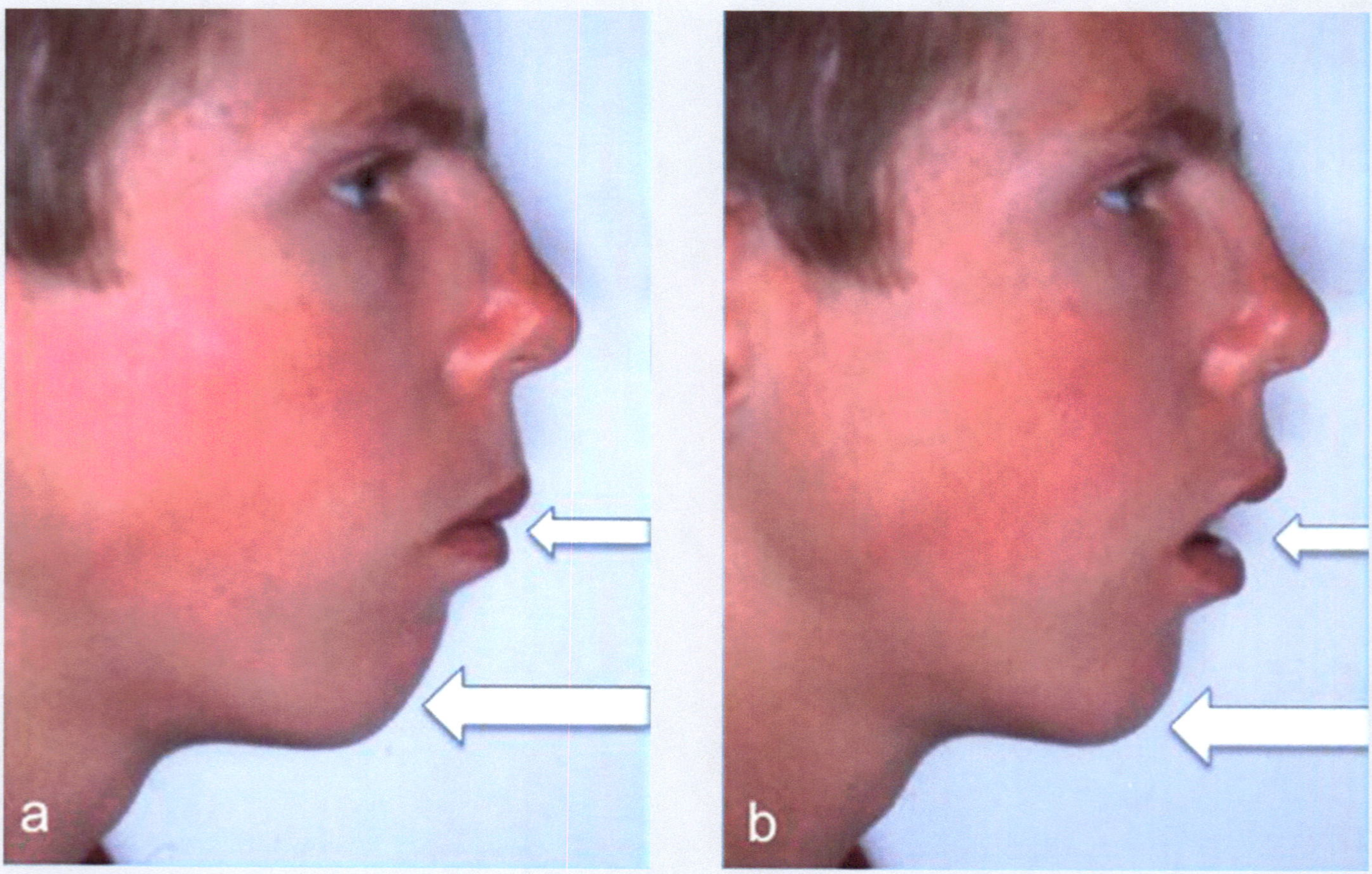

Figure 2.2 *A comparison between the two profile views of this patient reveals the change in labiomental fold, the lips and the shape of the chin with the lips strained (a) and the lips in repose and chin muscles relaxed (b) (arrows).*

Soft Tissue Evaluation - Frontal View Analysis

First, the general form of the face is assessed and categorized as round, oval, square, or long and the shape of the chin in relation to the facial form is correlated. At the same time, the characteristic facial differences between male and female faces should be considered. It is expected that females will have smaller, more rounded chins, whereas it is considered more attractive for males to have broad, square-shaped chins.

In general, two head shapes exist: the long, narrow head form (dolichocephalic) and the wide, short, globular head form (brachicephalic). The dolichocephalic form usually corresponds to a long, narrow, convex face with a narrow, pointed chin known as a leptoprosopic chin. Conversely, the brachicephalic form corresponds to a broad, box-like face and square chin known as the euryprosopic facial type *(Fig 2.3)*.[1] Ideal harmony between the facial structures results in facial beauty, thus shape, form, size, and position of the chin should be in harmony with the particular facial type.

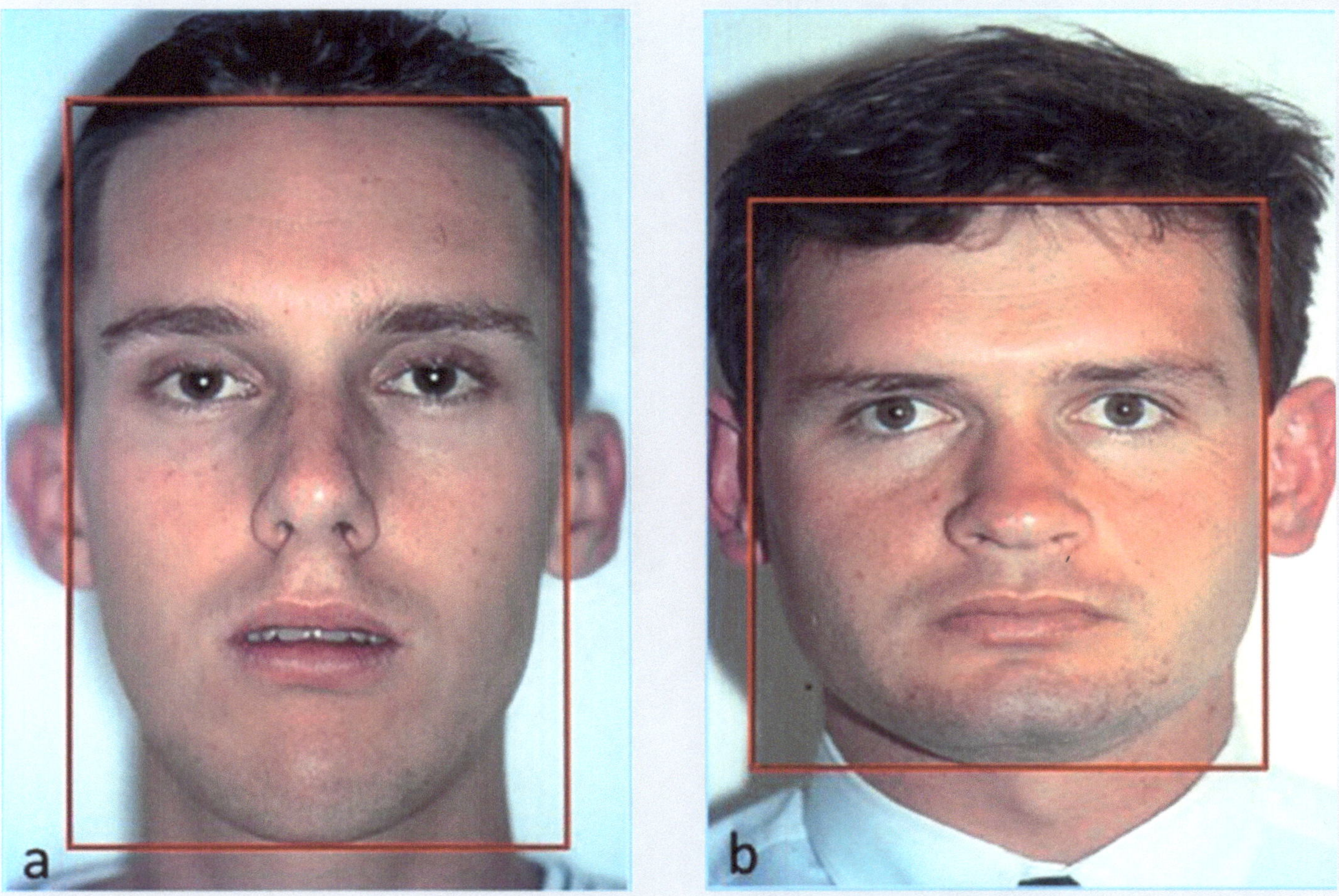

Figure 2.3 **a.** *A dolichocephalic head (narrow head form) with a leptoprosopic face (vertically long, convex face with a narrow chin), compared to a* **b.** *brachicephalic head (wide and square) with an euryprosopic face (broad and short). Note the difference in chin size and shape.*

The mandible should have a well-defined, smooth inferior border, from angle to chin, with a definite separation of the lower third of the face from the neck. *(Fig 2.4)* An ill-defined lower border of the mandible distracts from good chin–neck esthetics.

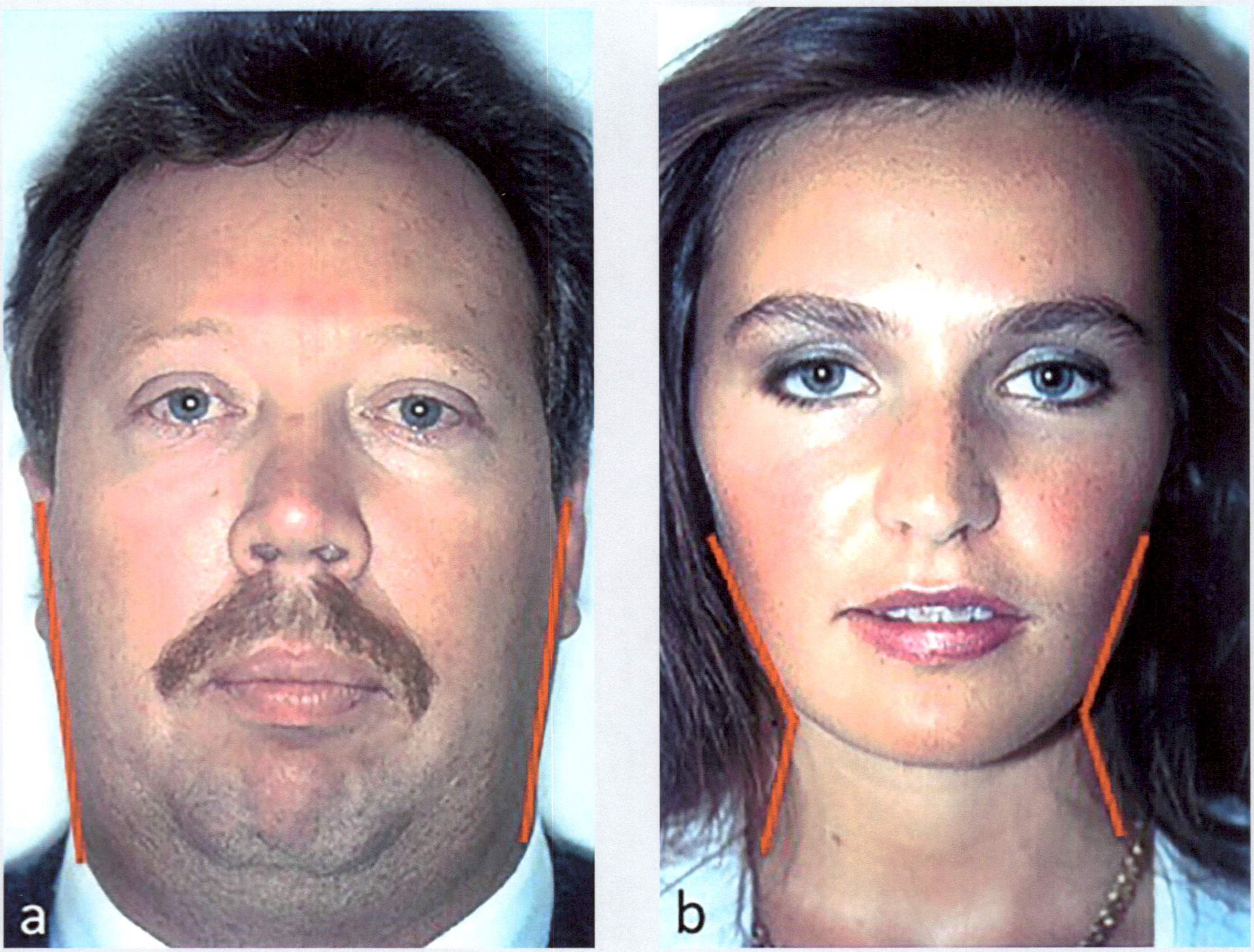

Figure 2.4 **a.** *An ill defined lower border of the mandible and the chin with poor separation between the neck and mandible is demonstrated.* **b.** *The mandible has a smooth well-defined lower border from angle to chin with a definite separation from the neck.*

Transverse dimension. The bigonial width of the face is approximately 30% less than the bizygomatic dimension, tapering down toward the chin, and the width of the chin should be in balance with the above transverse relation *(Fig 2.5)*.

Patients with leptoprosopic facial features also often have transversely deficient, "pointed" chins that seem separate from the mandible. For these patients, advancement of the chin by means of a traditional horizontal sliding osteotomy may improve the profile, however, it will accentuate the "pointiness" of the chin from the frontal view. For these patients, an advancement of the chin should be accompanied by simultaneous transverse augmentation for the best esthetic result.

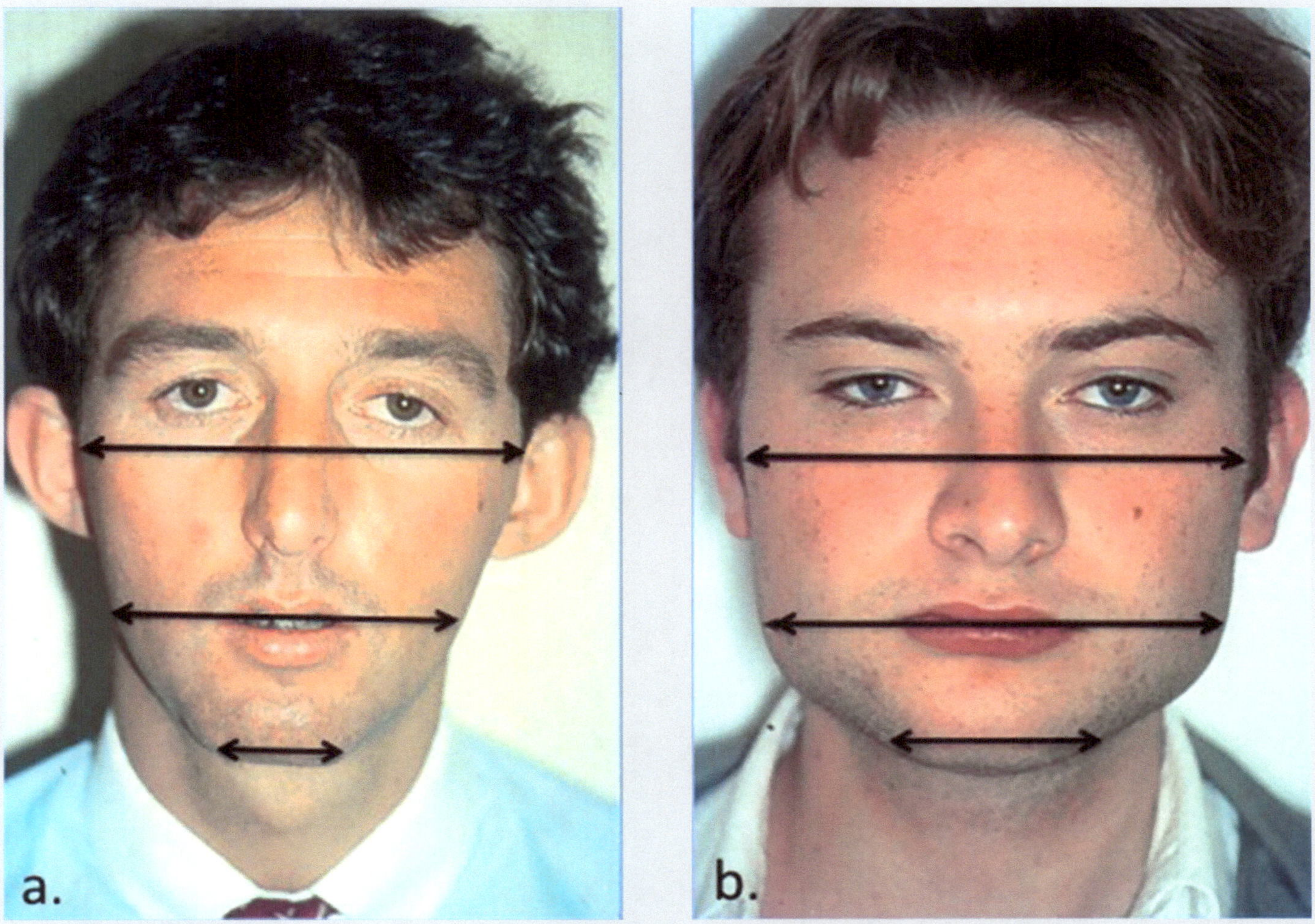

Figure 2.5 *The inter-zygomatic, bigonial width and the transverse dimension of the chin are narrow (arrows) (a), compared to the more rounded and broad transverse dimensions of the face in (arrows) (b).*

The esthetically pleasing chin should not have any parasymphyseal depressions or "marionette grooves," which often occurs accentuated with age.[2] *(Fig 2.6)* An advancement genioplasty without lateral augmentation will deepen these groves. Patients with broad, square chins, flat labiomental folds, and class III occlusions requiring mandibular setback procedures often need slight advancement of the chin to create a pleasing labiomental fold. Simultaneous narrowing of the chin should always be considered, especially for female patients, to reduce the strong square appearance. In all cases, the surgeon's objective should be to achieve a well-defined, smooth lower border of the mandible from the angle to the symphysis.

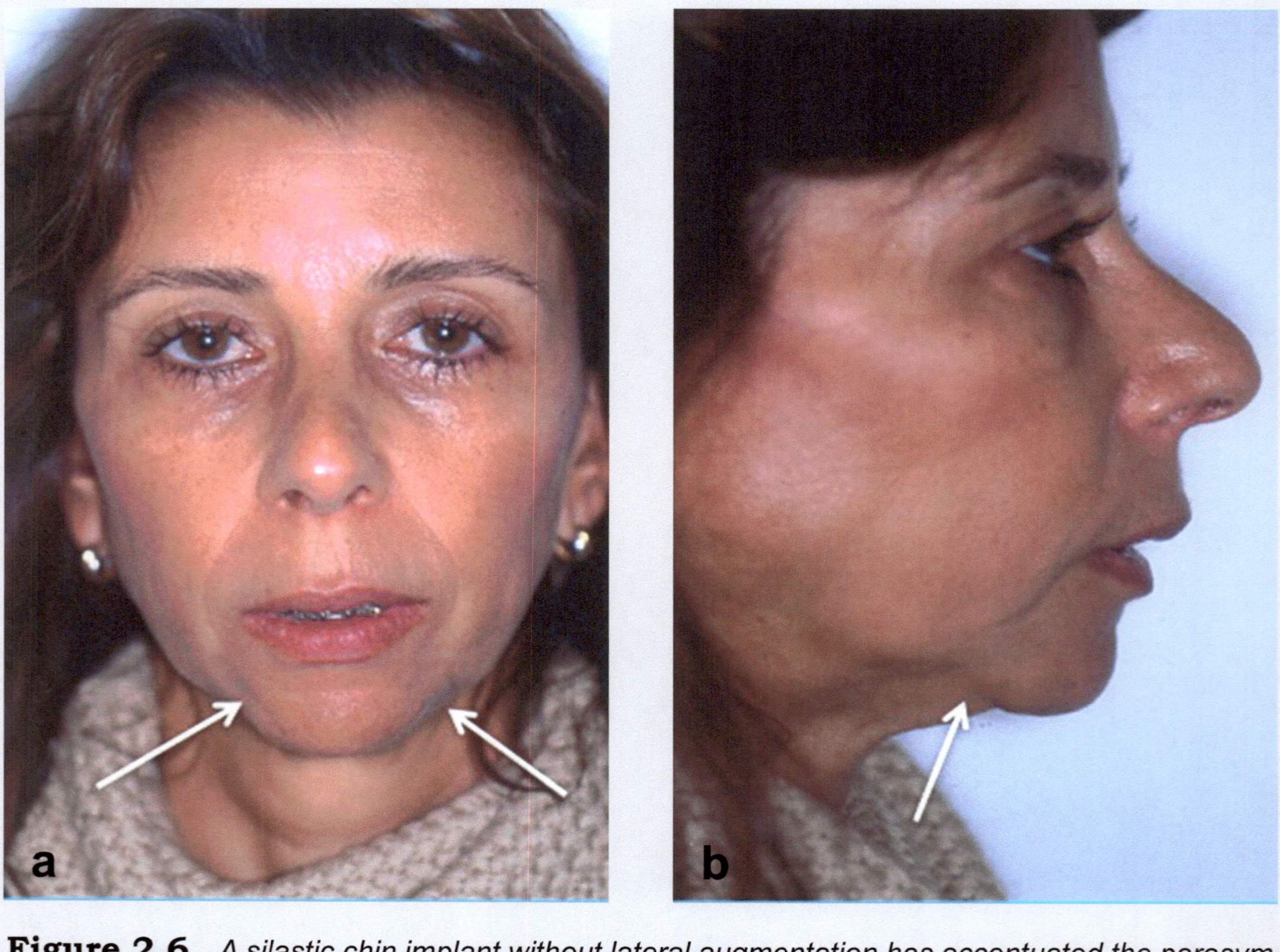

Figure 2.6 *A silastic chin implant without lateral augmentation has accentuated the parasymphyseal depressions (arrows).* **a.** *Frontal view* **b.** *Profile view*

Vertical dimensions. For the frontal vertical assessment, the following structures should be evaluated: the upper lip length, upper lip vermillion, lower lip vermillion, lower lip length, labiomental fold, chin button, and submental area. The part of the chin from the depth of the labiomental fold to the menton is called the chin button. Upper lip length (Sn – Stm[i]) should comprise one-third of the lower third facial height. Normal upper lip length is 20±2 mm for females and 22±2 mm for males. Upper lip vermillion exposure should be 25% less than the lower lip vermillion exposure. The amount of upper and lower lip vermillion exposure is influenced by upper and lower incisor teeth position. Maxillary dental protrusion will lead to increased upper lip vermillion exposure, whereas in maxillary anteroposterior-deficient cases, the upper lip vermillion will tend to be deficient.

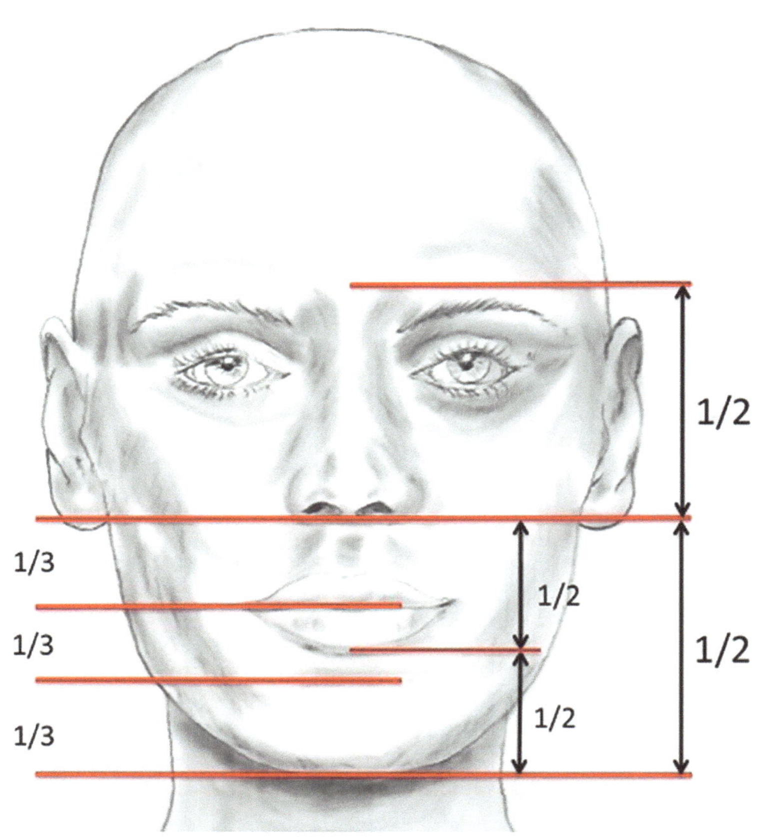

Figure 2.7 *The lower third of the face is divided in two halves, from subnasale to lower lip vermillion and from lower lip vermillion to soft tissue menton. This third of the face is also divided into thirds: from subnasale to stomion, stomion to labiomental fold and from labiomental fold to soft tissue menton. Vertical balance is more important than absolute dimensions when judging facial harmony.*

Due to the effect of the maxillary incisor teeth on the lower lip in Class II cases with increased overjet, the lower lip will be everted with excessive lower lip vermillion exposure and an acute labiomental fold. An attempt to correct an anteroposterior-deficient chin without correcting the increased overbite will deepen the labiomental fold and give the chin a "knobby" appearance with poor esthetics.

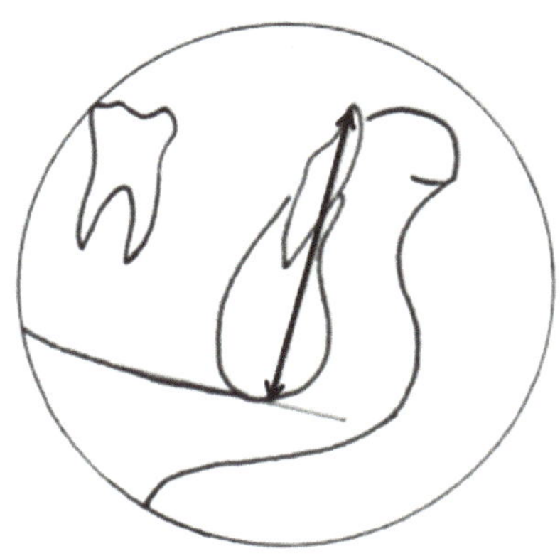

Figure 2.8 *The lower dental height is measured from lower incisor tip to menton (arrow) and should be ±42mm.*

The height of the lower lip stomion (Stm^s) to the labiomental fold should be equal to the distance from the depth of the labiomental fold to soft tissue menton (Me'). *(Fig 2.7)* The lower lip and chin should comprise two-thirds of the lower facial height with a length of 40±2 mm for females and 44±2 mm for males, measured from lower lip stomion (Stm^s) to soft tissue menton (Me'). *(Fig 2.7)* The lower lip length should also be related to the lower anterior dental height, and in deep bite cases, it should be evaluated with the teeth apart and the lips relaxed and just touching.[3] *(Fig 2.8)*

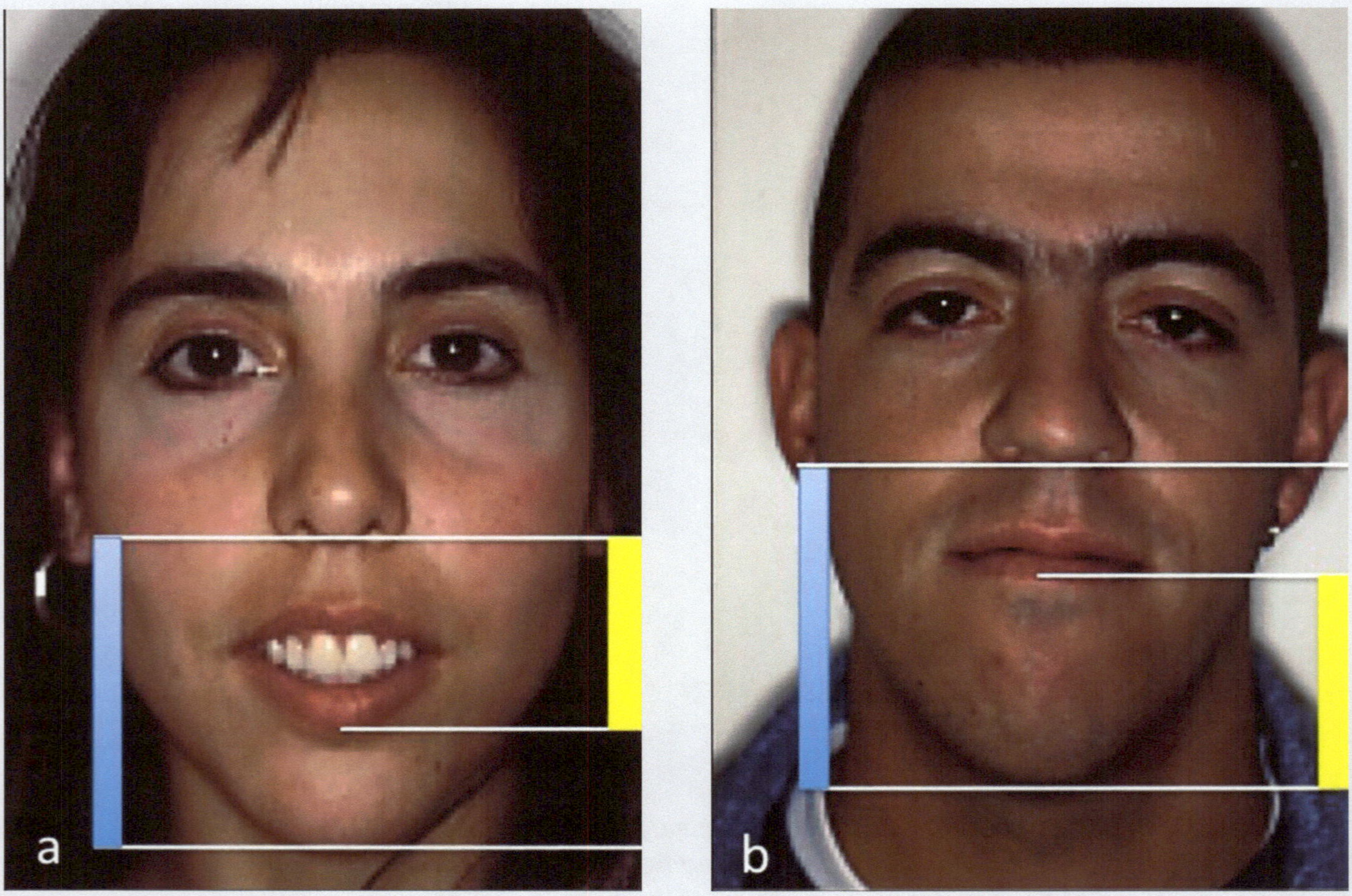

Figure 2.9 *Two examples of an increase of the lower facial third height* **a.** *The height of the lower facial third (blue) is influenced by vertical maxillary excess, the upper half of the lower facial third (yellow).* **b.** *The lower facial third height (blue) is increased due to vertical mandibular excess, a vertical increase of the chin (yellow).*

It has been emphasised that the chin should be examined with the soft tissue relaxed and lips in repose. Patients with vertical maxillary excess and an anterior open bite with increased interlabial gaps often have hyperactive mentalis muscle activity *(Fig 2.10).* This should be noted when the soft tissue thickness of the lips and chin are evaluated. Poor orbicularis oris muscle tone may contribute to an everted, procumbent lower lip that may expose the lower incisor teeth.

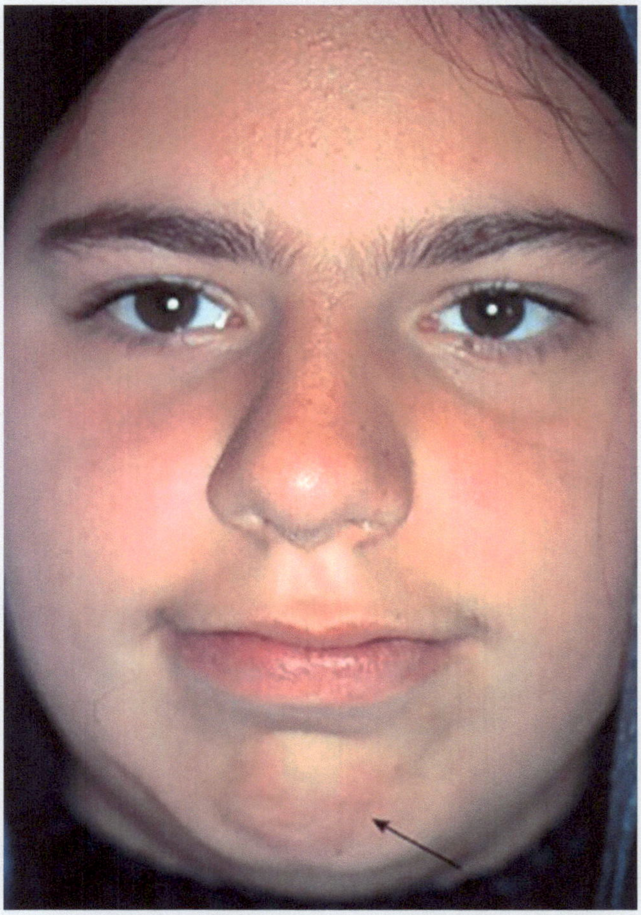

Figure 2.10 *The soft tissue thickness of the chin is distorted due to the hyperactivity of the mentalis muscle.*

Chin asymmetry. The symmetry of the chin should be assessed in relation to the facial midline as well as the dental midlines *(Fig 2.11)*.[5] If the chin is asymmetric to the facial midline and the midline of the lower incisors is coincident to the facial midline, the symmetry should be corrected by means of genioplasty. *(Fig 2.12)* If the chin is asymmetric to the facial midline and the midline of the lower incisors coincides with the midline of the chin and both are asymmetric, correction should be done by mandibular surgery. *(Fig 2.13)*

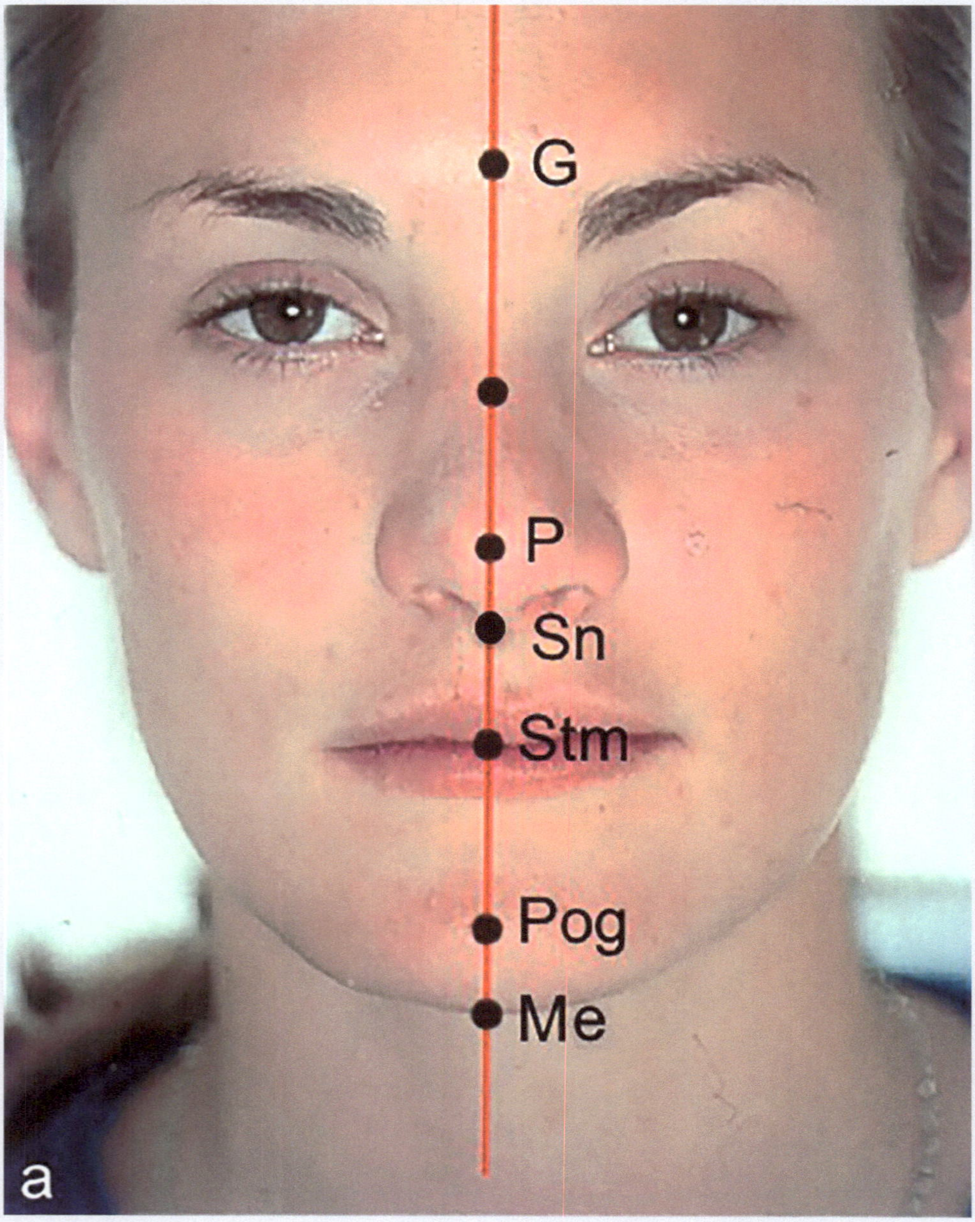

G - Glabella. *Most anterior point of the forehead.*

P - Pronasale. *The most anterior point of the nose.*

Sn - Subnasale. *The point at which the columella of the nose merges with the upper lip in the mid sagittal plane.*

Stm- Stomion *The center of the lips.*

Pog- Pogonion. *The most anterior point of the chin in the mid-sagittal plane.*

Me - Menton. *The lowest point on the contour of the soft tissue of the chin. Found by dropping a perpendicular line from horizontal through skeletal menton.*

Figure 2.11 *These soft tissue points should all fall on the same vertical line.*

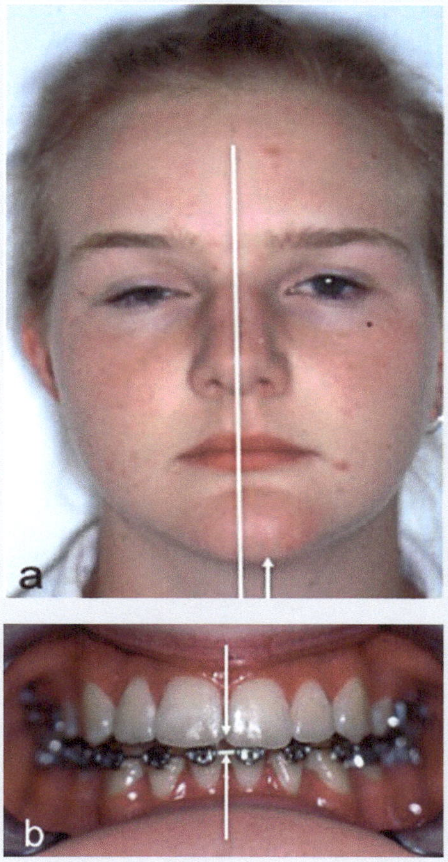

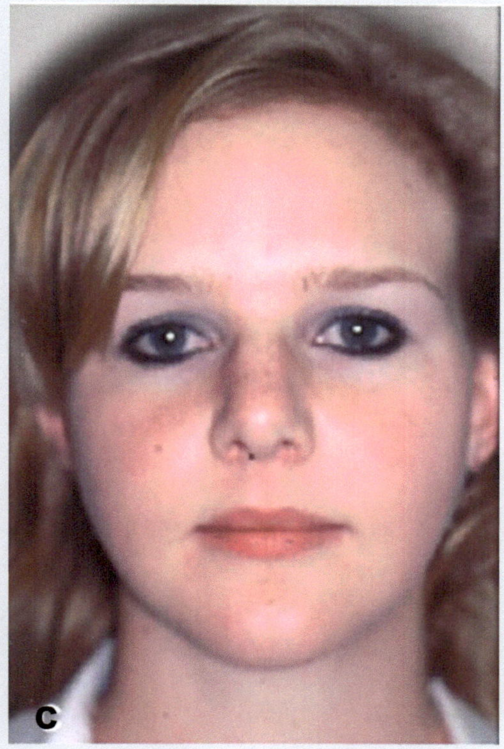

Figure 2.12

a. *Patient's chin was asymmetric to her left (arrow).*
b. *Her dental and facial midlines coincided and she had a skeletal Class II malocclusion.*
c. *Her mandible was surgically advanced, while her chin was setback and the chin asymmetry corrected with genioplasty.*

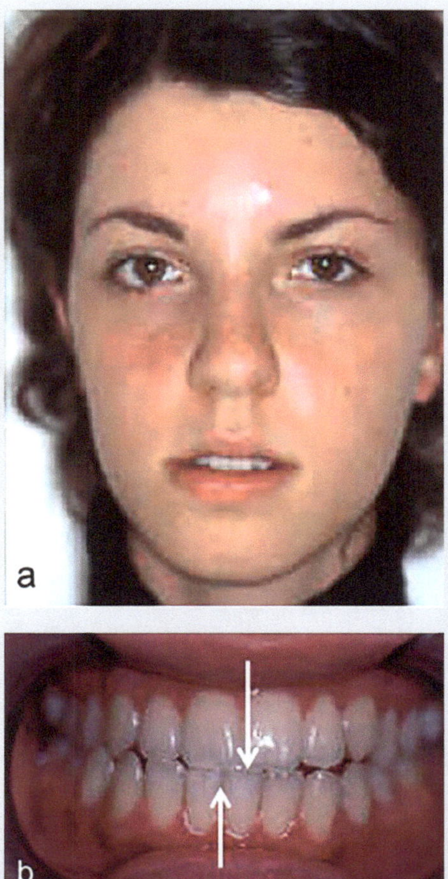

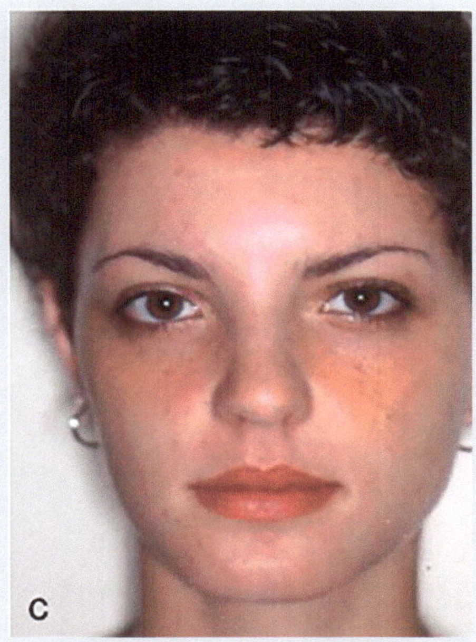

Figure 1.13

The lower incisor midline coincides with the mandibular (chin) midline, however, is asymmetric to the face. Correction was done by mandibular surgery only.

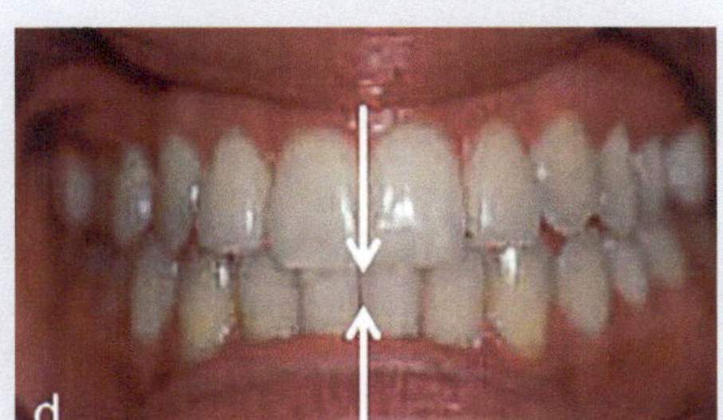

An important aspect that should be assessed is the cant of the lower border. Correction of chin asymmetry (midline of the chin in relation to the facial midline) without correction of an existing cant of the lower border is often not satisfactory. The cant should be related to the interpupillary line as well as the mandibular occlusal plane *(Fig 2.14).*

Keep in mind that correction of an occlusal cant by means of mandibular and maxillary surgery will have an effect on the transverse position of the dental midline, the chin, and the cant of the lower border of the chin. *(Fig 2.15)*

A cant of the lower border of the chin is often present in cases with unilateral condylar hyperplasia.[6] Various surgical techniques can be utiliszd for the correction of chin asymmetry and are described in Chapter 4.

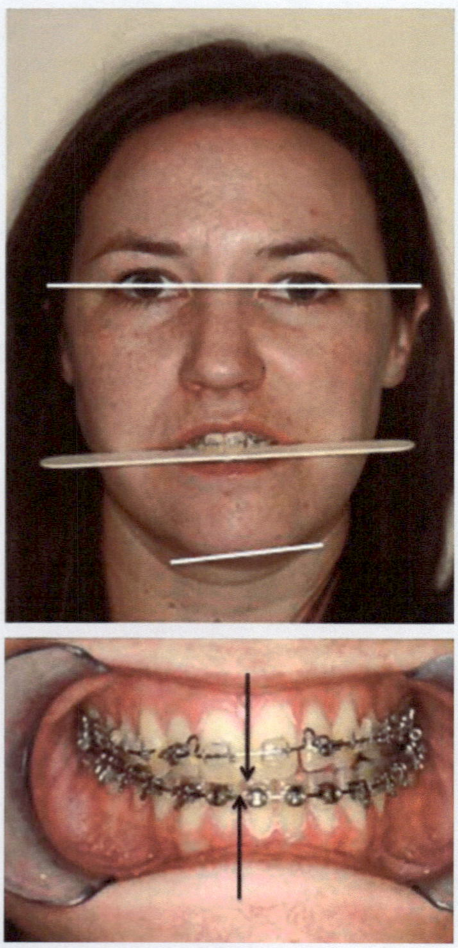

Left: Figure 2.14
Top: *A cant of the lower border of the chin should be assessed in relation to the inter-pupillary plane and the occlusal plane. Imaginary lines drawn on the lower border off the mandible are also helpful in assessing frontal symmetry of the face.*
Bottom: *The facial midline is indicated by the arrows whereas the dental and chin midline is the width of one incisor to the left.*

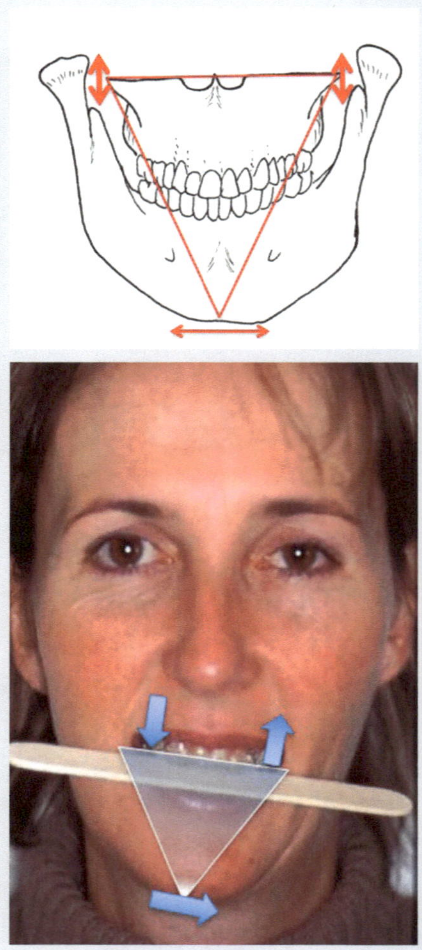

Right: Figure 2.15
Top: *By correcting a transverse occlusal cant the transverse chin position (symmetry) is inevitably effected. The constructed triangle illustrates this concept.*
Bottom: *A patient with facial asymmetry and a cant of her occlusal plane. By correcting the occlusal plane cant, her chin asymmetry will be corrected.*

Soft Tissue Evaluation - Profile View Analysis

During the profile evaluation of the chin, the lower third should be assessed in relation to the middle and upper third of the face. Again, it is emphasized that a sensible clinical examination can only be done when the teeth are in occlusion, the head posture is normal, and the lips are in repose.[7]

The actual numerical values for these relations may vary with age, gender, and race. In Caucasians, however, the ratio of the upper third [hairline (Tr) to glabella (G)], middle third [G to subnasale (Sn)], and lower facial third heights [Sn to menton (Me')] should be about equal. Any imbalances should be recorded and interpreted after all parameters are recorded *(Fig 2.17)*.

A systematic profile examination of the lower third of the face will include an evaluation of the lips, labiomental fold, chin projection, chin–neck angle, lip-chin–neck angle, and chin shape or contour. The nasal projection should be evaluated in relation to the chin projection.

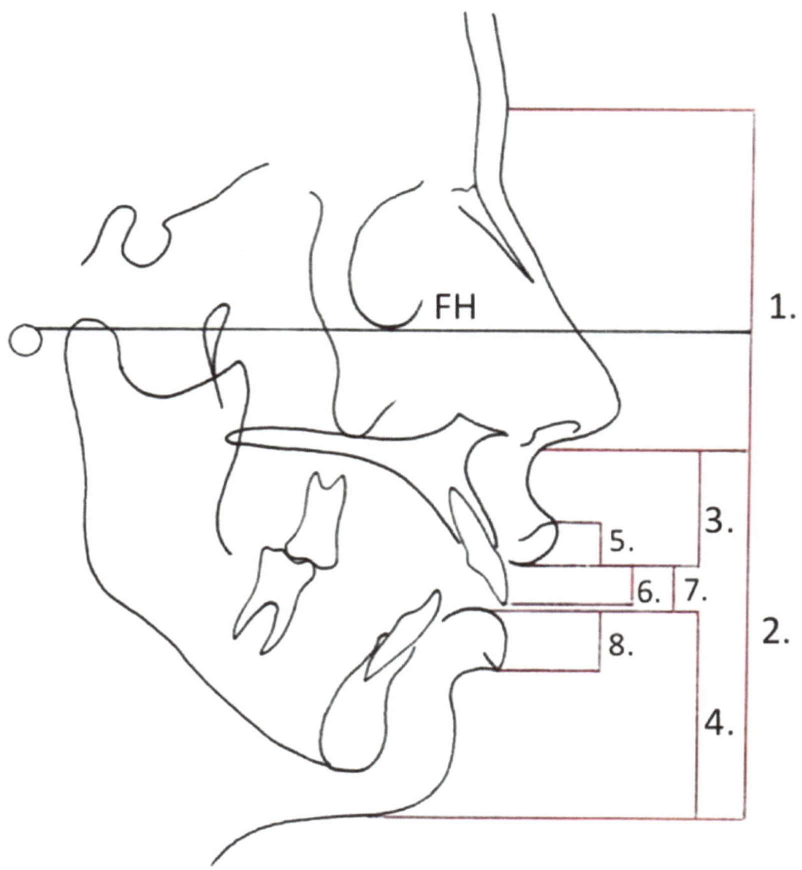

1. Middle facial third
2. Lower facial height
3. Upper lip length
4. Lower lip length
5. Upper lip vermillion
6. Upper incisor exposure
7. Inter-labial gap
8. Lower lip vermillion

Figure 2.17 *Soft tissue vertical evaluation. Vertical measurements are made to a line perpendicular to the FH plane.*

Lips. The anteroposterior position of the chin (chin projection) has a profound influence on the relative deficiency or prominence of the lips.[8,9] The upper lip [labrale superius (Ls)] usually projects slightly anterior to the lower lip [labrale inferius (Li)], while the lower lip vermillion exposure should be 25% more than the upper lip vermillion exposure. These relations will depend on the underlying dental position. It would be difficult to achieve harmonious balance between the lips and chin with a poor dental relationship, i.e., increased overjet, anterior crossbite, increased overbite, bimaxillary protrusion *(Fig 2.18a)*. Class II deep bite cases will result in excessive lower lip eversion with a deep labiomental fold *(Fig 2.18b)*, whereas less vermillion of the upper lip is exposed in Class III cases with an obtuse labiomental fold *(Fig 2.18c)*.

The anteroposterior position of the lips in relation to the chin may be assessed with the aid of the E-line (esthetic line) *(Fig 219a)* and S-line (Steiner line) as guidelines *(Fig 2.19b)*. A line drawn from the subnasale (Sn) to the pogonion (Po') is known as the lower facial plane and is also an important guide in assessing the lip position in relation to the lower face *(Fig 2.19c)*. The angle formed by the upper and lower facial plane (facial contour angle) is used to evaluate facial convexity and is another helpful guide for orthodontic positioning of the incisor teeth, as well as the surgical positioning of the maxilla, mandible, and chin *(Fig 2.20)*.

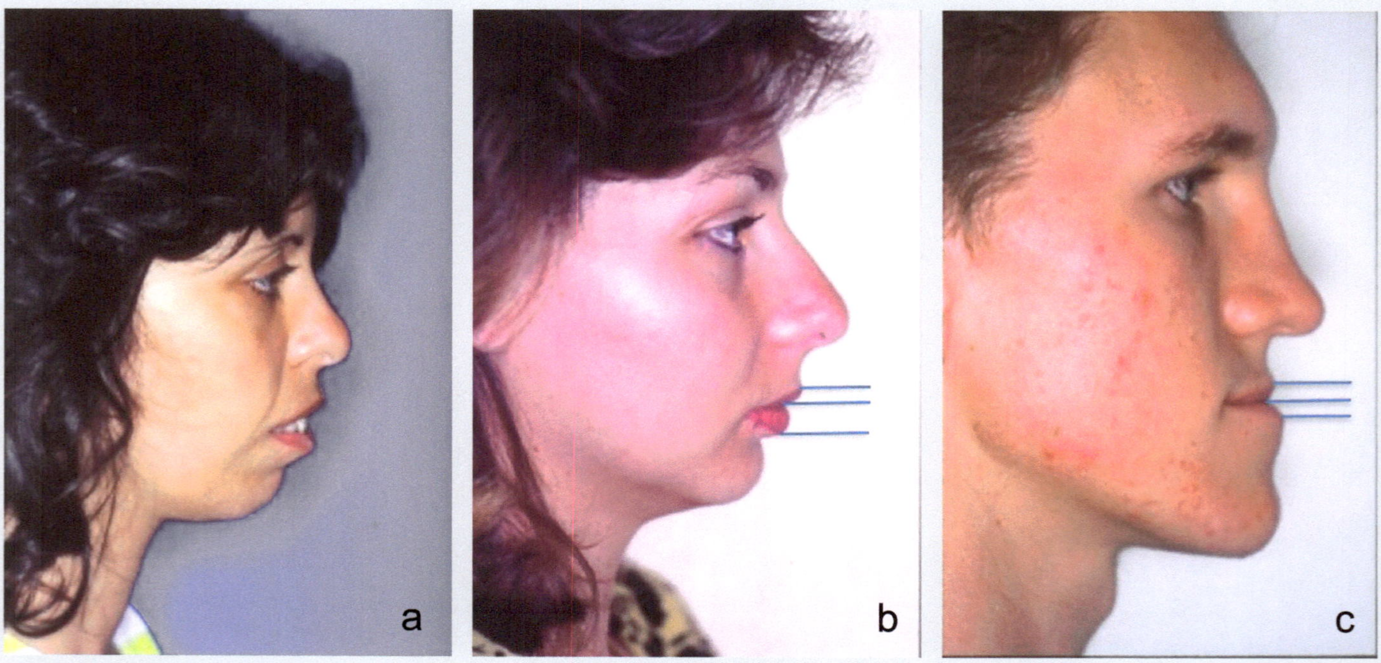

Figure 2.18a *The bimaxillary protrusion and lip protrusion of this patient will make it impossible to achieve facial balance without addressing the underlying dental situation.*

Figure 2.18b *The lower lip is everted (lower lip vermillion exposure increased) and the labio-mental fold is deep in this patient with a Class II deep bite malocclusion.*

Figure 2.18c *A patient with a Class III skeletal and dental relationship. The lower lip is ahead of the upper lip, the upper lip appears thin (decreased vermillion exposure) and the labio-mental fold is flat.*

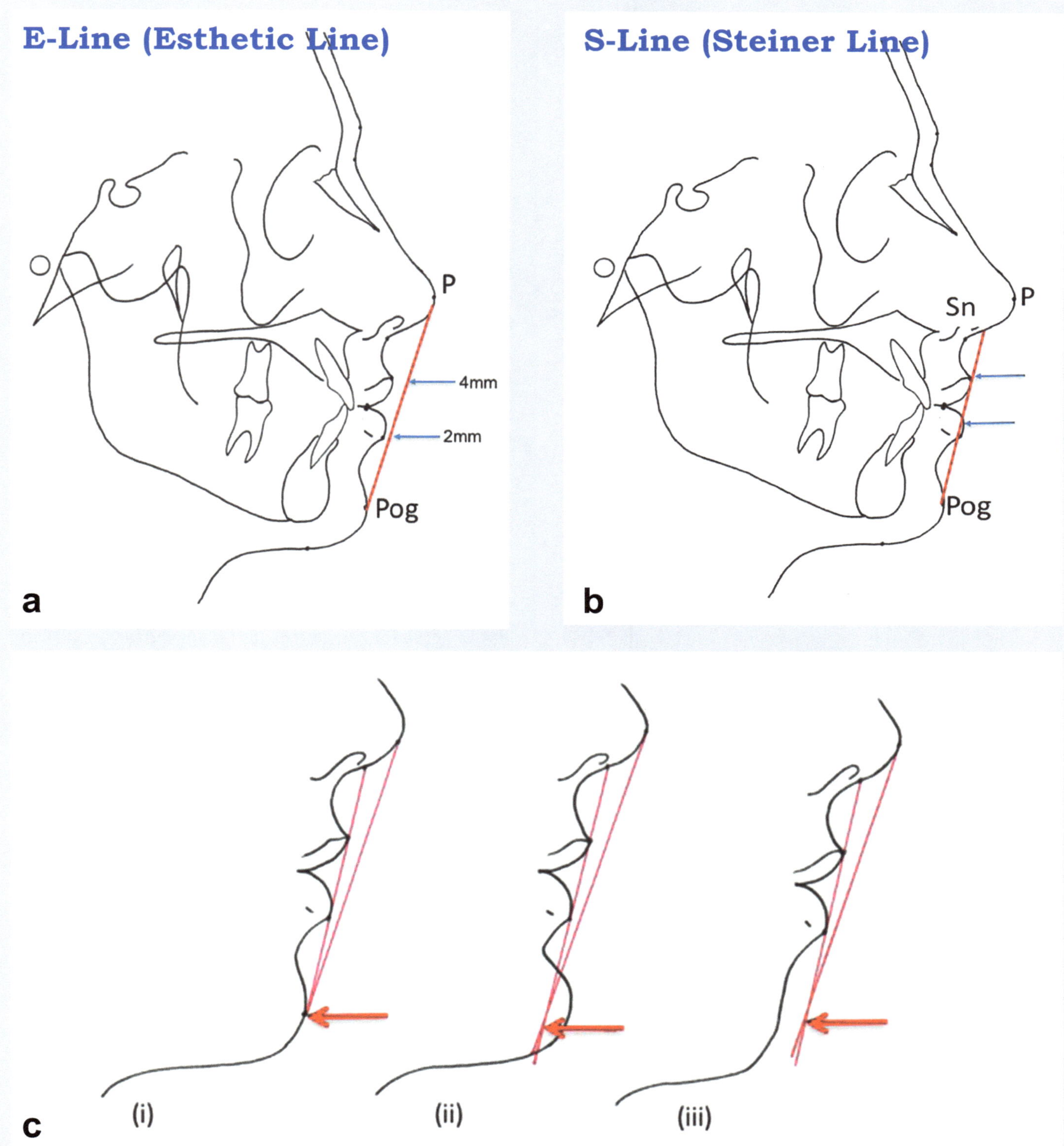

Figure 2.19a *The E-line (esthetic line) is a line drawn from the nasal tip (pronasale - P) to the most anterior surface of the chin (pogonion - Pog'). With the chin in ideal anteroposterior position to the lips, the upper lip should be 4mm and lower lip 2mm behind this line (arrows).*

Figure 2.19b *The S-line (Steiner line) connects pogonion and a point in the middle of the S-curve of the nose between the pronasale and subnasale. Taken the chin to be in ideal relationship to the lips, the upper and lower lip should touch the S-line (arrows).*

Figure 2.19c *A constructed S and E-line will assist evaluating the current chin position and in planning an ideal chin projection in relation to the lips (arrows).*

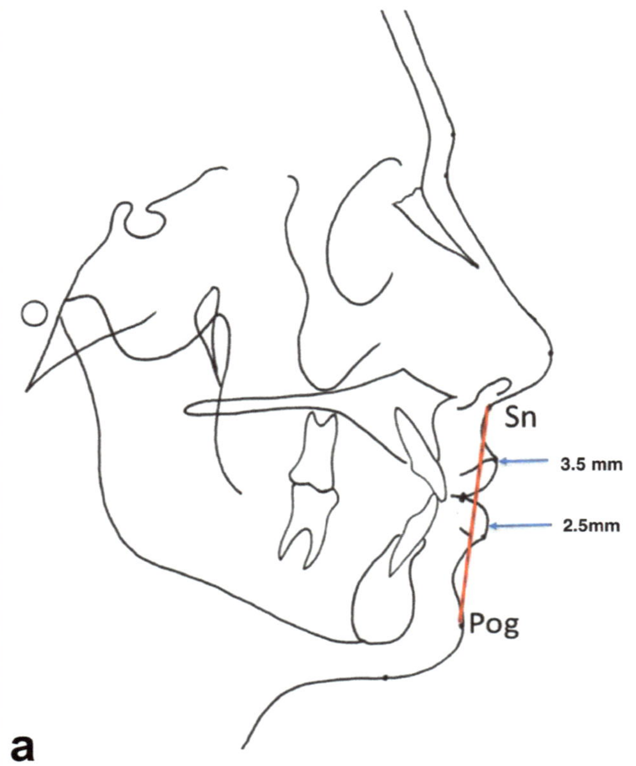

Figure 2.20a *Lower facial plane (Sn-Pog') relates the lip position to the chin projection. The lips are supported by the teeth and this plane can also be used as a guide to plan the orthodontic incisor positioning. With the lips in good relation to the rest of the face, the lower facial plane would indicate chin projection. When the chin is in good position the upper lip should be 3mm (±1) and the lower lip 2mm (±1) ahead of Sn-Po' (arrows).*

Figure 2.20b *Accepting the lips to be in ideal position, a lower facial plane can be constructed to assess the anteroposterior chin position.*

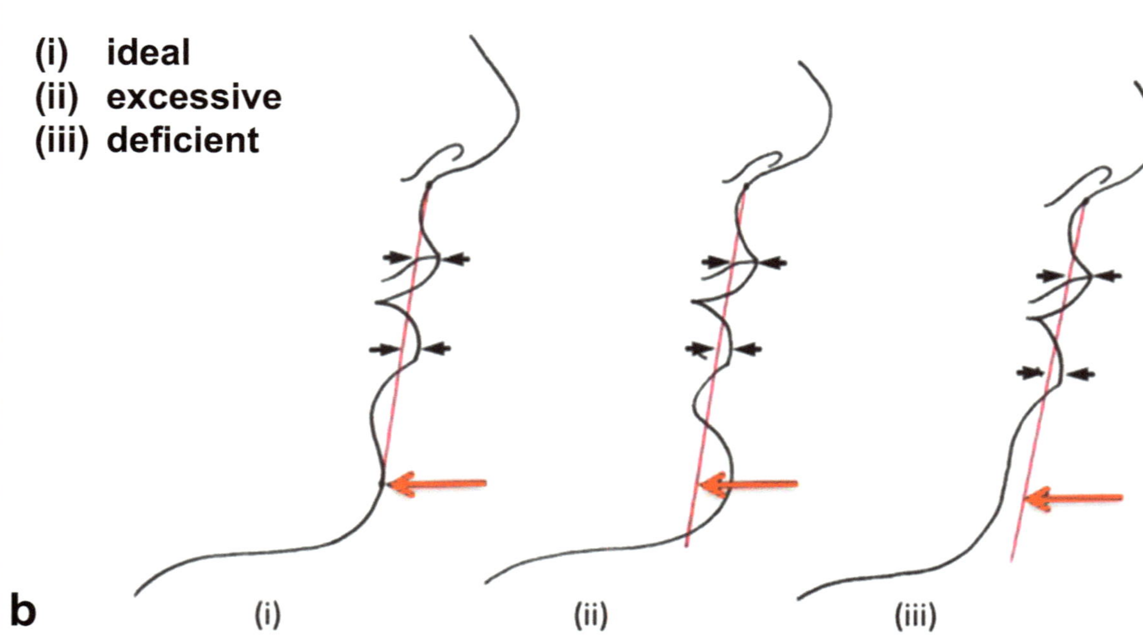

The lips and chins of patients with dento-facial deformities are often poorly related to each other as well as to the rest of the face. A constructed E-line, S-line and lower facial plane *(Fig 2.19a-b, Fig 2.20a & Fig 2.21)* are helpful guides to assess the chin's and the lip's position. These lines not only assist in diagnosis but can be constructed to assist in surgical visual treatment planning.

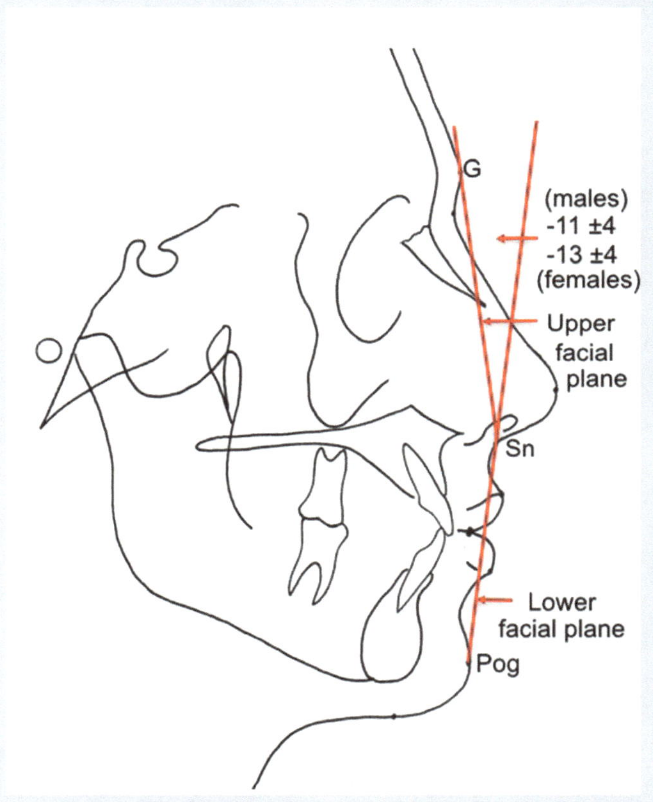

Figure 2.21 *The facial contour angle. The angle is formed between the upper facial plane (G'-Sn) and the lower facial plane (Sn-Pog'). When measured above Sn, a clockwise angle is expressed as positive, while an anticlockwise angle is negative. Males with a straight profile will have an angle of –11±4° (with Sn and G' in a relatively normal relation). Patients with convex profiles (chin deficient) would have a more negative angle (e.g. - 20°), while patients with more concave profiles (chin excessive) would have a less negative or even positive angle (e.g. -5°).*

Labiomental fold. The labiomental fold is an angle formed by the lower lip and a line tangent to the superior convexity of the chin and should be ±130°. The angle is usually acute in Class II cases and obtuse in Class III cases where the mandible is anteroposteriorly excessive *(Fig 2.22)*. The lower lip/chin contour should have a gentle S-curve and, when a genioplasty is planned, the clinician should not only concentrate on chin projection [anteroposterior position of the Pog'], but also pay careful attention to the depth and height of the labiomental fold, as well as the shape of the chin *(Fig 2.18)*.[10]

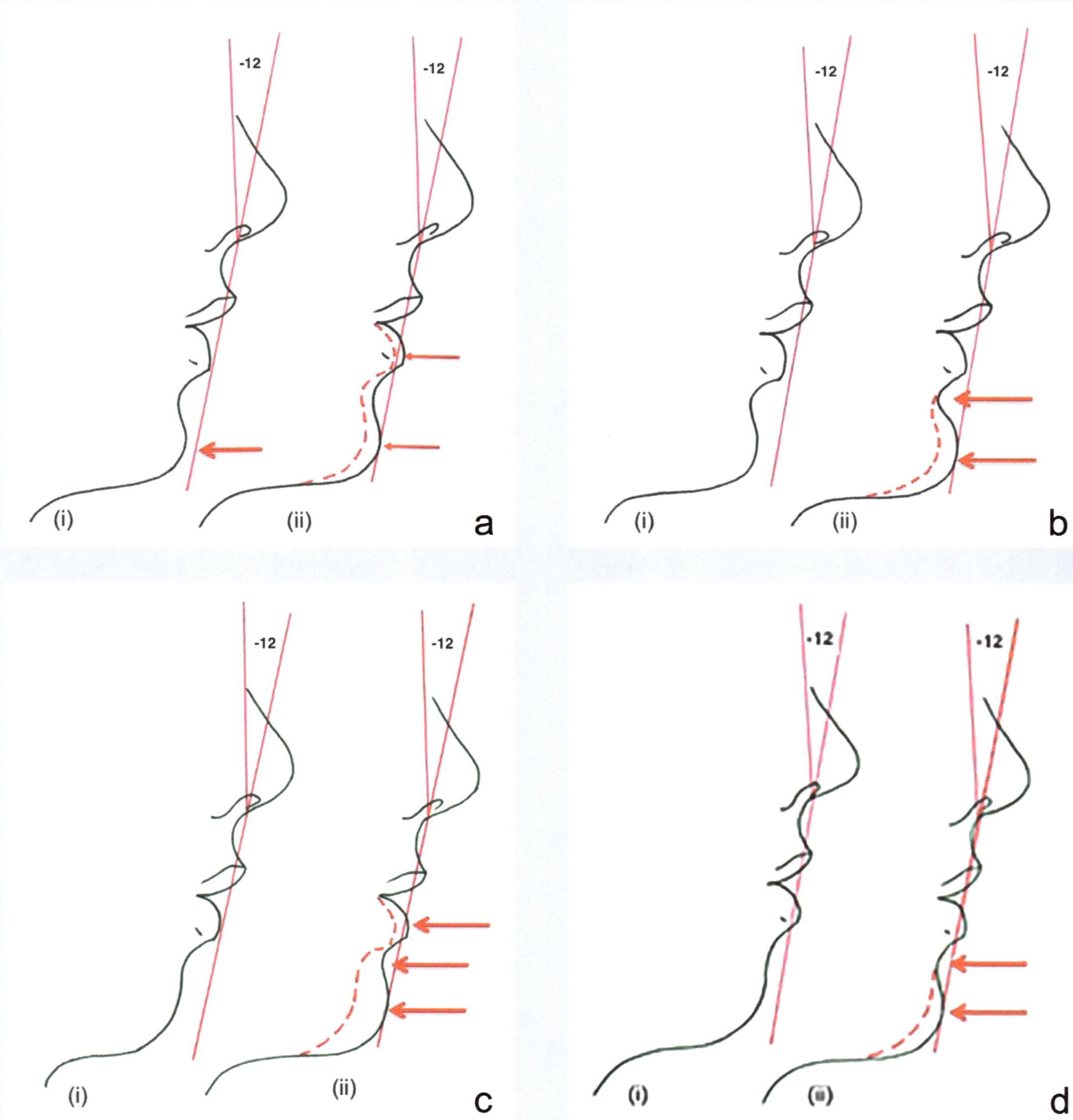

Figure 2.22: **a.** *i: A facial contour angle of -12° are constructed. Pogonion is in a retruded position, however, the shape of the chin is pleasing (arrow). ii: The lower lip is everted and the labio-mental fold is acute due to the influence of the maxillary incisors on the lower lip.The mandible should be advanced (arrows).* **b.** *i: In a case with a normal chin shape, ii: Augmentation genioplasty to achieve the required chin projection (pogonion position) will result in a "knobby" chin and an accentuated and deep labio-mental fold (arrows).* **c.** *i: Individuals with combined mandibular deficiency and microgenia, will require advancement of the mandible as well as the chin. ii: The increased lower lip dental support as well as chin projection is demonstrated (arrows).* **d.** *i: Microgenia with adequate lower lip support requires only ii: advancement genioplasty (arrows).*

Chin projection. The chin projection (anteroposterior position of the Pog') should be in good balance with the entire profile. Various soft tissue cephalometric analyses are available to assist in clinical evaluation and treatment planning. These cephalometric guidelines can often be used during the clinical examination of a patient by drawing imaginary lines on the face during assessment.

The reference line (Sn-Pog') is also called the lower facial plane and should form an angle of 12° to 16° (facial contour angle) with the upper facial plane (G'-Sn) *(Fig 2.22)*. The facial contour angle is an indicator of facial convexity. The greater the chin projection, the smaller the angle will become, while an angle of more than 18° would be indicative of an anteroposteriorly deficient position of Pog'. The retruded position of Pog' may be due to mandibular anteroposterior deficiency or microgenia and it is essential to differentiate between the two deformities. If Pog' is in an anteroposterior-deficient position, however, the shape of the chin is good, the mandible should be advanced. In cases where the labiomental fold is obtuse as a result of poor chin projection, the chin may have to be advanced in addition to mandibular advancement, whereas in cases with adequate lower lip support but anteropos-

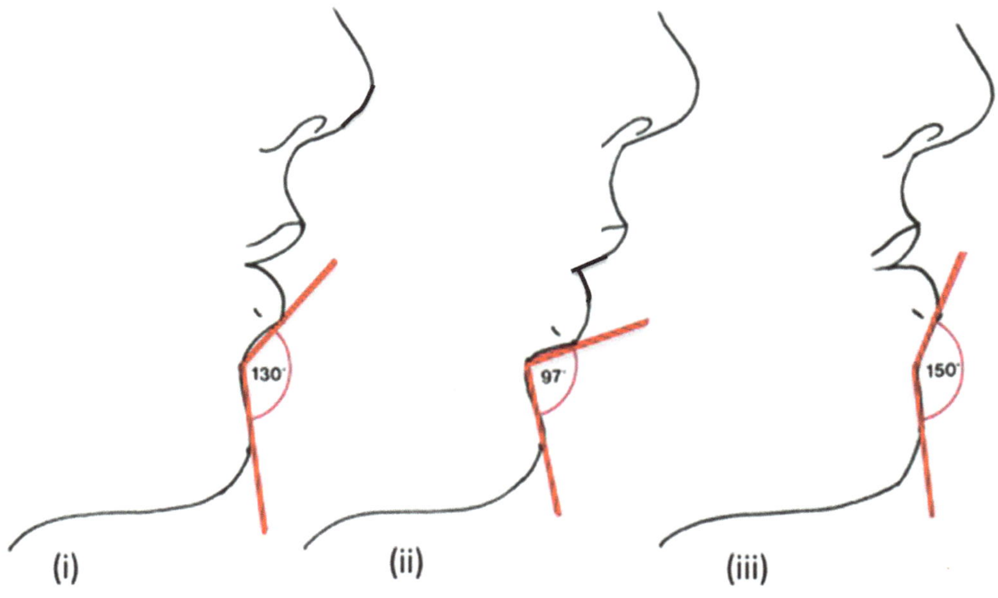

Figure 2.23 *The balance between the concavity of the labio-mental fold and the convexity of the chin plays and important part in the esthetic balance of the chin.* **i:** *An angle of 130° between the lower lip and a tangent to the superior aspect of the chin is considered normal.* **ii:** *Mandibular anteroposterior deficiency cases would tend to have acute labio-mental angles, mostly due to an everted lower lip.* **iii:** *Class III cases would have obtuse labio-mental angles, due to posterior rotation of the lower lip (the lip is not affected by the upper incisors and lack of lower dental support due to compensation of the incisors).*

terior chin deficiency, only an augmentation genioplasty would achieve the required aesthetic result *(Fig 2.23)*.

According to Legan and Burstone,[3] the upper lip should be 3.5±1.4 mm ahead and the lower lip 2.2±1.6 mm ahead of the lower facial plane. It is obvious that the anteroposterior chin position will have a profound influence on this assessment. On the other hand, this diagnostic line is a helpful guide during surgical planning of the anteroposterior chin position. Another valuable method of evaluating chin projection is to mask parts of the face with a card to evaluate the chin position independent of the rest of the facial structures *(Fig 2.24)*.

Chin shape or contour. In profile view, the main contributing factors responsible for an attractive chin shape or contour are the anteroposterior position of the lower lip, the depth, height, and shape of the labiomental fold, and last, the projection of the chin. A harmonious combination of the above three aspects will go a long way in achieving an attractive and esthetically pleasing chin. A smooth, well-defined contour of the lower border of the mandible will certainly contribute to the attractiveness of the chin. Correction of poor chin esthetics is difficult in cases with poor lower border contour and definition *(Fig 2.25)*.

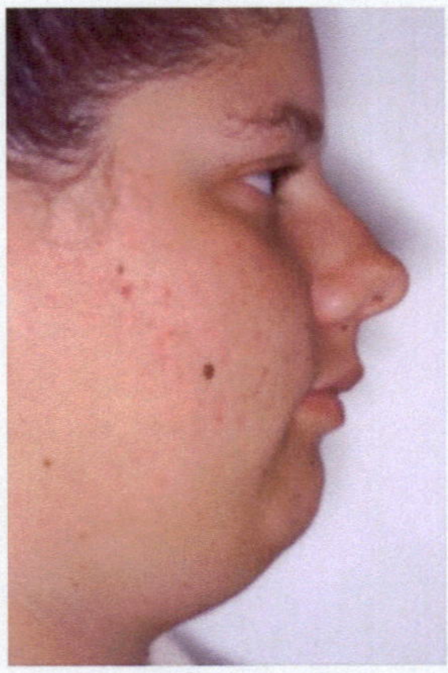

Figure 2.25 *The smooth, well defined lower border of the mandible enhances the chin esthetics, while the uneven, bulky line of the lower border and excessive lipid tissue will limit esthetic improvement by genioplasty.*

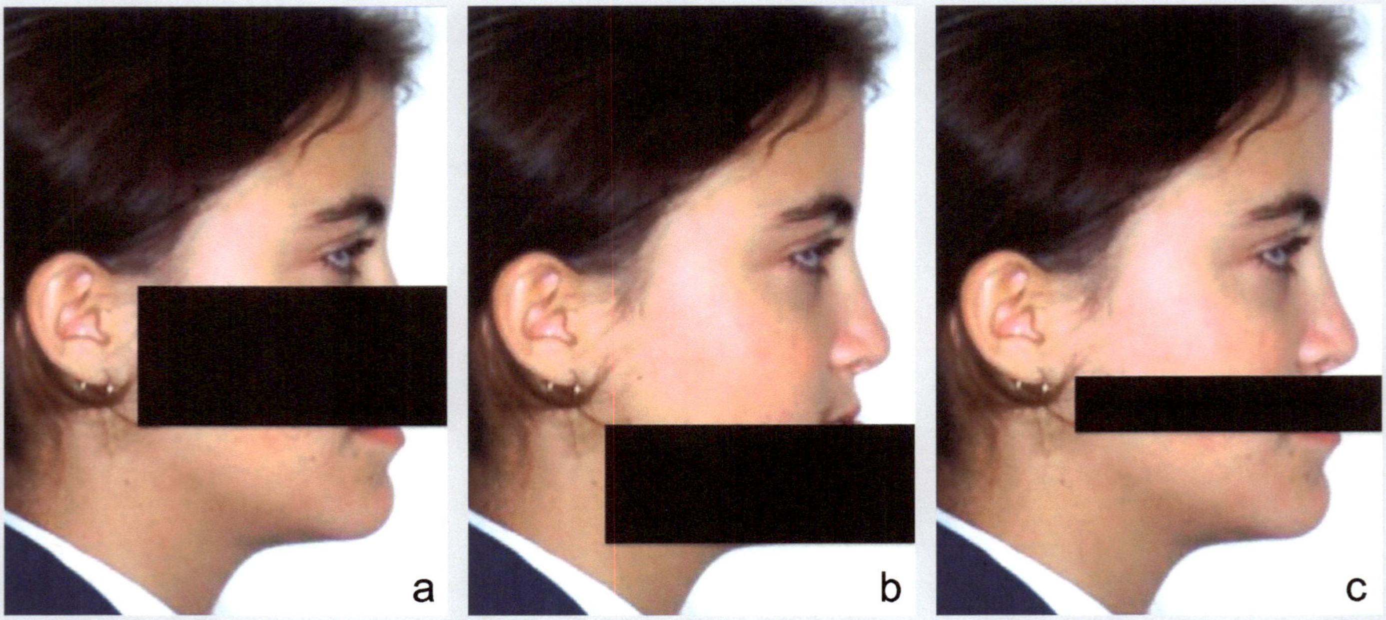

Figure 2.24. *To assist in the diagnosis,* **a:** *the midface is masked independently to relate the chin to the rest of the face.* **b:** *Then the chin is masked to evaluate the rest of the face independent to the chin.* **c:** *To further assist the clinician only the maxilla and upper lip may be blocked out.*

Chin–neck angle (cervicomental angle). Ensure that this assessment is made with the patient's head in a natural horizontal posture. The chin–neck angle (submental neck angle) is formed by a submental tangent and a neck tangent, which is preferably 126° in males and 121° in females *(Fig 2.26a).* The lower border of the mandible should form a smooth line from the angle to the chin, however, the angle and submental line are often influenced by submental fat deposits.[11] These observations are relevant when considering anteroposterior chin augmentation or reduction (mandibular advancement or setback), as well as submental liposuction. The poor definition of the lower border of the mandible and an obtuse chin–neck angle are demonstrated in Figure 2.26b.

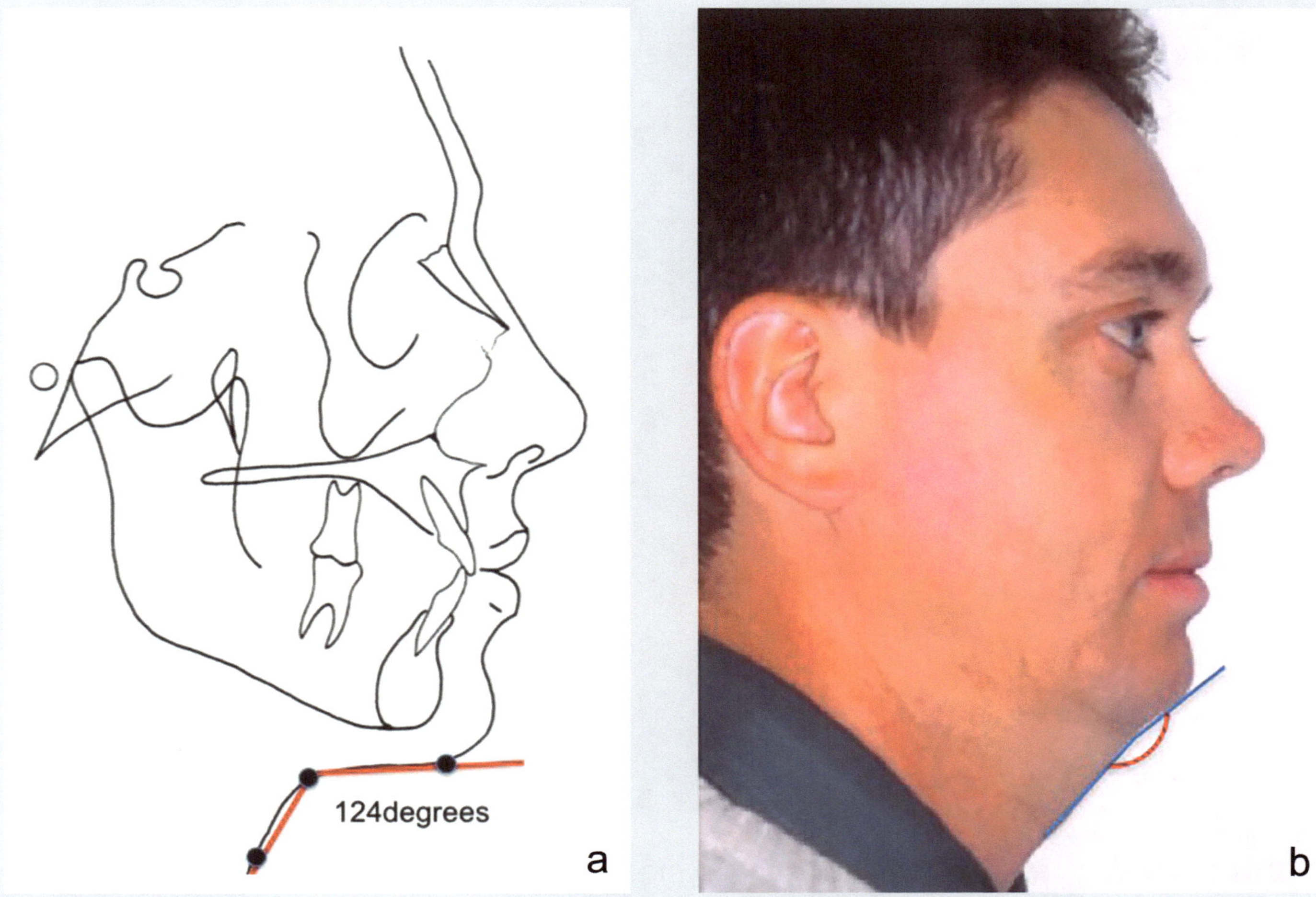

Figure 2.26 *The chin-neck angle (submental-neck angle).* **a:** *The angle between the submental tangent and the neck tangent should be ±126° for males and ±121° for females* **b:** *The angle is obtuse in mandibular or chin deficiencies and acute in mandibular excess or macrogenia. This angle is also influenced by submental fat deposits.*

Chin–neck length. The chin–neck length is an important aesthetic feature, but not easily quantifiable unless the head posture can be standardized. This measurement is made from the submental neck point (Smn) to soft tissue Me' and should be 42±4 mm *(Fig 2.27a).* Mandibular setback and reduction genioplasty procedures should be avoided in patients with short chin–neck lengths.

In patients with microgenia (or mandibular deficiency), the submental neck angle will be obtuse and the chin–neck length short, whereas patients with macrogenia (or mandibular excess) will most likely have an acute chin–neck angle and long chin-neck length *(Fig 2.27 b & c).*

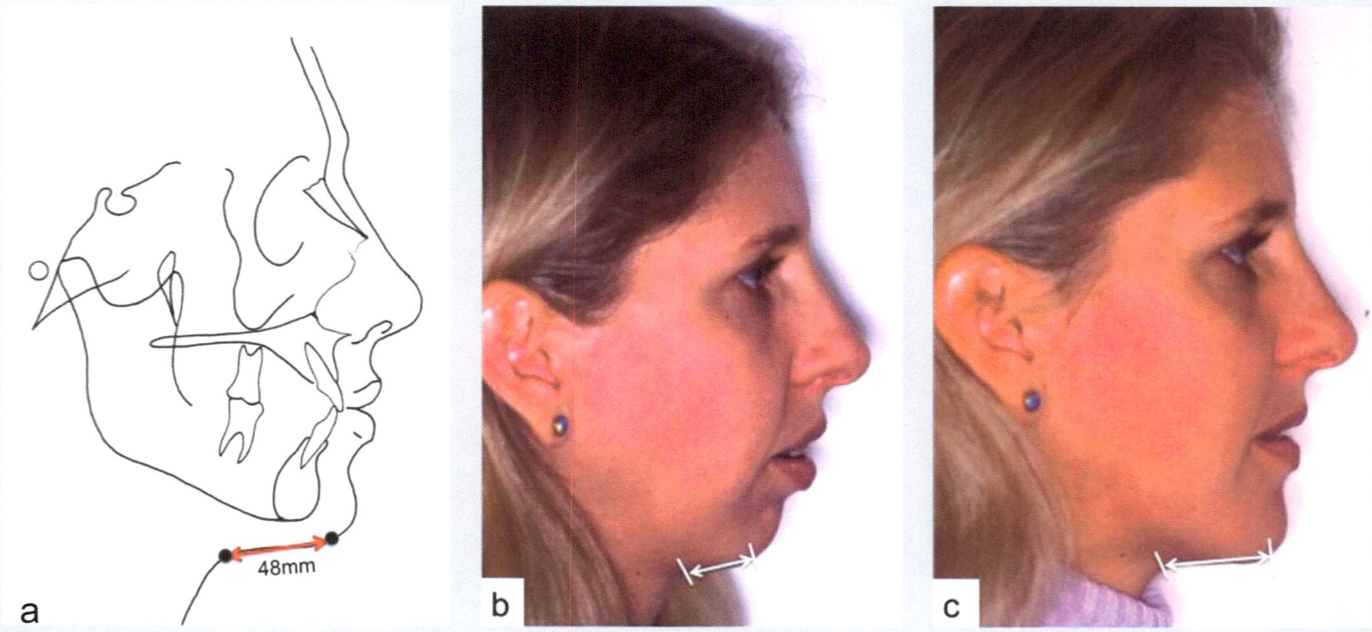

Figure 2.27: **a:** *The chin-neck length is measured from the submental neck point (Smn) to soft tissue menton (Me'). Mandibular setback procedures and reduction genioplasty is contra indicated in patients with short chin-neck lengths. Normal chin-neck length is 47mm ±4mm with the head in natural posture.* **b:** *A profile view of a patient with mandibular anteroposterior deficiency and microgenia. The chin-neck length is short.* **c:** *The increase in chin-neck length is well illustrated after mandibular advancement and advancement genioplasty.*

Lip–chin submental angle. This angle is formed by the lip–chin line (Li and Po') and a submental tangent line and should be 126° for males and 121° for females *(Fig 2.28a)*. This angle is obtuse in patients with deficient chins and acute in anteroposteriorly excessive chins, while lower lip procumbency will increase the lip–chin–submental angle. The effect that mandibular advancement and advancement genioplasty have on this angle is demonstrated in Figure 2.28b & c. Excessive submental fat will increase the bulk of the submental and neck area, increasing the angle *(Fig 2.28d)*.

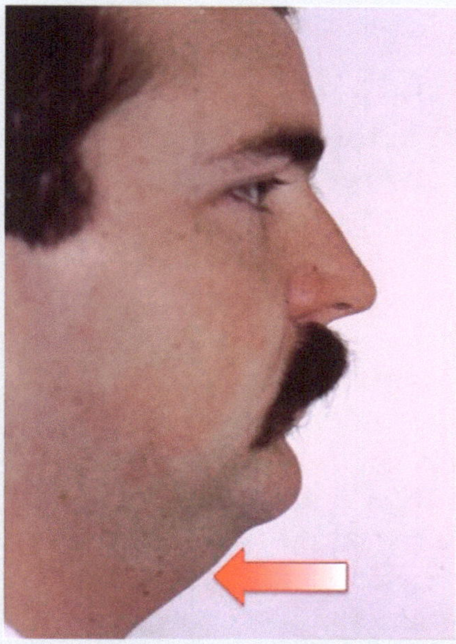

Figure 2.28d *Excessive submental fat will increase the lip-chin-submental angle, the submental-neck angle and the chin-throat length (arrow).*

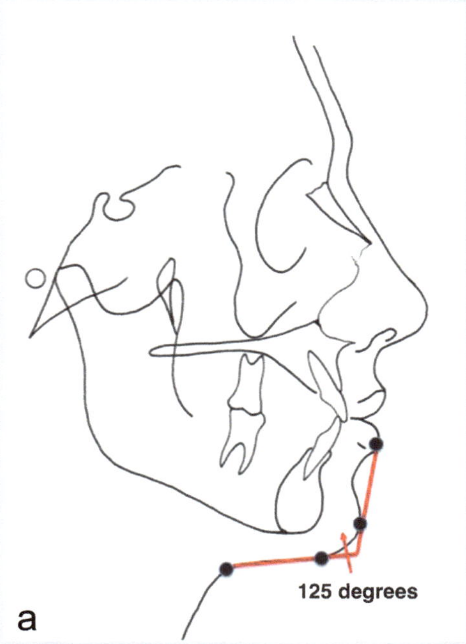

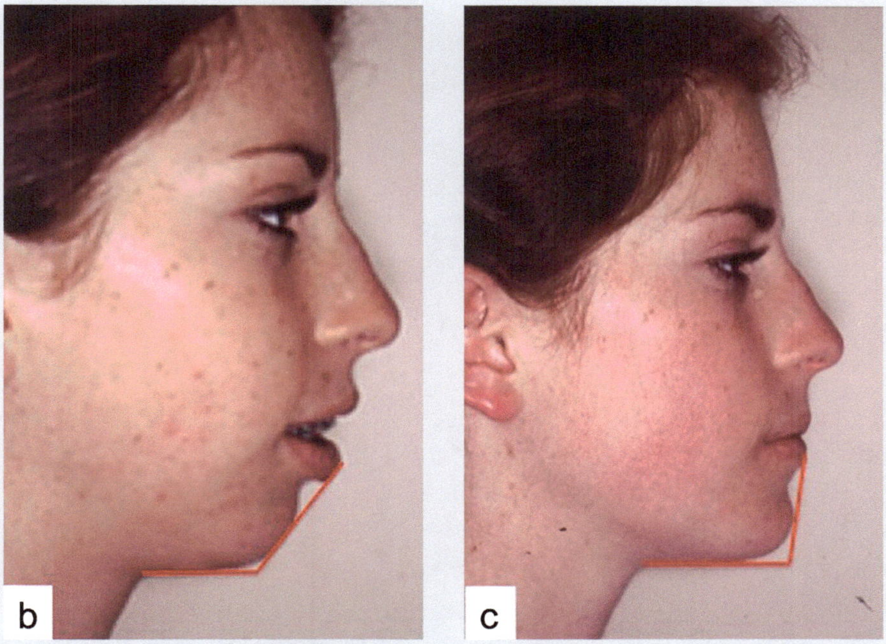

Figure 2.28: **a:** *The lip-chin-submental angle is acute in mandibular excess or macrogenia cases and obtuse in microgenia or mandibular deficient cases. This angle is influenced by the lower lip position and chin projection. An angle of 126° for males and 121° for females are considered normal.* **b:** *The lip-chin-submental angle is 129°* **c:** *The angle is changed to 116° by the advancement of the mandible and chin.*

There are various factors that may contribute to the anatomical structure of the chin–neck area such as excessive submental fat that, due to weight gain, has a substantial effect on the fullness of the submental line, leading to a double chin. Also, aging may lead to soft tissue sag of the cervicomental area once the elasticity of the skin is lost. Older individuals who are overweight will have a turkey gobbler appearance. Genioplasty alone will improve the esthetics very little for these patients. Chin augmentation for these individuals often has to be combined with submental liposuction, platysma plication and rhytidectomy (facelift).[11–14]

Double chins have been classified into three groups by Vinas et al:[13]

1. a redundancy of submental tissues with excess fat and skin;
2. soft tissue in the submental area appears normal; the skeletal chin is usually at fault;
3. a combination of Groups 1 and 2.[13]

The position of the hyoid bone also has an important role in the overall success of chin deformity correction. A low position of the hyoid bone is often an indication for sleep apnea. Low positioning of the hyoid bone (below the fourth cervical vertebrae) predisposes the patient to a less than ideal treatment result.[13,14] Both the submental–neck angle and lip–chin-submental angle would tend to be obtuse and will improve little with mandibular advancement and chin augmentation *(Fig 2.29)*. It is important to consider as well the chin–neck contour in treatment planning of various deformities involving the mandible and chin.[15–17]

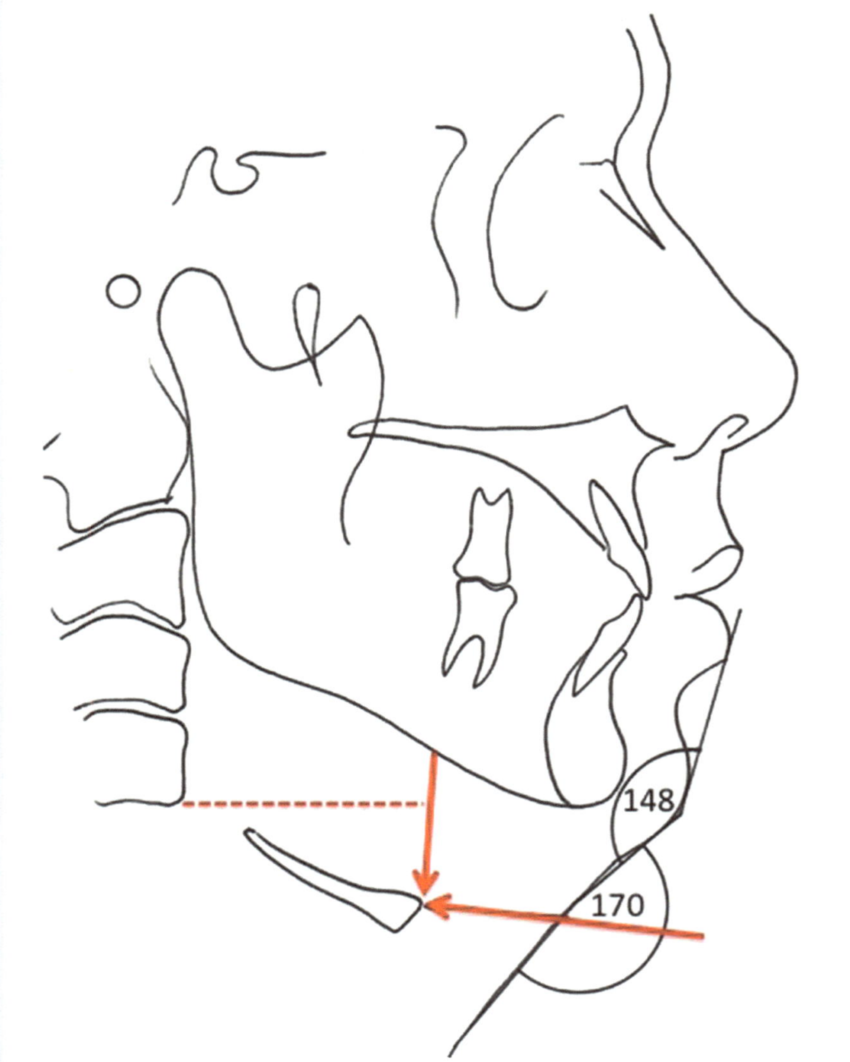

Figure 2.29 *The low position of the hyoid bone (below the fourth cervical vertebra) illustrated on a lateral cephalometric tracing (arrows). Note the obtuse lip-chin-submental (148°) and submental angles (170°). The low position of the hyoid bone renders esthetic improvement of the chin-neck area very difficult as seen on profile view.*

Radiographic Evaluation - Lateral Cephalometric Analysis

The information gained from the lateral cephalometric radiograph forms an important part of the database for orthognathic diagnosis and treatment planning. Analysis of the lateral cephalometric radiograph is essentially designed to measure relationships between various structures of the craniofacial complex. It is a helpful guide for diagnosis and treatment planning, predicting treatment results, and assessing soft and hard tissue changes resulting from treatment.

The lateral cephalometric radiograph should be obtained with the patient's head in a natural horizontal posture, the teeth in occlusion, and the lips in repose *(Fig 2.30a)*. When assessing the chin in Class II deep bite cases, it may be helpful to obtain an additional radiograph with the teeth apart and the lips just touching for more realistic soft tissue evaluation of the chin *(Fig 2.30b)*.

It must be emphasised that the primary soft tissue examination of the chin esthetics should be guided by cephalometric values. Cephalometric analysis and photographs of the patient should be part of the patient's permanent records because the controlled reliable notes of the clinical examination are imperative for accurate diagnosis, correct treatment planning, and meaningful assessment of treatment results.

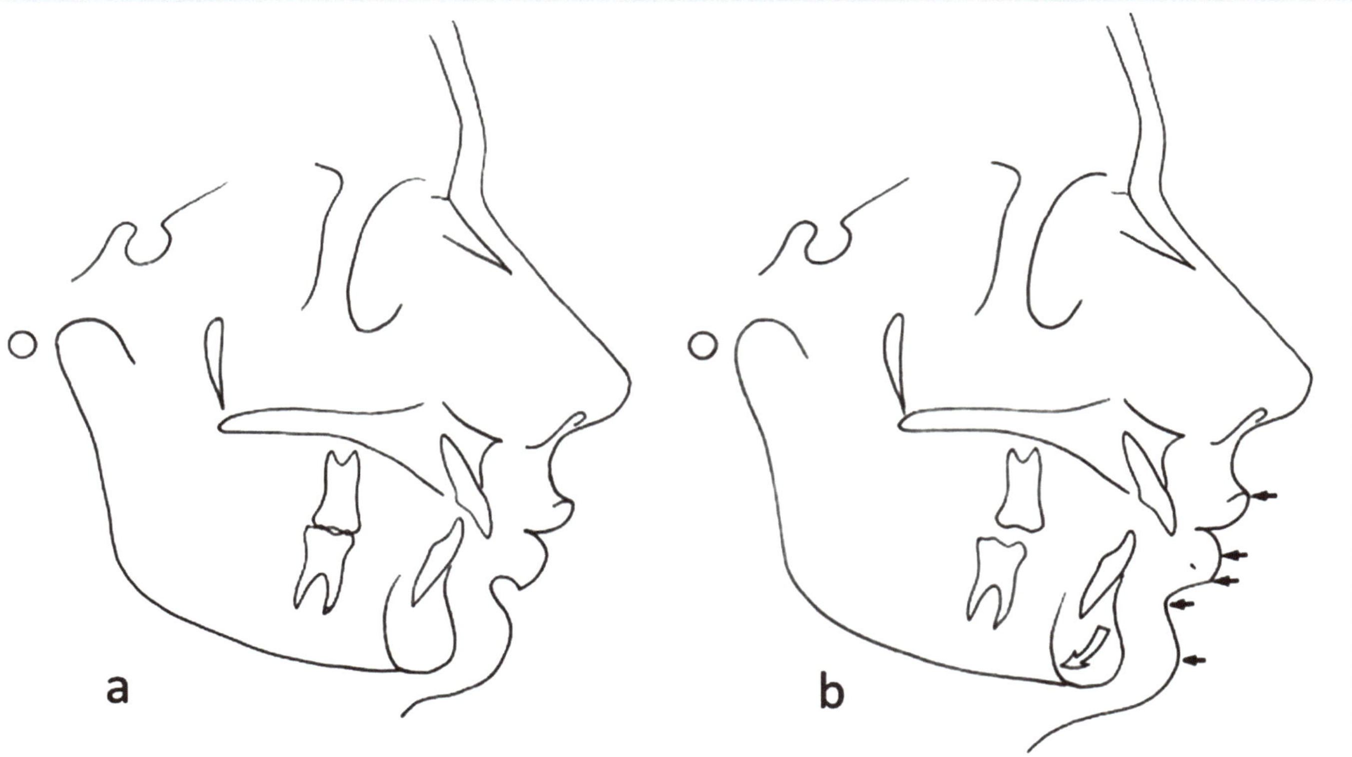

Figure 2.29 *A tracing of a lateral cephalometric radiograph of a patient with a Class II occlusion and deep bite.* **a:** *The teeth are in occlusion, lips in repose and the head in natural posture.* **b:** *The teeth are apart and the lips just touching on the lateral cephalometric tracing of the patient. The effect of the maxillary incisors on the lower lip is eliminated and the soft tissue changes are indicated by the arrows.*

Soft Tissue Vertical Analysis

The tracing of the lateral cephalometric radiograph below identifies the landmarks used to analyze the relationship between the various structures of the craniofacial complex *(Fig 2.31).*

Middle-to-Lower Facial Third Height Relation (MFH:LFH). The distance from G' to Sn (MFH) and Sn to Me' (LFH) is measured and the ratio should be approximately 1:1.

Interpretation: In most orthognathic surgical patient's, the abnormalities will be present in the lower third of their faces (Sn-Me'). In cases where the lower third is increased in relation to the upper third of the face, either vertical maxillary excess or an increase in the vertical anterior height of the mandible should be expected. A decrease in lower vertical height could be caused by either vertical maxillary deficiency, vertical deficiency of the anterior mandible, or an overclosed bite.

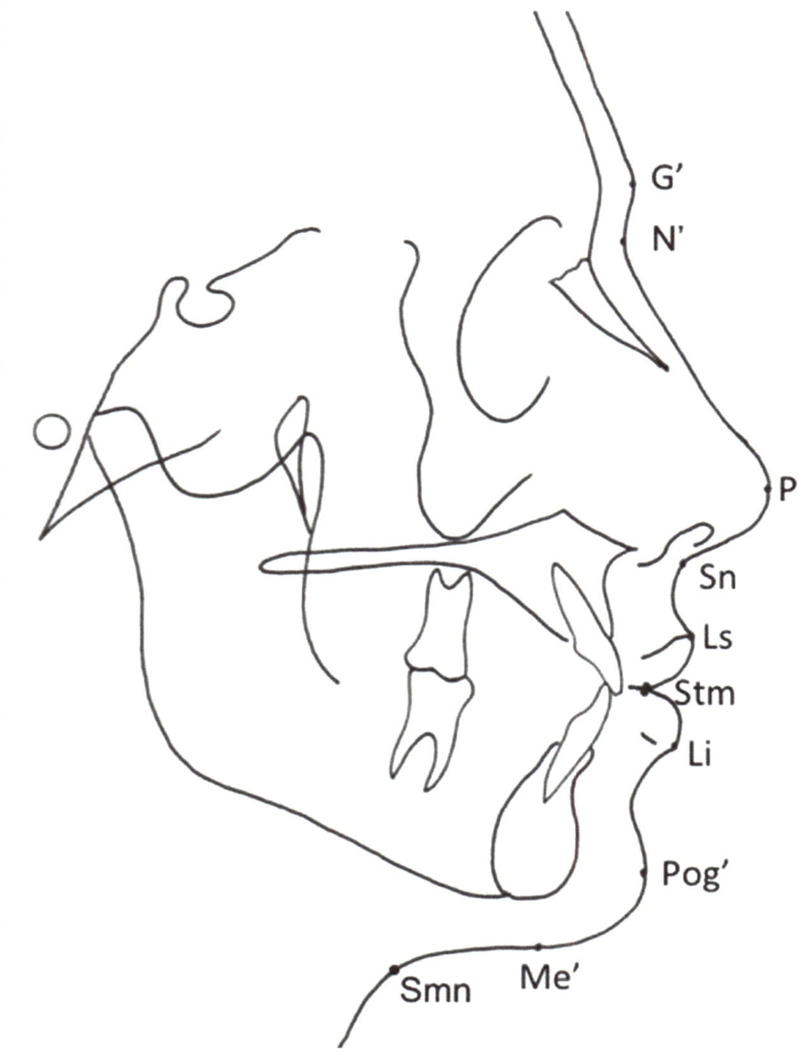

G' - Soft tissue glabella. *Most anterior point of the forehead.*

N - Soft tissue nasion for all points. *The deepest point of concavity in the midline between the forehead and the nose.*

P - Pronasale. *The most anterior point of the nose.*

Sn - Subnasale. *The point at which the columella of the nose merges with the upper lip in the mid sagittal plane.*

Ls - Labrale superius. *The mucocutaneous border of the upper lip vermillion.*

Stm^s- Stomion superius. *The lowest point of the vermillion of the upper lip.*

Stm^i- Stomion inferius. *The uppermost point of the lower lip vermillion.*

Li - Labrale inferius. *The mucocutaneous border of lower lip.*

Pog' - Soft tissue pogonion. *The most anterior point of the chin in the mid-sagittal plane.*

Me' - Soft tissue menton. *The lowest point on the contour of the soft tissue of the chin. Found by dropping a perpendicular line from horizontal through skeletal menton.*

Smn - Submental neck point. *Point where the submental tangent meets the neck tangent.*

Figure 2.31 *Soft tissue landmarks for lateral cephalometric analysis.*

Upper Lip-to-Lower Lip Length Ratio (ULL:LLL). The upper lip length (Sn – Stm^s) should be approximately one-half the length of the lower lip and chin (Stm^i – Me') *(Fig 2.32).*

Interpretation: A decrease in the vertical relation will either indicate a long upper lip or vertical deficiency of the anterior mandibular height. An increase in the ratio may be due to a short upper lip or vertical excess of the anterior mandible.

Interlabial Gap (ILG). When the lips are relaxed, they should just be touching; an interlabial gap of 1 to 3 mm is still considered normal *(Fig 2.32).*[7,18,19]

Interpretation: An increased interlabial gap (more than 4 mm) is usually an indication of lip incompetence due to vertical maxillary excess. Patients with short upper lips, however, will also tend to have an increased interlabial gap.[20–22]

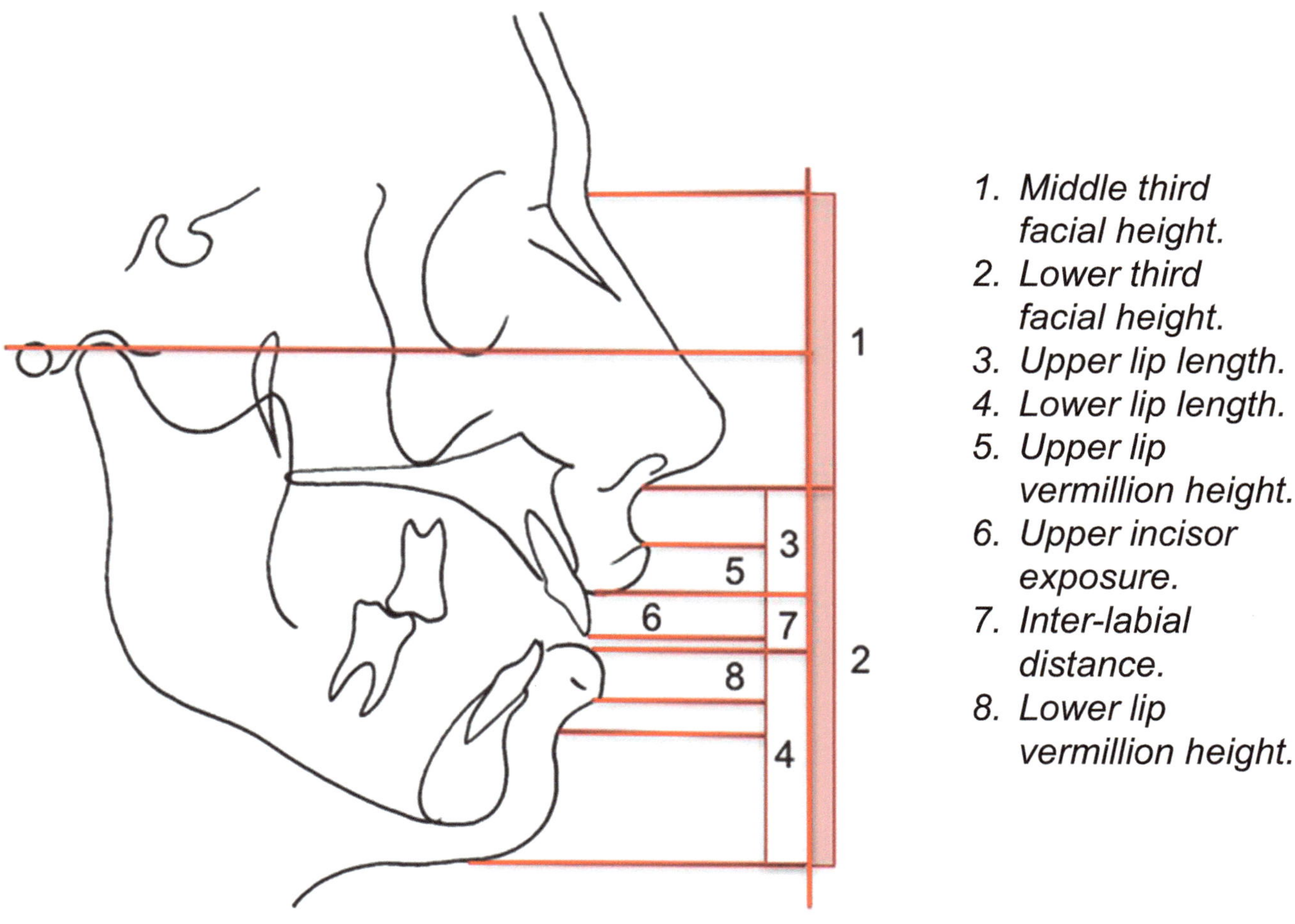

Figure 2.32 *Soft tissue vertical evaluation. Vertical measurements are made perpendicular to Frankfort horizontal.*

Upper Lip Length (ULL). ULL is measured from Sn to Stm^s and should be 22±2 mm for males and 20±2 mm for females *(Fig 2.32)*. Upper lip length tends to increase with age.

Interpretation: A patient with a relatively long upper lip will tend to have less maxillary incisor tooth exposure, whereas individuals with short upper lips will tend to have an increased interlabial gap with increased maxillary incisor tooth exposure. When vertical repositioning of the maxilla is contemplated, an important factor to consider is planning the correct amount of superior repositioning of the maxilla for each individual.

Lower Lip Length (LLL). Measured from Stm^i to Me', LLL should be 44+2 mm for males and 40±2 mm for females *(Fig 2.32)*.

Interpretation: An increase in the vertical dimension may indicate an increased anterior vertical height of the mandible, whereas a decrease may be indicative of a short anterior mandibular height. This dimension may also be decreased in deep bite cases where the lower lip will be everted and the labiomental fold acute.

Upper (ULV) and Lower Lip (LLV) Vermillion Height. The ULV height should be 25% less than the height of the LLV: Ls – Stm^s:Stm^i – Li = 3:4 *(Fig 2.32)*.

Interpretation: Vermillion heights are race specific, which should be kept in mind during evaluation. An increased LLV exposure may be because of lower lip evertion due to lip incompetence in patients with vertical maxillary excess. The lower lip is also often everted in Class II deep bite or Class II division 1 cases where the lower lip is rolled outward by the maxillary incisor teeth.

Vertical Soft Tissue Relation Summary

Vertical	Normal
Midfacial height (MFH) : lower facial height (LFH) G' – Sn:Sn – Me'	1:1
Upper lip length (ULL) (Sn – Stm^s)	20 ± 2 mm (female) 22 ± 2 mm (male)
Lower lip/chin length (LLL) (Stm^i – Me')	40 ± 2 mm (female) 44 ± 2 mm (male)
Upper lip length (ULL) : lower lip length (LLL) Sn – Stm^s:Stm^i – Me'	1:2
Sn – LLV:LLV – Me'	1:0.9
Interlabial distance (ILG)	0–3 mm
Maxillary tooth exposure (Stm^s – maxillary incisor tip)	1–4 mm
Upper lip (ULV) : lower lip vermillion (LLV) Ls-Stm^s:Stm^i – Li	3:4

Soft Tissue Anteroposterior Evaluation

Lip prominence I. A line is drawn from the Sn to soft tissue Pog' (lower facial plane). Burstone[18] estimates the perpendicular distance of the upper lip (Ls) ahead of this line to be 3±1 mm, while the labiale inferius (Li) should be 2±1 mm anterior to the lower facial plane (Sn – Pog') *(Fig 2.33).*

Interpretation: The anteroposterior position of the upper lip is an indication of soft tissue support by the maxillary incisors. The anteroposterior position of the maxillary incisors plays an important role in positioning of the upper lip and should be kept in mind during orthodontic and surgical treatment planning. The labiale inferius would tend to be further ahead of this line (Sn-Pog') in Class II cases or microgenia (with Pog' posteriorly situated) and behind the line in Class III cases or macrogenia (with Pog' anteriorly situated).[21]

Lip prominence II. If a vertical line (SnV) is drawn through the Sn perpendicular to the "true horizontal," the upper lip should be 1 to 2 mm ahead of this line. Bell et al.[20] estimate the lower lip to be on or just posterior of the Sn vertical line (SnV) *(Fig 2.34).*

Interpretation: In mandibular anteroposterior-deficient cases, the lower lip tends to be more than 1 mm posterior to the SnV vertical. In patients with mandibular anteroposterior excess and/or maxillary anteroposterior deficiency, the lower lip will be anterior to the SnV.

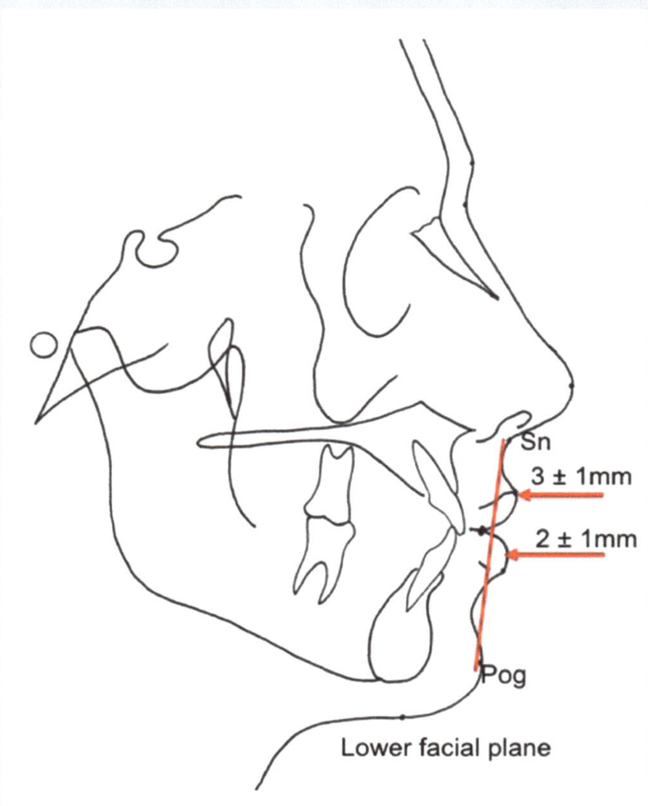

Figure 2.33 *Lip prominence. The distance from the upper lip (Ls) and lower lip (Li) is measured to the lower facial plane (LFP). Ls to LFP: 3±1mm. Li to LFP: 2±1mm.*

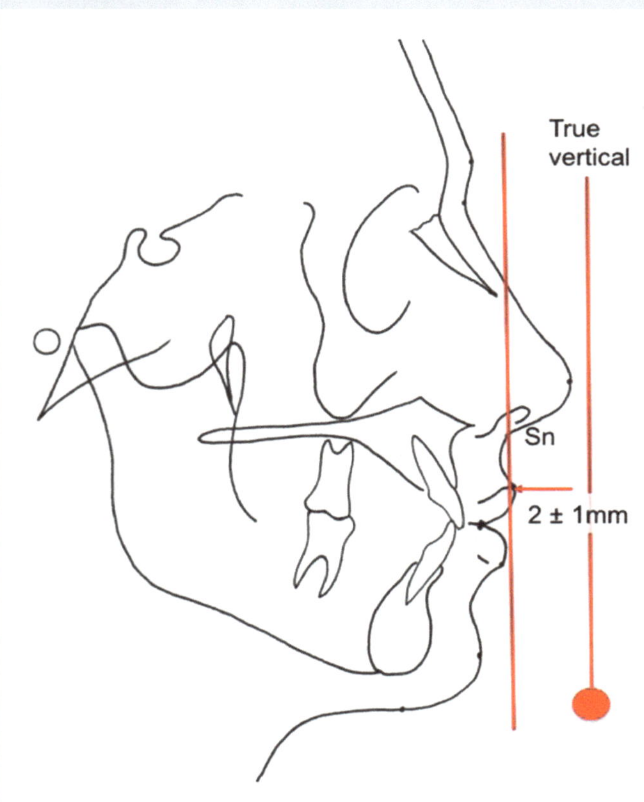

Figure 2.34 *Lip prominence. A line is drawn parallel to true vertical through Sn and distance from the upper lip (Ls) and lower lip (Li) measured to this line. Ls to SnV: 1-2mm. Li to SnV: 0mm.*

Lower lip prominence. The distance of the most prominent part of the lower lip is measured to the aesthetic line or E-line (P-Pog'). The lower lip should be 2±2 mm behind this line *(Fig 2.19a)*

Interpretation: This evaluation is influenced by the nose as well as the chin prominence and could also be used when planning the final chin position. The lower lip will tend to be ahead of this line in Class II mandibular anteroposterior-deficient individuals where Pog' is situated posteriorly and the lower lip will be everted.

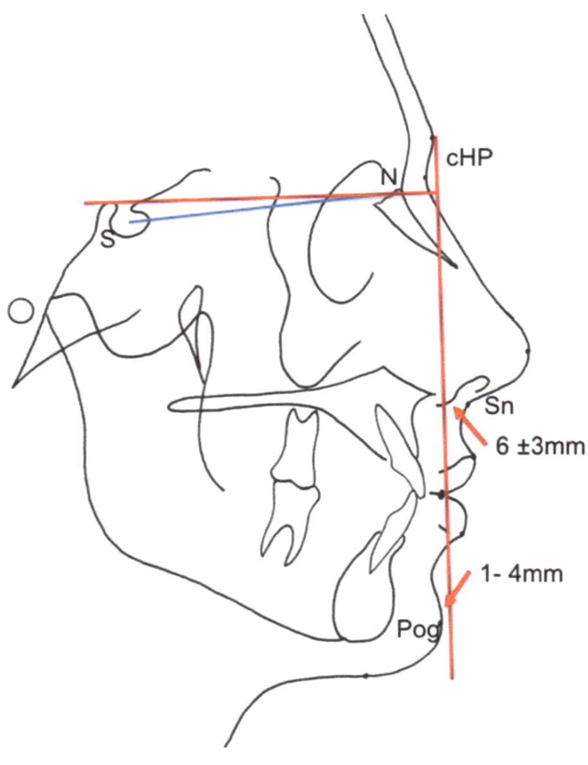

Figure 2.35 *Maxillary and mandibular anteroposterior position. Sn should be 6±3mm ahead and Pog' 1-4mm behind a vertical line through glabella (G'). The vertical line is perpendicular to a constructed horizontal (7° above Sn through N).*

Maxillary and mandibular anteroposterior position. A vertical line, perpendicular to the constructed horizontal (cHP), is drawn through the G'. Soft tissue pogonion (Pog') should be 1-4 mm behind the line. For maxillary anteroposterior assessment, the Sn should be 6±3 mm ahead of this line *(Fig 2.35)*.[20]

Interpretation: In maxillary anteroposterior deficiency cases, Sn will be less than 3 mm ahead of the line or in severe cases even behind the line. Pog' ahead of the line indicates possible mandibular anteroposterior excess, whereas in mandibular anteroposterior deficiency, Pog' will be more than 4 mm behind the line. It is, however, important to evaluate anteroposterior position of the chin in conjunction with other features (most importantly, the shape of the chin) to distinguish between microgenia, macrogenia, prognathia, or retrognathia.

Chin prominence. Soft tissue chin prominence can be evaluated by measuring the distance to a line drawn through soft tissue nasion perpendicular to Frankfort horizontal (FH). This line is also known as the O° meridian and Pog' should be 0±2 mm from this line *(Fig 2.36)*.[22]

Interpretation: The more prominent chin would be more than 2 mm ahead of the 0° meridian, whereas a horizontally deficient chin would be more than 2 mm posterior to the line.

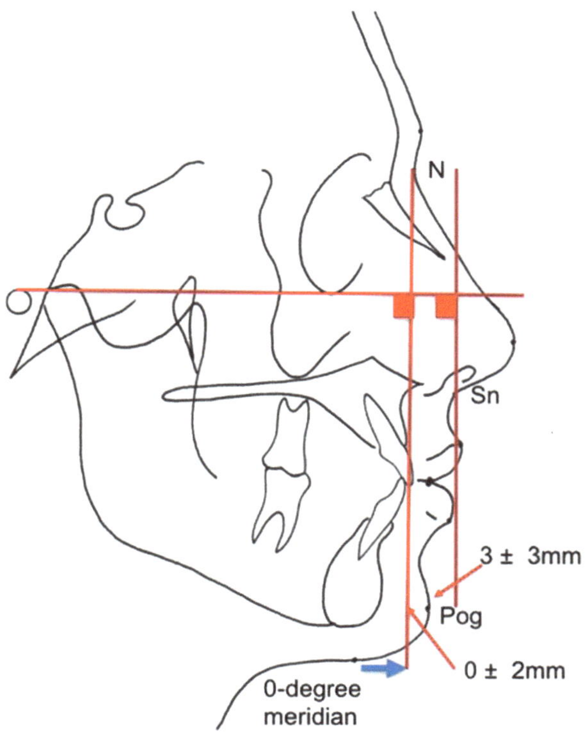

Figure 2.36 *Chin prominence. Anteroposterior evaluation of the chin to 0° meridian and a perpendicular line to Frankfort horizontal through Sn. Pog' to 0° meridian: 0±2mm ahead, and Pog' to Sn vertical line: 3±3mm behind.*

Another vertical line that is helpful in assessing the horizontal prominence of the chin is a line drawn perpendicular to FH through Sn. Pog' should be 3±3 mm behind this line *(Fig 2.36)*.

Interpretation: A horizontally excessive chin would be on or ahead of the vertical line, whereas a deficient chin would be more than 6 mm posterior. It is, however, important to use the above measurements only as a guide when assessing the chin position. Chin prominence must be evaluated in conjunction with other factors such as chin shape, depth of the labiomental fold, microgenia, macrogenia, lower lip position, and mandibular anteroposterior excess or deficiency.

Lower lip–chin submental angle. This angle is contained between a line drawn from Li to Pog' and a submental tangent line. An angulation of 110±8° is considered normal. For the submental assessment, it is paramount that the radiograph be obtained in a natural head posture *(Fig 2.37)*.

Interpretation: This angle will be more acute in mandibular anteroposterior excess cases and/or patients with macrogenia and more obtuse in mandibular anteroposterior deficiency and/or microgenia cases.

Chin–throat Length. This distance is measured from the Smn point to soft tissue Me' *(Fig 2.38)*. A distance of 42±6 mm is considered normal. This measurement is only meaningful with the patient's head is in a natural head posture.[23]

Interpretation: The distance will be excessive in mandibular prognathism or macrogenia and short in mandibular recessive or microgenia cases. When differentiating between mandibular anteroposterior excess and maxillary deficiency, this measurement is significant. Mandibular setback or chin reduction would obviously reduce this length with esthetic consequences.

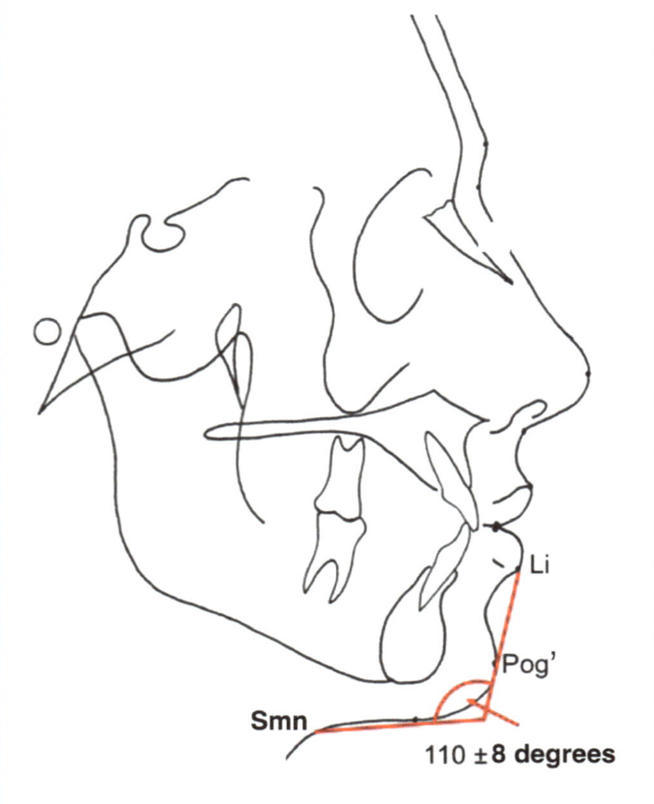

Figure 2.37 *Lower lip-chin-throat angle.*

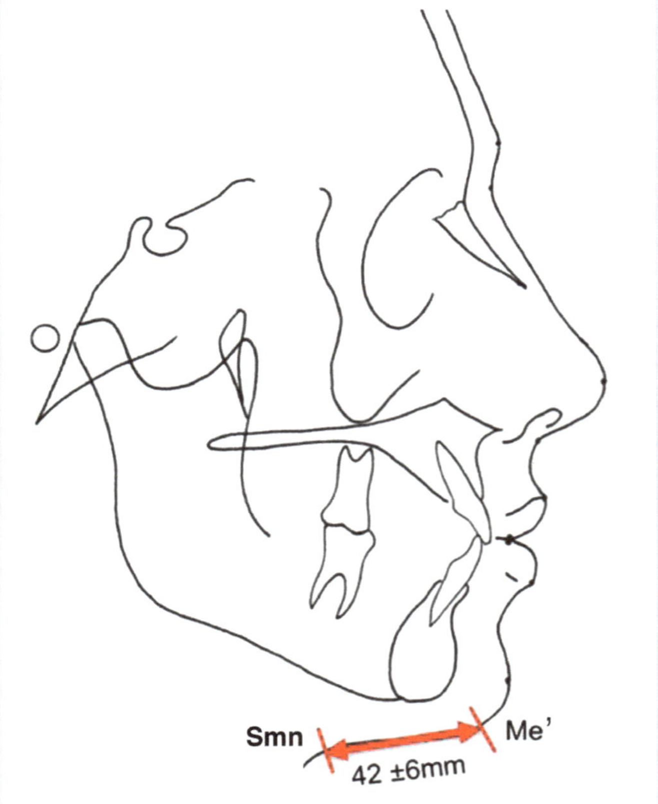

Figure 2.38 *Chin-throat length.*

Facial contour angle. The angle of facial convexity is formed by lines drawn from G' to the Sn [comprising the upper facial plane (UFP)] and from the Sn through soft tissue Pog' [comprising the lower facial plane (LFP)]. The mean angulation is estimated to be −12°.[3,7] A clockwise angle is expressed as positive, while an anti-clockwise angle expressed as negative. Males tend to have a straight profile (−11±4°), while a slightly more convex profile is considered esthetically pleasing for females (−13±4°) *(Fig 2.39)*. It is, however, important to differentiate between the various facial deformities that may produce the same facial contour angle. The value of the angle does not reveal the localization of the deformity.[5]

E-line (Esthetic Plane) – Rickets. The E-line is drawn from nasal tip (Pn) to soft tissue chin (Pog') *(Fig 2.40)*.[21] The upper lip should be ~4 mm behind the line, while the lower lip lies ~2 mm behind it. The profile contained by this line should form a symmetrical "cupid's bow."

Interpretation: Dental support for upper and lower lips, the depth of the labiomental fold, and the chin projection will affect these values and distort the shape of the cupids bow. The affect of an anteroposterior-deficient or -excessive chin position on the relationship of the lips and labiomental fold should therefore be kept in mind with this assessment.

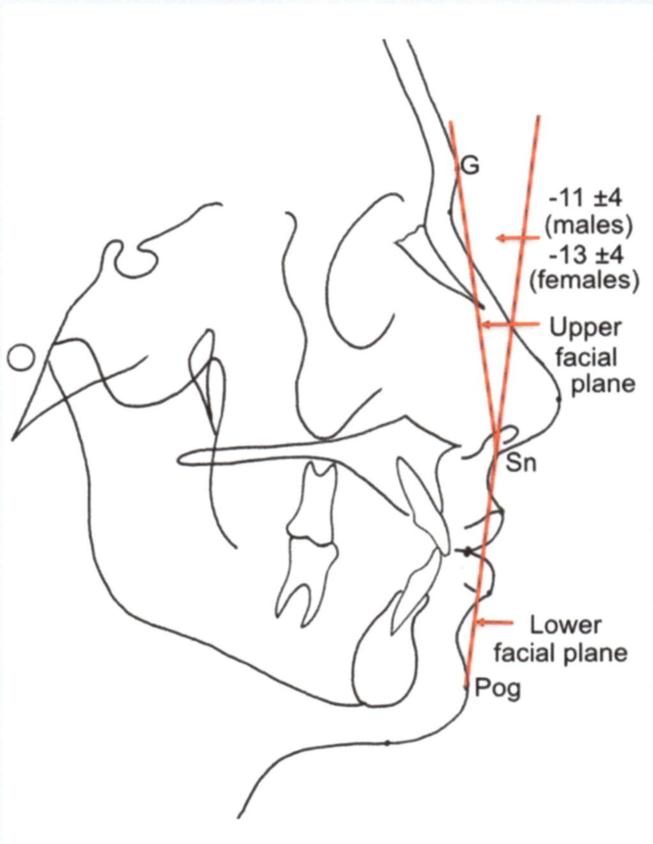

Figure 2.39 *Facial contour angle.*

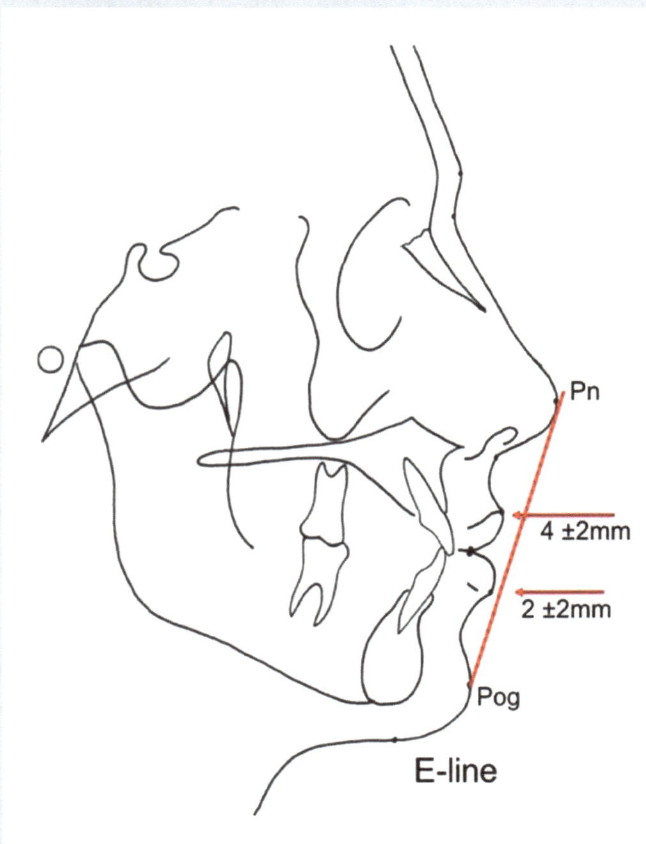

Figure 2.40 *Esthetic line.*

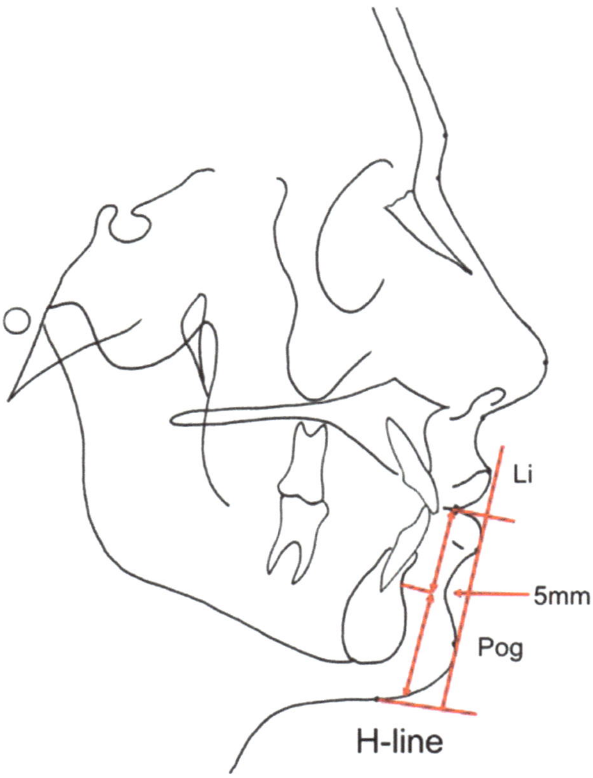

Figure 2.41 *The H-line. The anteroposterior position of the lips in combination with the depth and height of the labiomental fold plays an important role in the esthetic balance of the lower facial third.*

H-line (The Harmony Line). The H-line is tangent to Pog' and the Ls. The depth of the labiomental fold is measured at the point of deepest curvature between the lower lip and the chin and should be 5 mm. The deepest point of the labiomental fold should be one-half the lower two-thirds of the lower third of the face *(Fig 2.41).*[10,22]

The anteroposterior position of the lips in combination with the depth and height of the labiomental fold plays an important role in the esthetic balance of the lower facial third. In Class II division 1 cases with an increased overjet, the upper incisor teeth evert the lower lip and deepen the labiomental fold. Dental compensation by proclination of the lower incisors will inevitably worsen the soft tissue balance by increasing the lip fullness and deepening the labiomental fold *(Fig 2.42a & b).* Retroclination of the lower incisors in Class III cases will reduce lower lip support and flatten the labiomental fold, worsening the esthetics *(Fig 2.42c).*

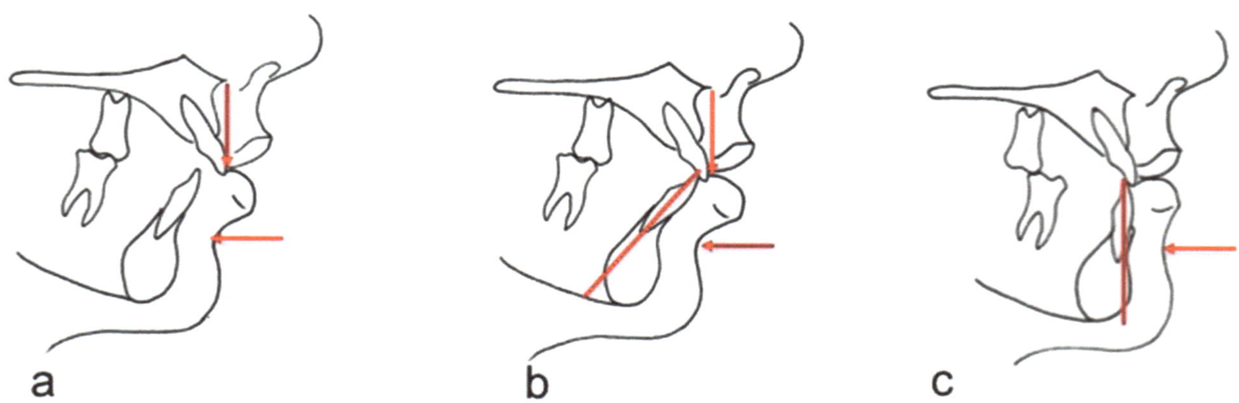

Figure 2.42 **a.** *The lower lip is everted and the labiomental fold accentuated by the upper incisor (arrows).* **b.** *Proclination of the incisors will inevitably disturb the soft tissue balance by increasing the lip fullness and deepen the labiomental fold (arrows).* **c.** *Retroclination (compensation) of the lower incisors in Class III cases will flatten the labiomental fold (arrow). Compromised correction by surgical reduction of the chin position in Class III cases without addressing the dental problem will result in poor esthetics.*

Interpretation: The sulcus will be deep when the lower lip is everted, e.g., Class II deep bite cases or excessive chin projection. In Class III cases with retroclined incisors (compensated), the lower lip tends to roll back, leading to an obtuse labiomental sulcus.

S-line (Steiner line). The S line is drawn from soft tissue chin (Pog') to the midpoint of the S-shaped curve between the Sn and the nasal tip (Pn) *(Fig 2.43)*. The upper and lower lips should touch this line with the chin in an ideal anteroposterior position.[24]

Interpretation: Lips behind this line may indicate a lack of lip support by the incisor teeth or a prominent chin. Lips ahead of this line may be due to dental protrusion or a deficient chin.

Merryfield's Z-Angle. The angle formed by the intersection of the FH and a line connecting soft tissue chin (Pog') and the most protrusive lip point (upper or lower) *(Fig 2.44)*. Average: 80±9°.[25]

Interpretation: An angle of more than 80° is indicative of mandibular anteroposterior excess, while an angle of less than 80° suggests an anteroposterior deficiency of the mandible. It also indicates the relationship of the lips to the chin as well as possible chin prominence or deficiency.

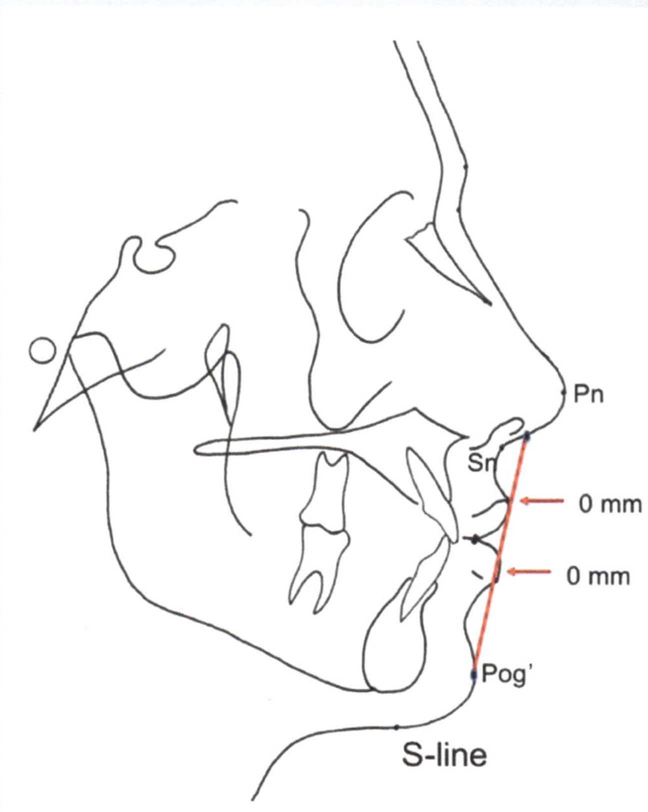

Figure 2.43 *S-line.*

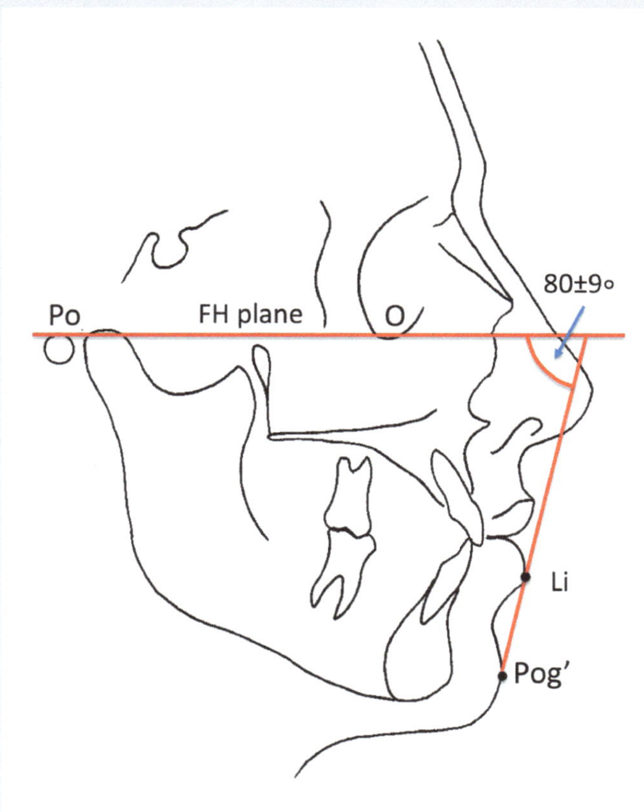

Figure 2.44 *Merryfields Z-angle.*

Soft Tissue Thickness. The thickness of the soft tissue of the chin is measured from the bone to the facial surface and should be 10 to 12 mm from the lower lip superior to gnathion inferior where the soft tissue will become thinner inferiorly *(Fig 2.45)*.[7,26–29]

Interpretation: Mentalis muscle hyperfunction will distort the harmonious tissue thickness and can be recognized on the lateral cephalometric radiograph by a flat, thin area of tissue at the inferior one-half of the chin, elevation of the lower lip above the lower incisor edges, and a flattened labiomental fold. Proclination of the incisors may result in lower lip strain, causing it to be thinner than the rest of the soft tissue covering the chin. Fat deposits in the soft tissues of the chin will increase the soft tissue thickness over the bony chin and should be noted, as removal of the fat may be part of the treatment plan. Fat in this area will also influence the soft tissue reaction to hard tissue change, making soft tissue prediction less reliable.

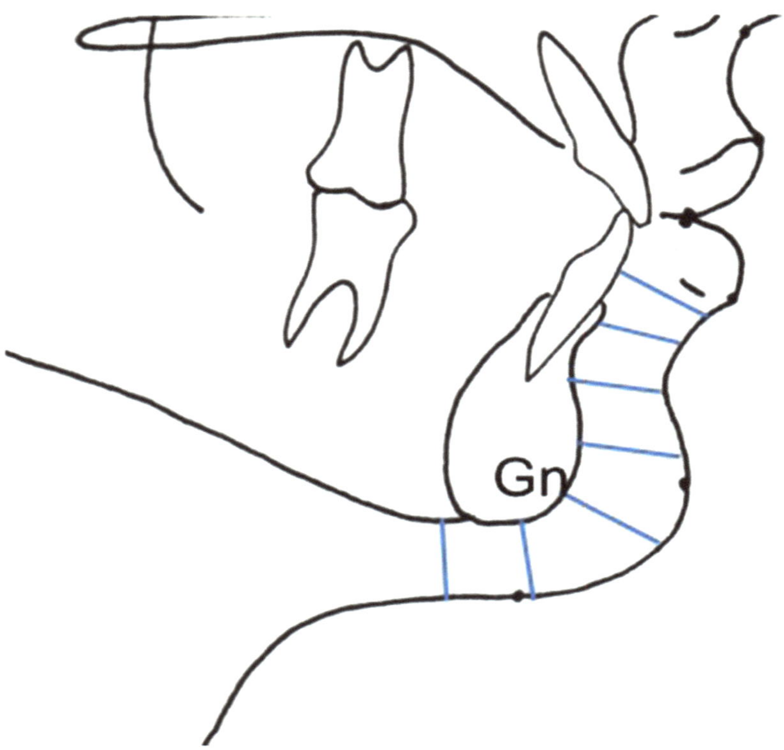

Figure 2.45 *Soft tissue thickness. The thickness of the lower lip and soft tissue covering the chin should be the same from the lip to gnathion (10-12 mm). Proclination of the lower incisors often causes lipstrain and hyperactive mentalis muscles distort the smooth and even soft tissue contour of the chin. Excessive thickness of the soft tissue covering the bony chin is indicative of fat deposit in this area.*

Anteroposterior Soft Tissue Relations Summary

Anteroposterior		Normal
Lip prominence:	Sn – Pog' to: Ls Sn – Pog' to: Li SnV to: Ls SnV to: Li	3 ± 1 mm ahead 2 ± 1 mm ahead 1–2 mm ahead 0 mm
Chin prominence:	0°meridian to Pog' Sn perpendicular to FH to Pog'	0 ± 2 mm 3 ± 3 mm behind
Lower lip – Chin–Submental Angle		110 ± 8°
Chin Neck Length		42 ± 6 mm
Facial contour angle		−11 ± 4 male −13 ± 4 female
E – line:	to Ls to Li	−4 mm −2 mm
S – line:	to Ls to Li	0 mm 0 mm
Merryfields Z-angle		80 ± 9°
Soft tissue thickness		10–12 mm

Skeletal Analysis

A - Subspinale.
Most posterior midline point in the concavity where the lower front edge of the anterior nasal spine meets the alveolar bone overlying the maxillary incisors.

ANS- Anterior nasal Spine.
Anterior tip of the nasal spine.

B - Supramentale.
Most posterior midline point in the concavity of the mandible between the alveolar bone overlying the lower incisors (infra dentale) and pogonion.

Co - Condylion.
Most posterosuperior point on the head of the condyle.

G - Glabella. *The most anterior point of the frontal bone.*

Go - Gonion.
Point located on the curvature of the mandible defined by bisecting the angle formed by two lines, one tangent to the inferior border of the mandible and the other tangent to the posterior border of the ramus.

Gn - Gnathion.
The lowest, most anterior midline point on the symphysis of the mandible (midway between menton and pogonion).

Me - Menton.
The most inferior point on the symphysis of the mandible in the midline.

N - Nasion.
The most anterior point on the frontal nasal suture in the mid-sagittal plane.

O - Orbitale.
The lowest point on the inferior orbital rim.

PNS - Posterior Nasal Spine.
The most posterior aspect of the palatine bone.

Pog - Pogonion.
The most anterior point of the chin.

Pr - Porion.
The most superior point of the external auditory meatus (anatomical point). Machine porion is the uppermost point on the outline of the rods of the cephalometer.

Ptm - Pterygomaxillare.
The apex of the teardrop-shaped pterygo-maxillary fissure (lowest point of the opening).

S - Sella (sella turcica).
The center of the sella as on the lateral cephalogram and is located by inspection.

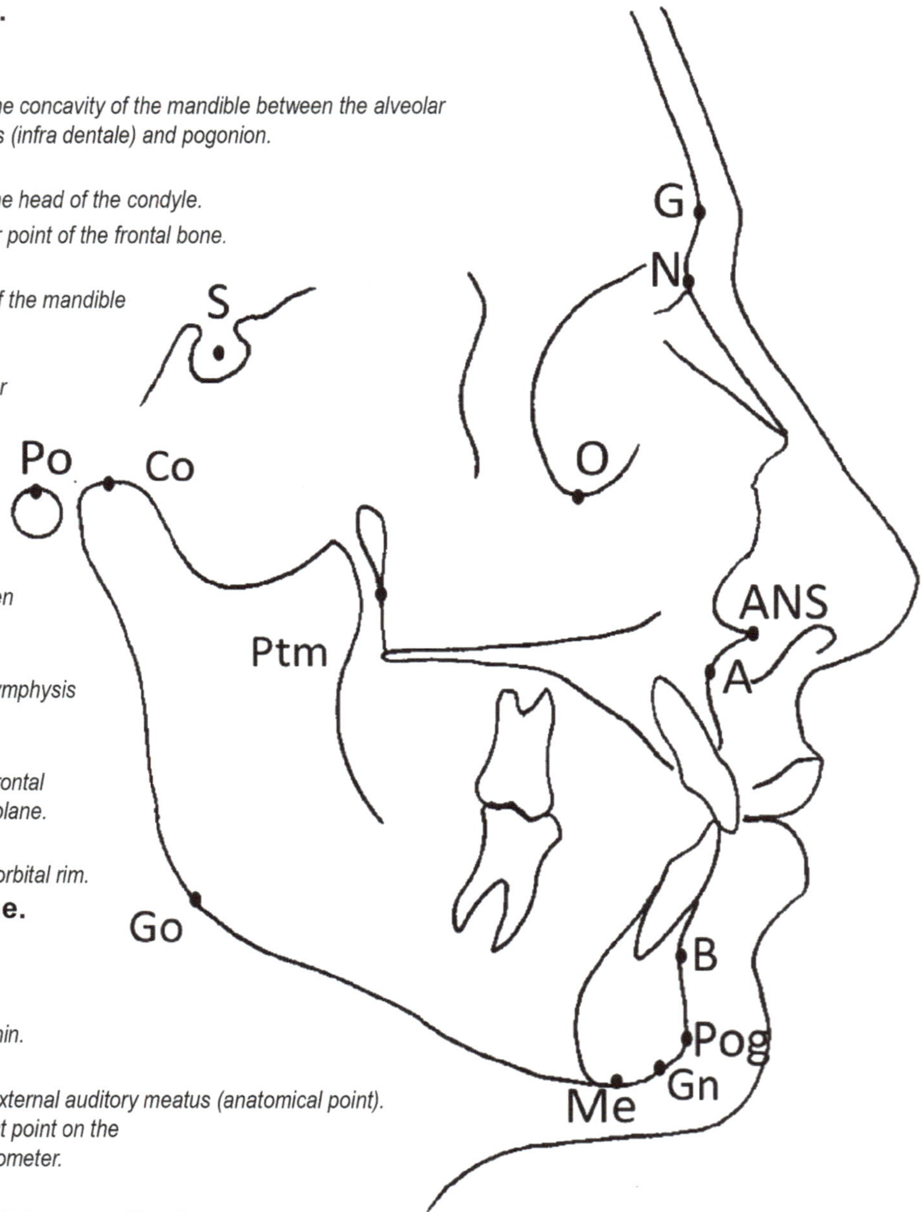

Figure 2.46 *Hard tissue landmarks*

Anteroposterior Evaluation

The clinician should differentiate between mandibular anteroposterior excess and macrogenia as well as mandibular anteroposterior deficiency and microgenia. An attempt to correct mandibular anteroposterior excess by chin reduction or mandibular anteroposterior deficiency by chin augmentation will lead to poor aesthetic results.

Facial angle (Downs's). The facial angle is the inferior inside angle in which the facial plane (N-Pog) intersects the FH. Mean: 82 to 95° *(Fig 2.47a)*.[30] A line perpendicular to the FH through B-point should be 4 mm behind the facial plane (N-Pog), indicating the amount of chin projection. Figure 2.47b and c shows patients with macrogenia (B-point perpendicular ahead of the facial plane) and microgenia (B-point perpendicular more than 4 mm behind the facial plane).

Interpretation: The facial angle indicates the relative anteroposterior position of the mandible to the cranium.

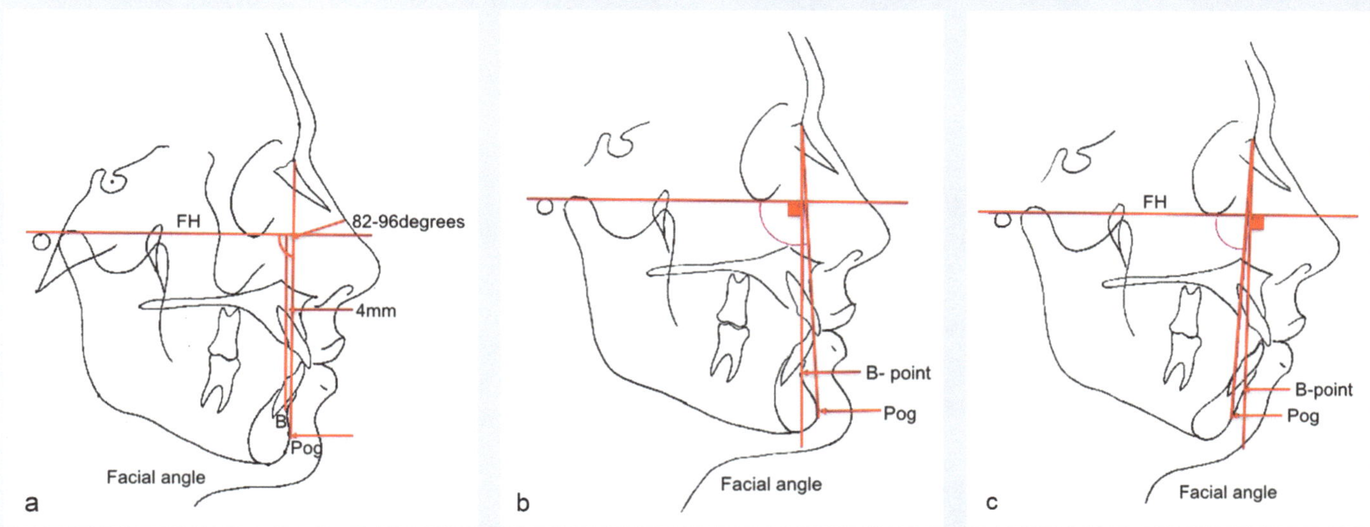

Figure 2.47 *Facial angle. Mean: 82 to 96°* **a.** *By relating B-point to the N-Pog line one can distinguish between mandibular anteroposterior excess and macrogenia.* **b.** *When the mandible is anteroposterior excessive the chin projection ahead of the N-Pog line will be normal (4mm) or slightly increased, while when the chin is excessive this distance will be increased. When microgenia is present, B-point will be less than 4mm behind the N-Pog line or even ahead of the line.* **c.** *In cases where the mandible is anteroposteriorly deficient, B-point and the N-Pog line would be normal or close to normal relationship (B-point 4mm behind N-Pog line).*

Facial Depth Angle. This angle is formed by the facial line (Nasion – A-point) and the FH plane (the posteroinferior angle) and should be ±90° *(Fig 2.48)*. Pog should be 4 mm ahead of an in.ferior extension of the facial line (N-A).[31,32]

Interpretation: The facial angle indicates the relative anteroposterior position of the mandible (or chin) to the cranium and maxilla. The discrepancy between the facial plane and the B-point perpendicular to the FH is an indication of the chin projection.

Lower Incisor Lip and Chin Relation. The lower incisor is responsible for lower lip support, while the hard tissue of the chin (position of Pog) determines the soft tissue chin projection.[33] The degree of chin prominence is one of the factors that will influence the orthodontic positioning of the lower incisor teeth in the mandibular arch. The balance between the incisor position and chin projection will determine the depth of the labiomental sulcus. According to Haldaway,[32] the distance of the labial surface of the lower incisor and Pog to the N-B line should be equal (i.e., 4 mm) *(Fig 2.49)*.

Interpretation: If a discrepancy between these two measurements exceeds 4 mm, corrective measures are indicated. Corrective measures would include orthodontic correction of the lower incisor angulation, surgical repositioning of the chin, or both.

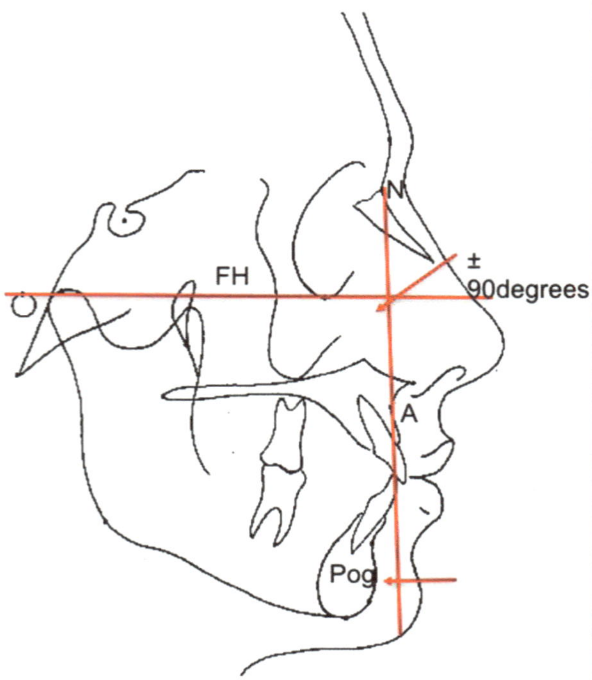

Figure 2.48 *Facial depth angle.*

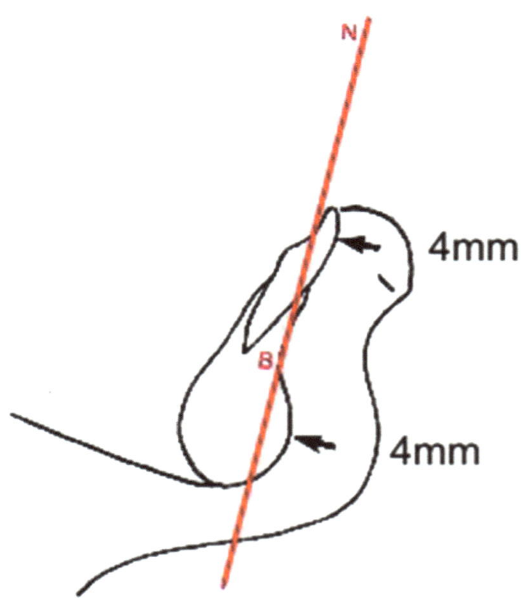

Figure 2.49 *Lower incisor lip and chin relation. Pogonion and the labial surface of the lower incisor is 4mm ahead of the Nasion B-point line.*

Vertical Evaluation

Skeletal Vertical Relations Mid- to Lower Face Skeletal Height. The skeletal mid-facial height is measured from N to anterior nasal spine (ANS) and the lower facial height from ANS to Me. A vertical line is drawn perpendicular to the FH plane anterior to the face. In turn, perpendicular lines are drawn to the vertical line from the N, ANS, and Me and the distance measured from N to ANS and from ANS to Me *(Fig 2.50).* The normal values are considered to be 53 mm from N to ANS and 65 mm from ANS to Me. However, the relationship between the vertical heights is more important than the actual measurement. A ratio of 5 to 6 is normal.[7,22]

Interpretation: In most individuals with vertical dentofacial deformities, the lower facial height (ANS – Me) will be affected. ANS – Me will be increased in individuals with vertical maxillary excess, vertical mandibular excess, and open bites. The lower facial height (ANS – Me) will be decreased in individuals with vertical maxillary deficiency, deep bites, and vertical mandibular deficiency.

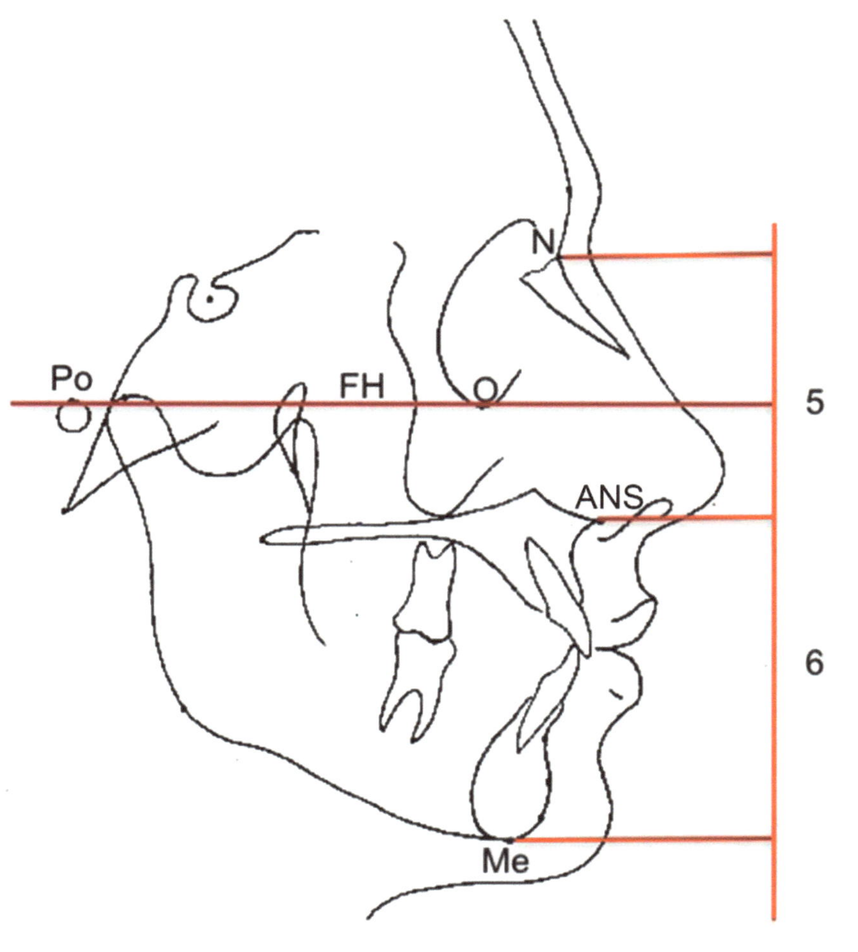

Figure 2.50 *Mid-and lower face skeletal heights.*

Lower Anterior Dental Height. The average lower dental height for males is 44±2 mm and for females is 40±2 mm and is measured from mandibular incisor tip to the inferior border of the mandible *(Fig 2.51)*. The average length of the lower incisor and canine teeth is more important because to assure tooth vitality, the horizontal osteotomy should be performed at least 5 mm below the tooth apexes. The average length of the lower incisor is 21.4 mm, the length of the lower lateral incisor is 23.2 mm, and the length of the canine is 25.4 mm.

Interpretation: With an increase in the lower vertical height of the face, normal upper lip length, and normal maxillary incisor exposure, the anterior vertical height of the mandible may be increased. Vertical reduction genioplasty may be indicated. The amount of bone below the incisors and canine teeth will dictate the amount of bone that can be removed safely in individuals that require vertical reduction of the chin. When simultaneous vertical reduction and anteroposterior chin augmentation is indicated, both of these dimensional changes may be achieved by changing the angulation of the horizontal osteotomy.

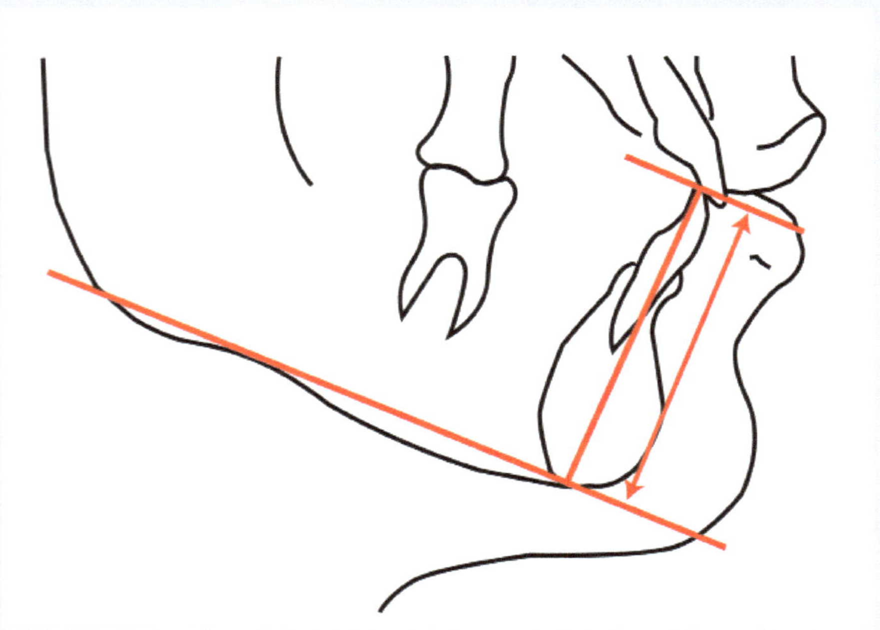

Figure 2.51 *Lower anterior dental height.*

Posteroanterior Cephalometric Analysis

Individuals with facial asymmetry require a posteroanterior radiograph of the facial bones in addition to a lateral cephalometric radiograph. This radiograph assists in differentiating between asymmetry of the various facial structures, the dimensions involved, and the severity of the asymmetry.[7,34–36] Computer-generated scan digital images have certainly become a state-of-the-art requirement for the accurate assessment of complex cases, i.e., facial asymmetry and syndromic cases *(Fig 2.52)*.

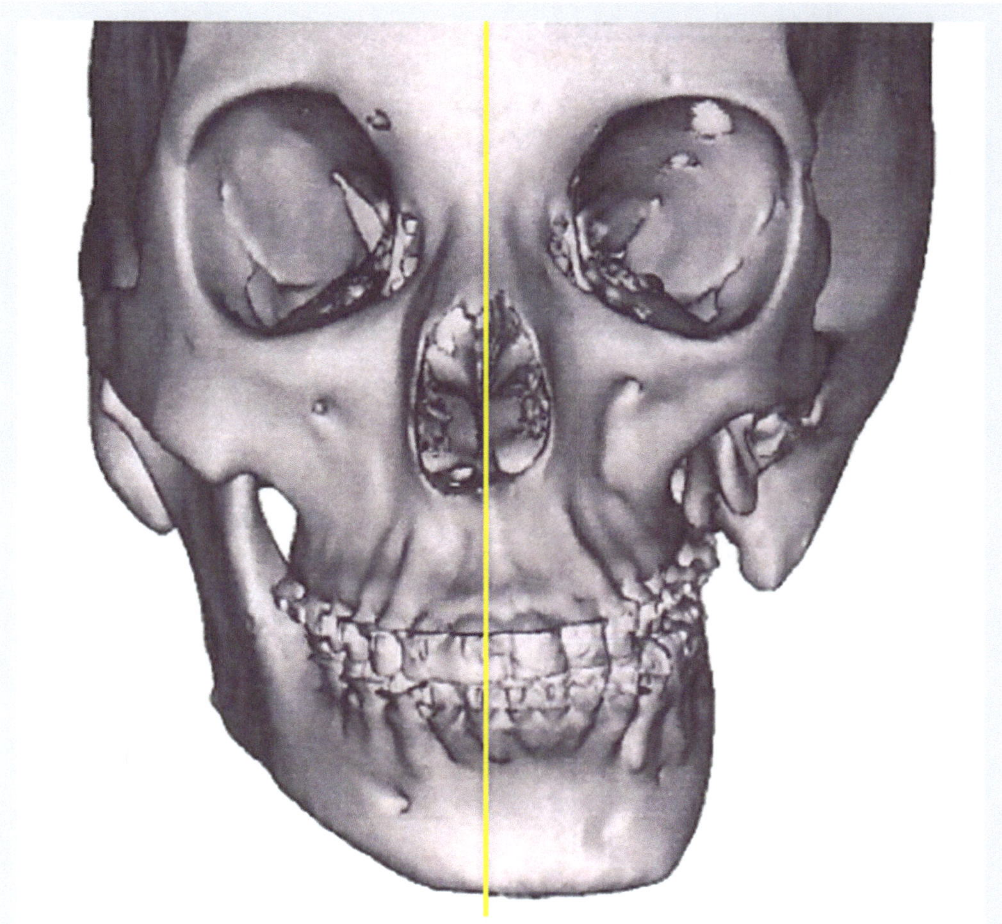

Figure 2.52 *A Postero-anterior computer generated 3D scan of the facial skeleton of an individual with Kaban type III hemifacial microsomia. This image allows for virtual surgical planning.*

Hard Tissue Posteroanterior Landmarks

A - *Contact area between the maxillary incisor teeth.*

ANS- Anterior Nasal Spine.
The center point at the base of the nose.

B - *Contact area between the mandibular incisor teeth.*

CH - Chin Plate.
Most inferior lateral point on the anterior inferior border of the mandible: CHL left & CHR right.

Go - Gonion.
Most inferior posterior point at the angle of the mandible.

J - Jugelare.
Most superior and medial point on the zygomatic buttress.

M - Mastoid.
The most inferior point on the mastoid bone.

Me - Menton.
The most inferior point at the anterior mandibular area.

SF - Sphenoid Fissure.
Where the smaller wing of the sphenoid bone crosses the medial orbital ridge.

Y - *Most lateral point on the buccal surface area of the first maxillary molar tooth.*

Z - *Most lateral point on the buccal surface area of the first mandibular molar tooth.*

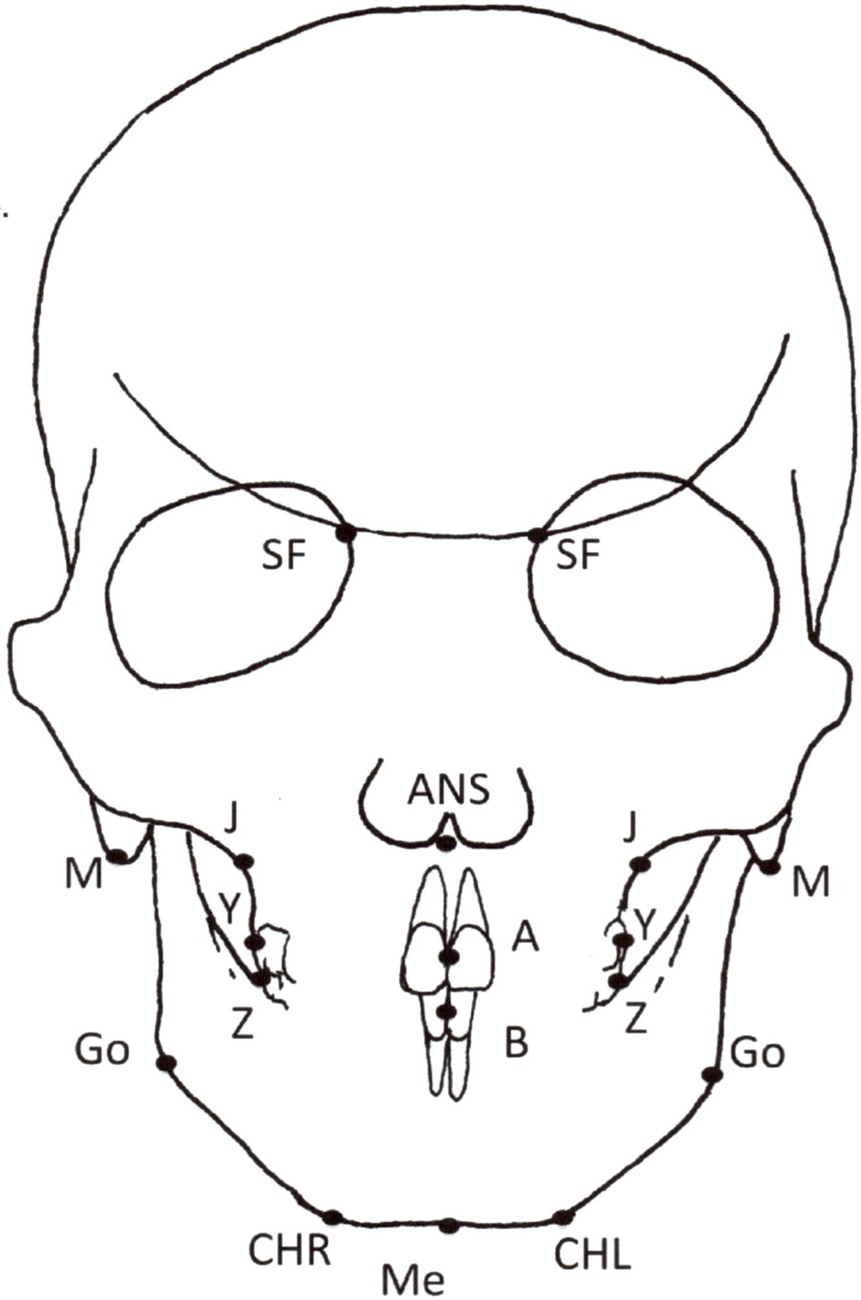

Figure 2.53. *Posteroanterior cephalometric landmarks*

Transverse and Vertical Planes

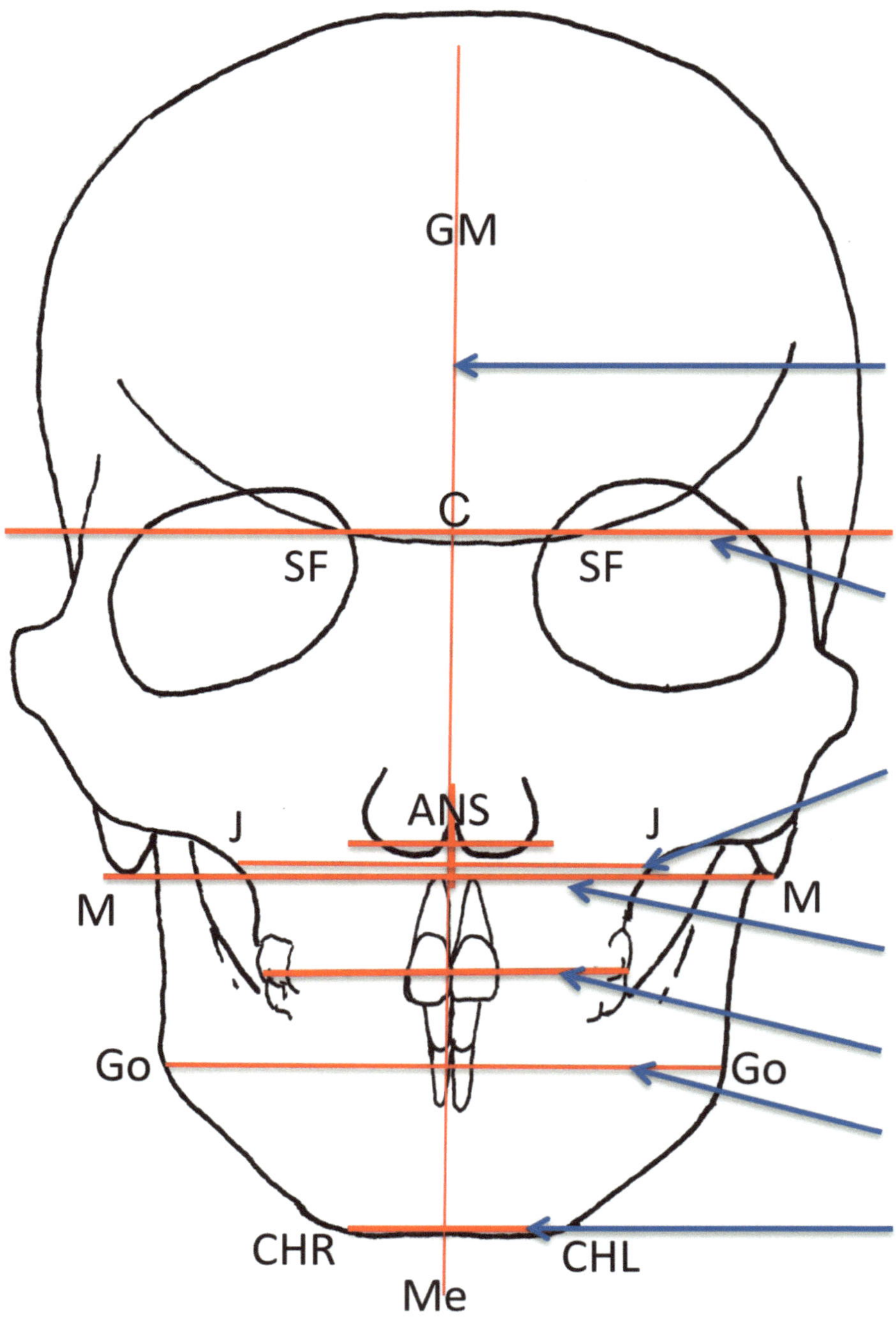

ANS- Ant. Nasal Spine
CHL- Chin Left
CHR- Chin Right
GM - Geometric Axis
Go - Gonion
J - Jugelare
M - Mastoid
Me - Menton
SF - Sphenoid Fissure

Geometric axis
Constructed by dividing the C-plane and the S-plane, connecting these two midpoints, and extending this line to the chin.

C-plane
Cranial Base Plane.Horizontal line connecting the left and right SF points extending laterally to the cranium.

C - *The midpoint between the left and right SF points*

J-plane
Line connecting left and right J-point divided in two halves by GM.

Mastoid plane
Line connecting left and right mastoid points.

Occlusal plane
Line connecting occluding points of the maxillary mandibular buccal cusps.

S-plane
Line connecting left and right Gonion (Go) of the mandible.

Chin plane
The inferior border of the chin at maximum bone contact through Me.

Figure 2.54 *Posteroanterior transverse and vertical planes.*

Facial Triangles

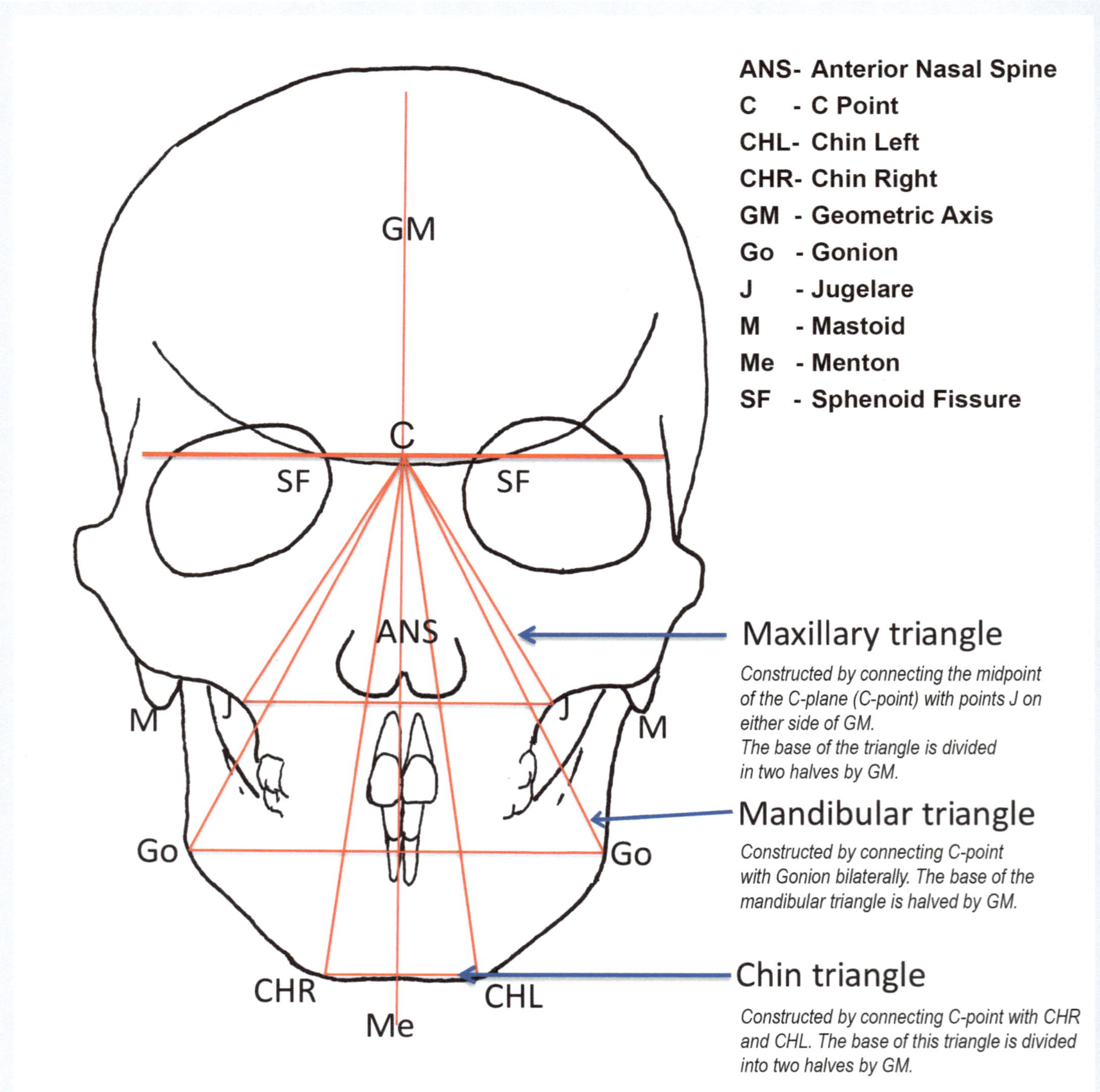

Figure 2.55 *Construction of posteroanterior facial triangles.*

The Maxillary Triangle is formed by connecting C-point with left and right J-points. The base of the triangle indicates the cant of the base of the maxilla as well as transverse symmetry of the maxilla *(Fig 2.55).*

The Mandibular Triangle is formed by connecting C-point with the left and right side of the S-plane (left and right gonion). This triangle is helpful when assessing mandibular asymmetry *(Fig 2.55).*

The Chin Triangle is formed by connecting the left and right side of the chin plane (CHR and CHL) with C-point. Draw a line from B-point perpendicular to CH to evaluate the mandibular incisor midline in relation to the midline of the chin *(Fig 2.55).*

Treatment planning is assisted by relating the base of the triangle with the horizontal plane and the occlusal plane. It is important to differentiate between, mandibular asymmetry, dental asymmetry, occlusal cant, lower border cant and chin midline asymmetry or any combination of the above.

Interpretation: By measuring the long legs of the triangles, cants in the maxilla, mandible, and chin can be evaluated in relation to the cranial base as well as to each other. By comparing the left and right sides of the bases of the triangles, transverse discrepancies on rotations can be assessed. Midline asymmetries of the nasal spine, menton, and dental midlines should be also evaluated. Discrepancies between the mandibular dental midline and the midpoint of the chin should be evaluated by using the vertical line.

When a discrepancy exists between the lower dental midline and the midline of the chin, correction should include genioplasty. The cant of the lower border of the chin (CHR-CHL) should be related to the occlusal plane. A transverse cant in the occlusal plane often exists in patients with condylar hyper- or hypoplasia and surgical correction for these deformities will include correction of the occlusal cant. If the cant of the lower border is parallel to the occlusal cant of the mandible, it will be corrected as a consequence of the correction of the occlusal cant. In cases where the cants differ, surgical correction of the lower border is indicated. *(See Chapter 4, Surgical Technique.)*

Panoramic Radiograph

A panoramic radiograph is an excellent means to establish the position of anatomic structures involved during the genioplasty procedure, e.g., the position of the mental foramina and the root apices of the lower incisor and canine teeth *(Fig 2.55).*

The osteotomy should be performed at least 5 mm below the apices of the teeth and the mental foramen. The mental foramen lies halfway between the upper and lower borders of the mandible and between the premolar teeth in the dentate patient where it allows exit to the inferior alveolar nerve now called the mental nerve. The foramen faces backward and slightly upward. The mental nerve is a sensory nerve and supplies the skin of the lower lip and chin and the adjacent mucous membrane and gingiva. This information will assist in the design of the genioplasty osteotomy as well as the performance of the surgery safely without damage to the nerve.[37] *(See Chapter 4, Surgical Technique.)*

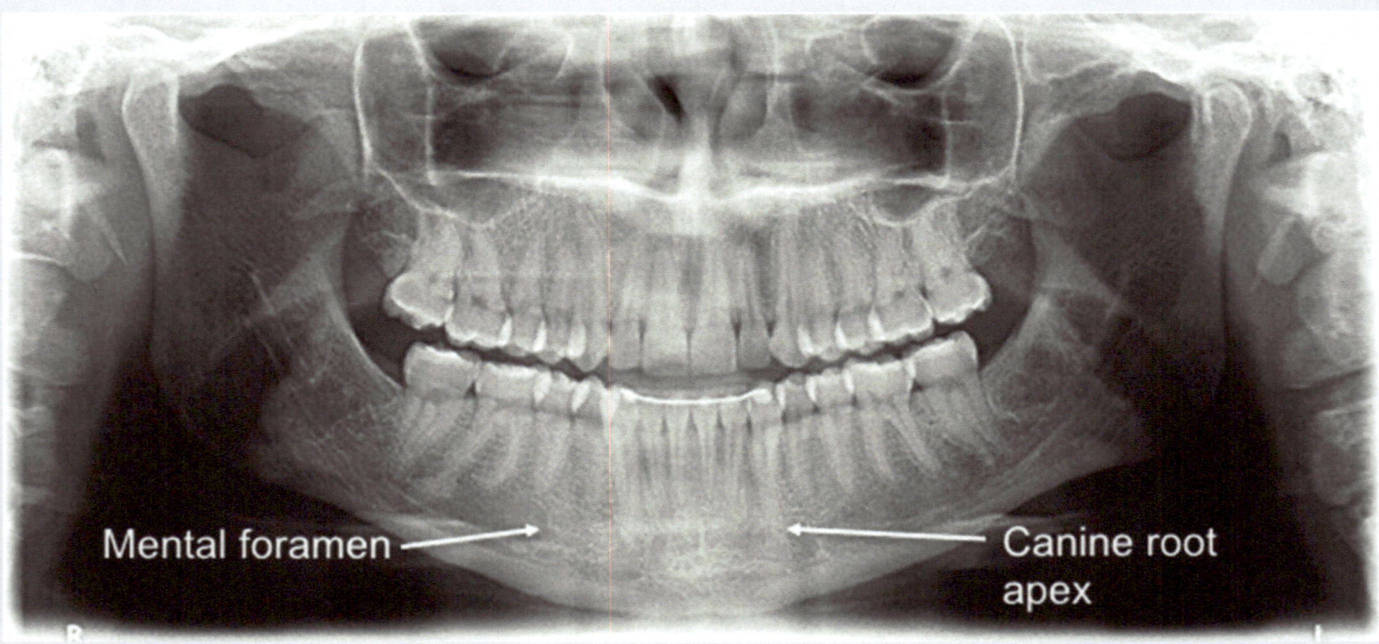

Figure 2.56 *Panoramic radiograph. Note: The position of the mental foramen and inferior alveolar canal (arrow) and the length of the canines and lower incisor teeth (arrow).*

Chapter 3 - Development of the Visual Treatment Objective

Genioplasty may be performed as a single procedure for the correction of a chin deformity. However, it more often forms part of the orthognathic surgical correction of a dentofacial deformity. The planning for a genioplasty procedure is therefore often done in conjunction with other surgical procedures to establish optimal functional and esthetic results. The visual treatment objectives are developed from a lateral cephalometric radiograph tracing and are used in conjunction with all the data obtained from the systematic patient evaluation to make the visual objectives as accurate and realistic as possible.[1–6]

The prediction tracing (PT) has become an integral part of the treatment planning and the assessment of post-treatment results. It is done with three questions in mind:

1. Will the surgical procedure produce the required soft tissue esthetic changes?
2. In cases where orthodontic tooth movement is contemplated, how will the tooth movement influence the lip position, which in turn will influence the soft tissue balance of the chin?
3. How will other orthognathic surgical procedures, contemplated in conjunction with genioplasty, influence the facial balance in relation to the chin?

Numerous studies have produced average ratios relating soft tissue response to hard tissue change.[7–15] Clinicians realized, however, that these ratios were averages and individual variabilities are significant. Soft tissue response is influenced not only by skeletal repositioning but also by surgical technique and respectful control of hard and soft tissue during surgery. In 1970, J.M. Ferrer wrote, "It must be recognized that at every operation the surgeon inevitably injures the patient; this injury can and must be minimized by the use of careful, gentle and accurate surgical technique."

The visual treatment objective has several advantages:

- It can accurately predict the soft tissue result following skeletal repositioning of the chin. The predicted soft tissue result can be assessed and the treatment plan adjusted if necessary.
- It enables the clinician to investigate various treatment options and to evaluate the advantages of each option before treatment, e.g., should a Class II occlusion be treated orthodontically and the mandible be advanced or should an existing occlusion be excepted and the chin advanced by means of a genioplasty.
- The post-surgical skeletal and soft tissue result can be assessed and compared to the predicted objectives.
- It acts as a communication between the surgeon and the patient as well as between the surgeon and the orthodontist.

When genioplasty is performed as part of other orthognathic surgical corrections, the planning of the hard and soft tissue prediction of the chin is done last.

The development of the visual treatment objectives for chin surgery are discussed here, assuming that all other facial hard and soft tissue structures are in an ideal position or have surgically been placed in their planned (ideal) position on the visual treatment objective.

It is emphasized that during the esthetic planning of the soft tissue of the chin, consideration should not only be given to horizontal (profile) changes, but also to the transverse and vertical dimension and the shape of the chin. This is then related to the overall esthetics of the face. The following factors should be considered when planning the final chin esthetics:

- the height of the chin
- lower lip length
- lower lip vermillion exposure
- depth of labiomental angle
- submental–neck angle
- submental length
- curvature of the chin
- the relationship between the chin, lips, and nose
- anterior and posterior width of the chin
- the cant of the lower border

Step by Step Development of a Visual Treatment Objective for Genioplasty

Prediction Tracing For Advancement Genioplasty

STEP 1. Obtain a lateral cephalometric radiograph with the patient's teeth in centric occlusion, a natural head posture, and the lips in repose. Establish an original tracing (OT) by tracing the hard and soft tissue structures without analysis lines on a separate sheet of acetate paper *(Fig 3.1).*

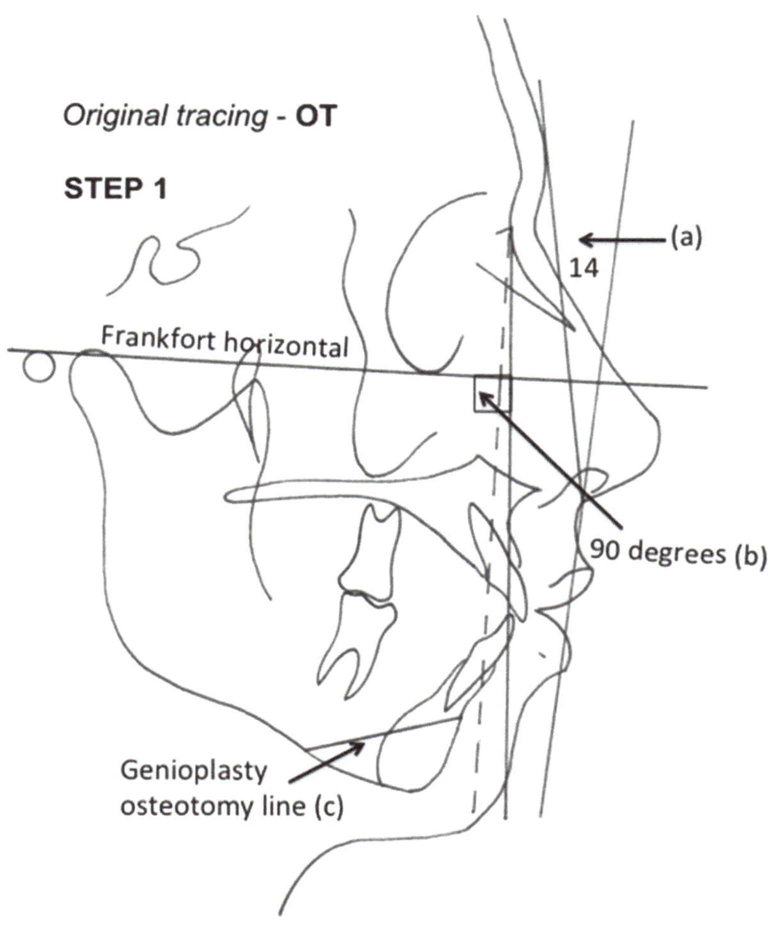

Figure 3.1 - STEP 1 *Prediction for an advancement genioplasty. The original tracing (OT).* **a.** *Draw a facial contour angle of -14° (soft tissue).* **b.** *Draw a facial depth angle of 90° (predicted hard tissue).* **c.** *Draw a line representing the planned osteotomy line.*

Various cephalometric analysis in combination with the data obtained during the clinical examination and the clinicians artistic flare may now be used to establish the ideal hard tissue and soft tissue pogonion positions, respectively. In this case, the constructed facial depth angle and facial contour angle are used as indicators for the ideal anteroposterior hard and soft tissue positions, respectively.

The facial depth angle is formed by drawing a line from nasion (N) through the A-point crossing the FH plane. The posteroinferior angle of the line to the FH should be 90° for males and 86° for females. An extension of the N-A line should go through pogonion (Pog') and acts as a guide for the desired hard tissue chin projection.[5] In this case, the current facial depth angle is 94°. A line through N perpendicular to the FH is constructed (dotted line) at an angle of 90° to represent the desired hard tissue (Pog) position. The soft tissue chin projection (Pog') may be indicated by the construction of an "ideal" facial contour angle (males 11-15° and females 13-17°). The facial contour angle is formed between the upper facial plane (G'-Sn) and the lower facial plane (Sn-Pog').[6]

In Figure 3.1, the facial line (N-A) is constructed through N at 90°

to the FH and the lower facial plane constructed at an angle of 14° (considered to be esthetically pleasing for this specific patient).

Now, also draw the intended osteotomy line on the anterior mandible where the genioplasty will be performed. Anatomical structures such as the mental nerve (mental foramen) and the apices of the incisor and canine teeth should be considered. *See Chapter 4, Surgical Technique.)*

The Genioplasty Osteotomy Line. The height as well as the angulation of the osteotomy play important roles in the esthetic outcome. In Chapter 4 (Surgical Technique), the esthetic effect obtained with advancement of the chin along a steep angle compared to a more horizontal angle and a high and low horizontal osteotomy is discussed. The shape of the chin, and to a lesser extent, the depth and position of the labiomental fold, can be influenced by varying the height of the osteotomy. In Chapter 4, Figure 4.46d illustrates the difference in soft tissue outcome that can be expected by varying the osteotomy height.

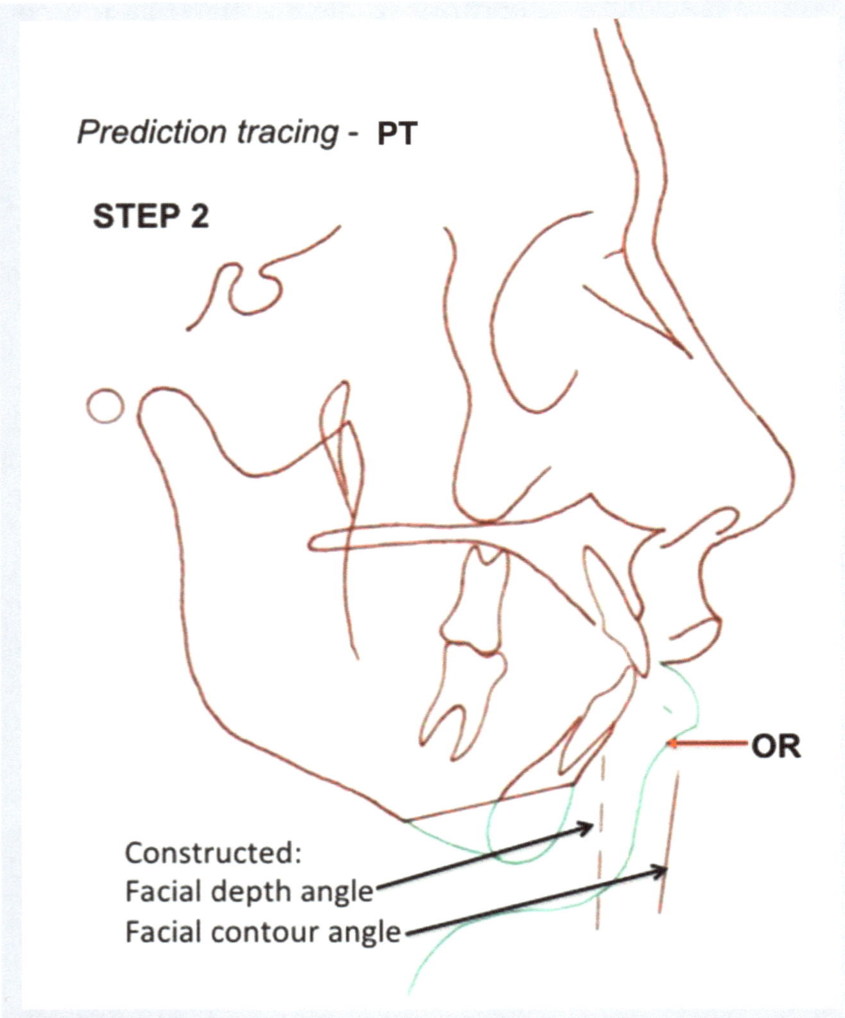

Figure 3.2 - STEP 2 *Place a clean piece of tracing paper over the OT. The tracing will be called the prediction tracing (PT). All structures not to be influenced by the genioplasty are traced in red (the soft tissue below stomion and hard tissue below the osteotomy line). The constructed N-A line and the LFP in the chin area are also traced.*

STEP 2. Start the PT on a clean piece of acetate paper by tracing (in red) all the soft and hard tissue structures that will not be influenced by the genioplasty. It is assumed that all other facial structures are in good balance *(Fig 3.2).*

The hard tissue below the genioplasty osteotomy line, and the soft tissue of the lower lip, chin, and submental area are not traced. Also, trace part of the facial plane line (N-A) and lower facial plane (LFP) constructed on the OT in the chin area.

STEP 3. Draw the lower lip and the ideal soft tissue of the chin on the PT guided (in this instance) by the constructed lower facial plane at −14° for chin projection. Complete the soft tissue by drawing the submental area. The lower lip, labiomental sulcus, and chin should be in balance and should form a smooth S-curve. Create a symmetric "cupid's bow" *(Fig 3.3)*.

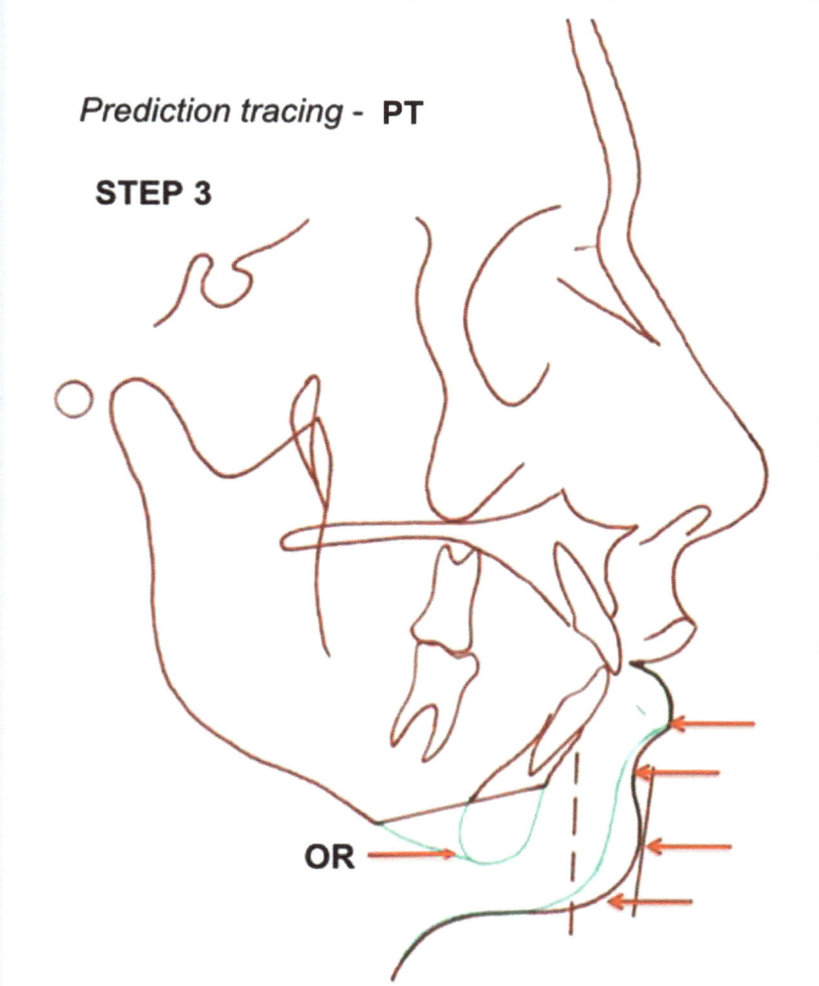

Figure 3.3 - STEP 3 *Utilize the LFP and the clinician's artistic flare to draw the desired soft tissue of the chin in red (arrows).*

STEP 4. Numerous investigators have found a consistent relationship between hard tissue surgical advancement of the chin and soft tissue response *(Fig 3.4)*.[7–15]

Hard Tissue:Soft Tissue = 1:0.9

Slide the PT to the left. The OT will move to the right relative to the PT. Move the PT until the soft tissue of the chin on the OT and PT coincide *(Fig 3.4)*. Evaluate the osteotomy lines of the OT and PT; If the two lines coincide, it is an indication that an advancement of the chin along this osteotomy line would produce the predicted soft tissue result. In case the lines do not coincide, a change in angulation of the osteotomy, a change in the height of the osteotomy, a vertical reduction or augmentation, or the soft tissue prediction should be reconsidered. The soft tissue shape should be reasonably compatible with the soft tissue shape of the OT. With the knowledge of the soft tissue response to the hard tissue change, it can now be calculated how far the hard tissue chin has to be advanced to affect the predicted soft tissue esthetics. *(Refer to Table 1.)* In this case, the planned soft tissue changes are 6 mm and will require 6.5 mm of hard tissue advancement. The facial line constructed in this instance is also an indication of hard tissue pogonion position *(arrow)*.

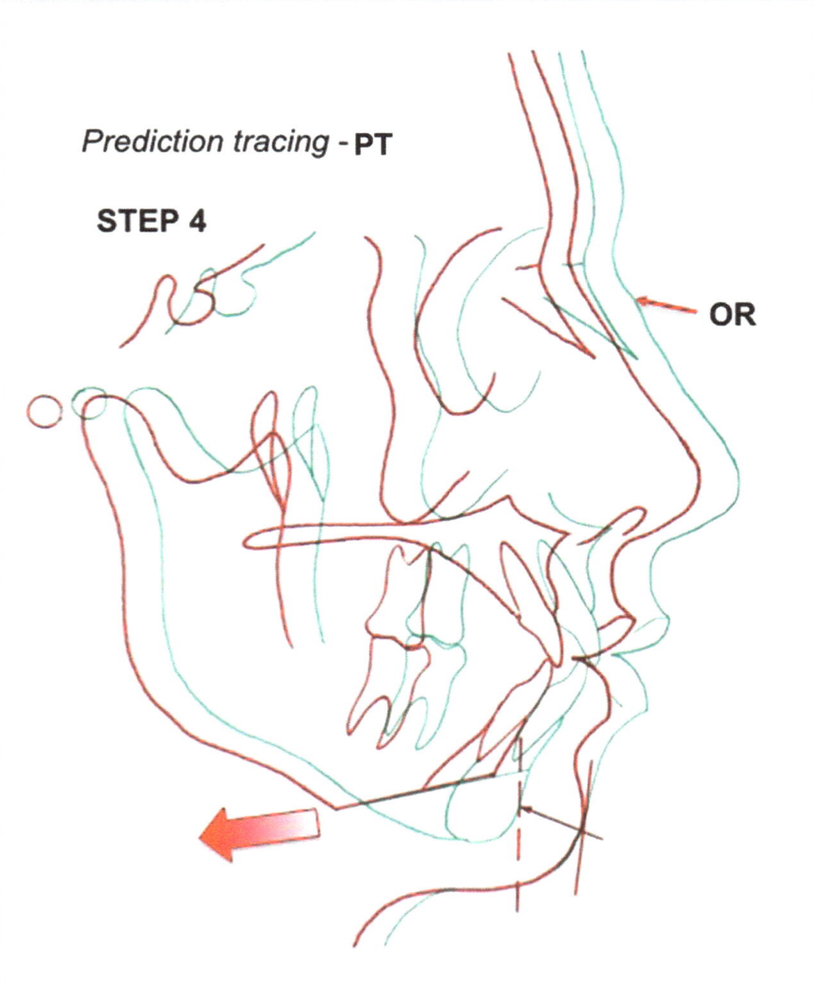

Figure 3.4 - STEP 4 *Slide the prediction tracing (PT) to the left along the osteotomyline. The hard tissue of the chin on the OT will effectively move to the right on the PT. The expected soft tissue reaction in relation to the hard tissue repositioning is summarized in Table 1. Draw the hard tissue of the chin.*

The hard tissue of the chin below the osteotomy line is now traced from the OT. If no vertical change is contemplated, the lines should coincide. In some cases where simultaneous vertical change is required, a change of the angulation of the osteotomy should be considered. By performing the osteotomy on a steeper plane, the anterior height of the chin can be reduced as it is advanced. When a vertical increase of the chin is contemplated, the chin should be down-grafted. The final PT is demonstrated in Figure 3.5.

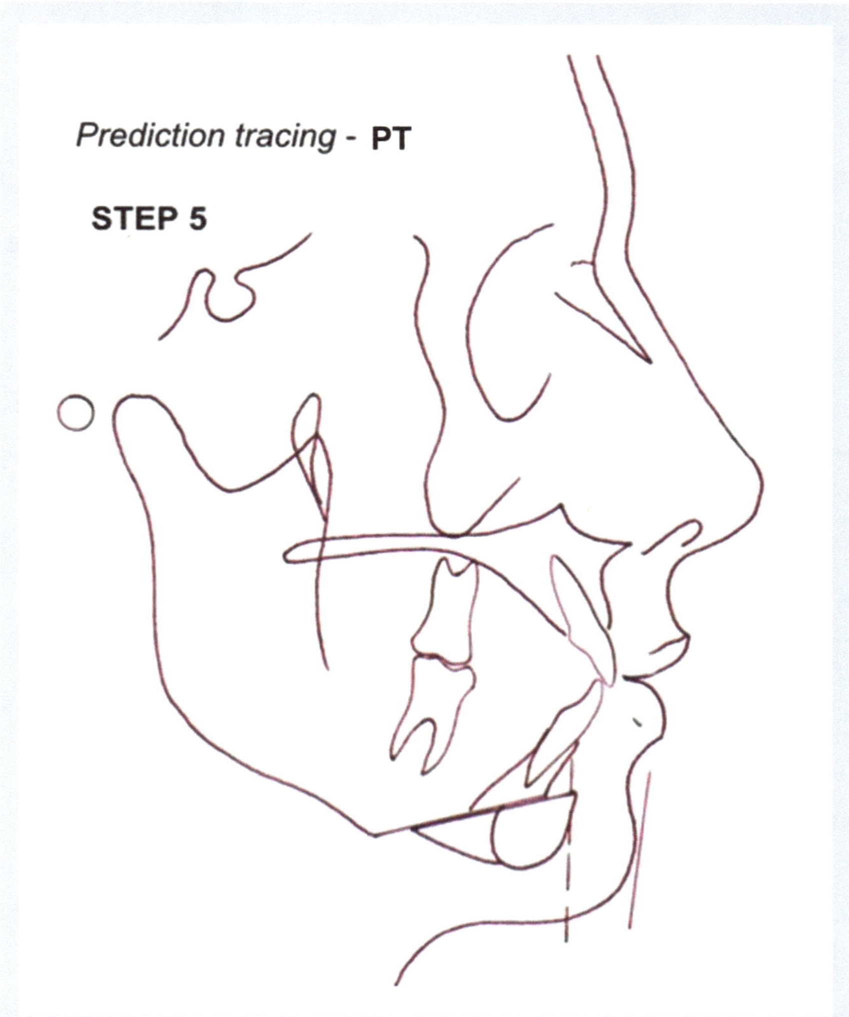

Figure 3.5 *The final prediction tracing.*

Soft Tissue Changes. Many studies have been carried out regarding soft tissue change in relation to skeletal repositioning of the chin.[7–15] Total stripping of the periosteum off the chin segment will not only result in increased bone resorbtion of the repositioned chin, but will also decrease the soft tissue predictability.[12-14] Minimal periosteal stripping, respect for soft and hard tissue during surgery, and accurate surgical technique enhances soft tissue predictability and ultimately improved esthetic results.
(See Table 1.)

Soft Tissue Changes Associated With Advancement Genioplasty

Chin(H)	0.57:1	Po':Po Ant.Sliding	Bell, Dann (1973)[7]
Chin(H)	0.75:1	Po':Po Horizontal (some Multistep)	McDonnel (1977)[8]
Chin(H)	0.67:1		Proffit, Epker (1980)[4]
Chin(H)	approx 1:1	Horizontal (broad pedicle)	Bell (1981)[9]
Chin(H)	0.97:1	Po':Po Horizontal w/broad pedicle (IVRO setback)	Scheideman (1981)[10]
Chin(H)	0.85:1	Horizontal (broad pedicle)	Bell (1983)[11]
Chin(H)	0.93:1	Po':Po Adv. and vertical reduction Horizontal sliding (broad pedicle)	Gallagher (1984)[12]
Chin(H)	0.7:1	Horizontal	Epker (1986)[13]
Chin(H)	0.97:1	Po':Po Horizontal (broad pedicle)	Park, Ellis (1989)[14]
Chin(H)	0.95:1	Po':Po Horizontal (broad pedicle)	Reyneke, van Eeden (1993)[15]

TABLE 1.

Prediction Tracing For Horizontal Reduction Genioplasty

This prediction is performed in the same manner as for advancement genioplasty, however, the soft tissue change in relation to hard tissue repositioning is less predictable *(Refer to Table 2)*. Great care should be taken to critically assess the predicted soft tissue result as horizontal reduction genioplasty may have undesirable effects on the labiomental sulcus (flattening) and worsen the submental contour.

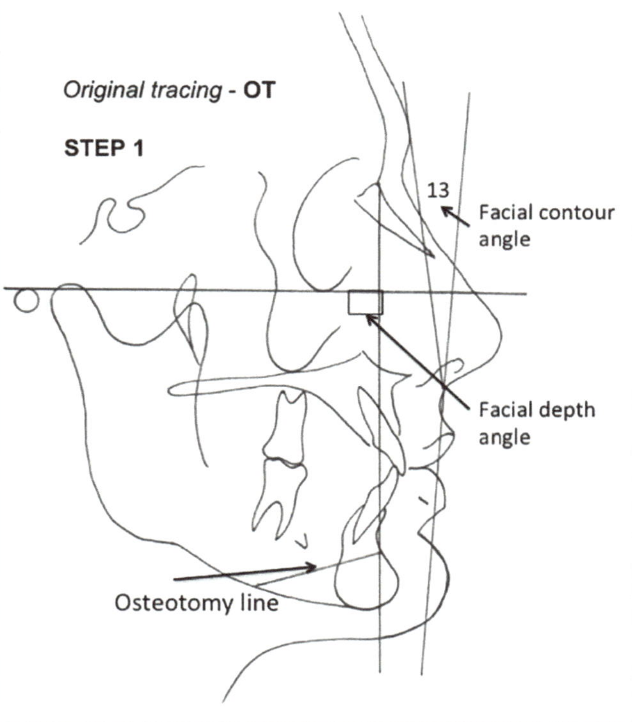

Figure 3.6 - STEP 1 *Prediction for anteroposterior reduction genioplasty. The original tracing (OT). A facial depth angle of 90° (hard tissue prediction) and a facial contour angle of 13° (soft tissue prediction) are constructed. A genioplasty osteotomy line is drawn.*

Figures 3.6 to 3.10 illustrate the method of predicting the soft tissue results when the chin is horizontally reduced. In Figure 3.9, the arrows indicate the predicted soft tissue change. Note the slight increase in height due to the chin segment sliding slightly downward on the downward-angled horizontal osteotomy. Note the surgical contouring of the superior aspect of the anterior mandible to enhance the labiomental fold in Figure 3.10. The posteromedial aspect of the chin segment is also contoured to prevent a palpable step on the inferior border and poor lower border contour *(Fig 3.10, arrows 1 & 2)*. In Figure 3.10, arrow 3 indicates the chin segment positioned behind the facial plane to achieve the predicted anteroposterior soft tissue position.

The soft tissue change in response to chin setback ratio is:

Soft Tissue:Hard Tissue = ±2:3

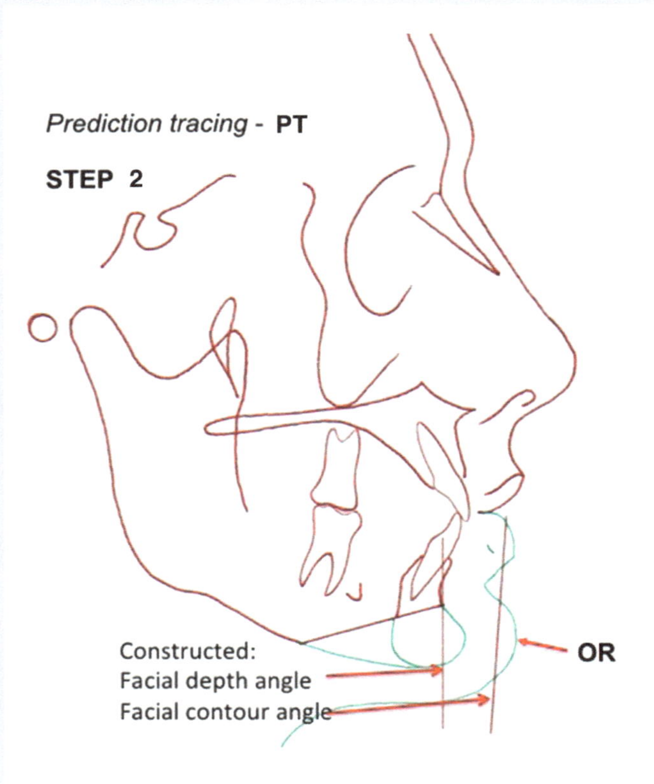

Figure 3.7 - STEP 2 *The hard and soft tissue structures not influenced by the surgery are traced in red (PT). The N-A line and the LFP is also traced as indicators of the desired hard and soft tissue.*

Figure 3.8 - STEP 3 *Utilize the LFP and the clinician's artistic "flare" to draw the desired soft tissue of the chin in red (arrows).*

Figure 3.9 - STEP 4 *Slide the prediction tracing (PT) to the right along the osteotomy line. The hard tissue of the chin on the OT will effectively move to the left on the PT. The expected soft tissue reaction in relation to the hard tissue repositioning is summarized in Table 2. Keep in mind that the soft tissue change in relation to hard tissue repositioning is less predictable. Draw the hard tissue of the chin.*

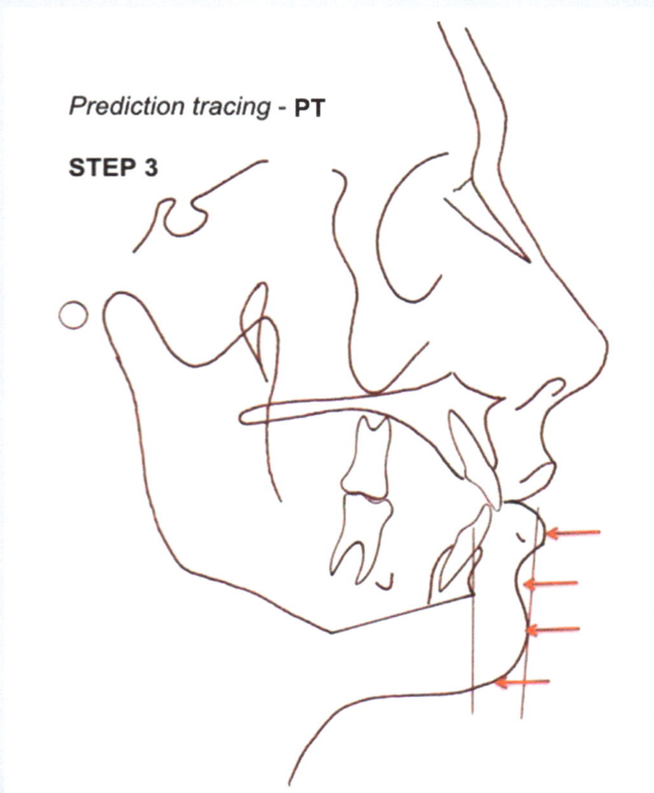

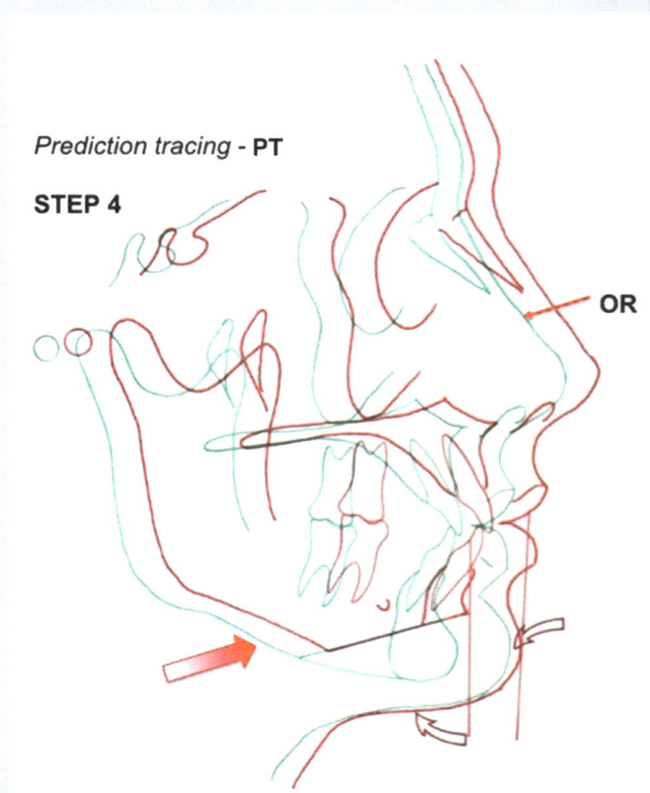

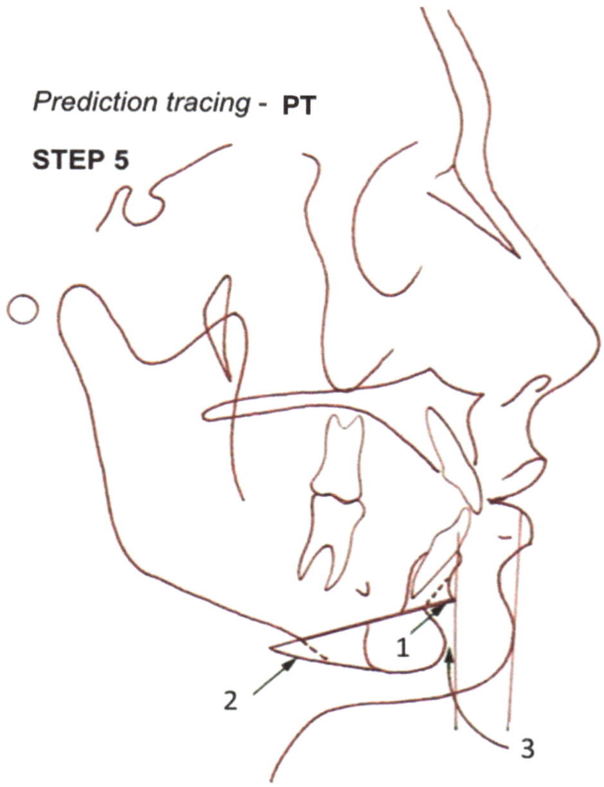

Figure 3.10 *The final prediction tracing. The depth of the labiomental fold (1) and lower border contour (2) can be controlled. Note that the soft tissue of the chin reacts less than the genial segment's repositioning (3).*

Soft Tissue Changes Associated With Reduction Genioplasty

Chin(H)	−0.33:1	Pog':Pog Ant. Recontouring; degloving dissection	Hohl, Epker (1976)16
Chin(H)	−0.58:1	Pog':Pog Horizontal	Bell (1981)9
Chin(H)	−0.62:1	Pog':Pog Horizontal	Reyneke (unpubl)

TABLE 2.

Prediction Tracing For Vertical Chin Augmentation

STEP 1. Prepare an OT and in addition to the cephalometric parameters for antero-posterior relations, various vertical guidelines may be utilized to generate the best balance *(Fig 3.11)*. Vertical cephalometric parameters that may be of assistance when planning the correct amount of augmentation are:

Vertical Relation Between Middle:Lower Facial Third = 1:1

Stms-Labial Fold:Labial Fold-Menton = 1:2

Sn-Li : Li –Me' = 1:1

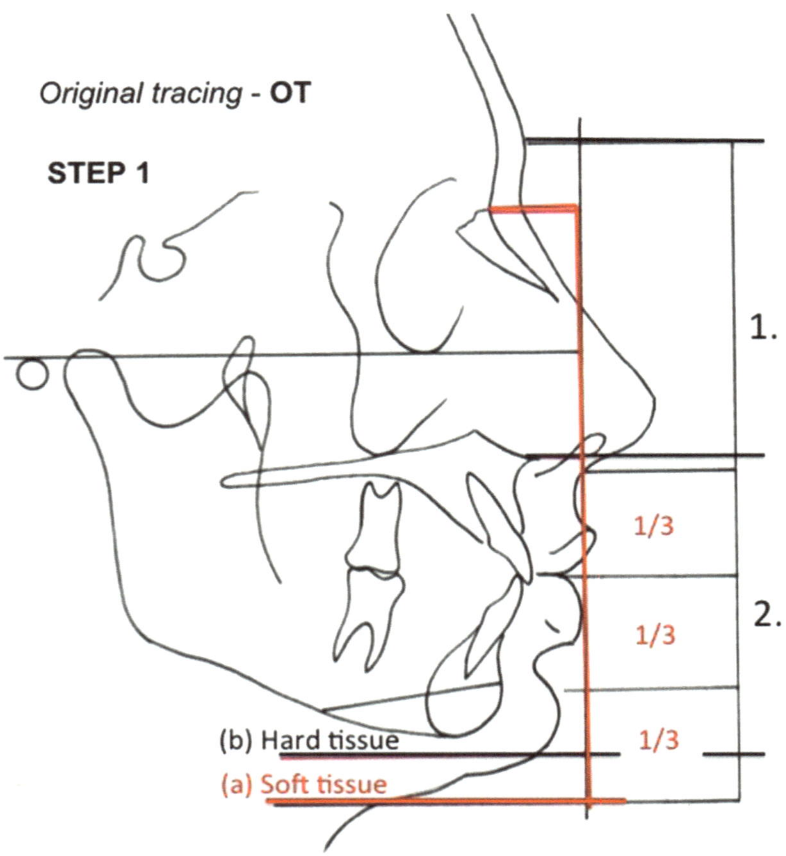

Figure 3.11 - STEP 1 *Prediction tracing for vertical augmentation genioplasty. The original tracing (OT). Vertical guidelines are constructed to increase the chin height. For soft tissue prediction, a horizontal line indicating a lower facial height equal to the middle facial height is drawn. The upper lip (1/3) to lower lip (2/3) can also be used as a guide* **(a)**. *For a guide to the hard tissue height, a horizontal line is drawn at a ratio of 5 (middle third) to 6 (lower third)* **(b)**.

STEP 2. Trace a PT as before in Step 2. The arrow indicates the ideal height of the deepest point of the labiomental fold *(Fig 3.12)*.

STEP 3. Draw an ideal lip and chin and increase the height of the chin to achieve the best esthetic balance. Use the constructed lines as guides *(Fig 3.13)*.

STEP 4. The PT should now be moved superiorly over the OT until the soft tissue of the PT and the OT coincide *(Fig 3.14)*. For vertical augmentation of the chin, the soft tissue will follow the hard tissue change quite closely, similar to horizontal augmentation (0.1-0.9) *(Refer to Table 3)*.

The hard tissue chin repositioning can now be calculated and traced in *(Fig 3.15)*. The distance (defect) between the osteotomy lines indicates the required amount of down grafting (arrow). It also indicates the shape of the graft. Various patterns of vertical repositioning of the chin to achieve different esthetic outcomes are discussed in Chapter 4, Surgical Technique.

Figure 3.12 - STEP 2 *The prediction tracing (PT). The hard and soft tissue structures not influenced by the surgery are traced in red (PT). Also trace the vertical guidelines (a) and (b).*

Figure 3.13 - STEP 3 *Draw the desired soft tissue of the chin in red (arrows). Use the horizontal line indicating the desired soft tissue height of the chin (b).*

Figure 3.14 - STEP 4 *Slide the PT superior (arrow) over the OT until the soft tissue of the PT co-enside with the soft tissue line. The chin on the OT will effectively move inferior relative to the PT. The relative soft tissue change to hard tissue repositioning is about 1:1 (table 3). Trace the hard tissue chin in red (arrow).*

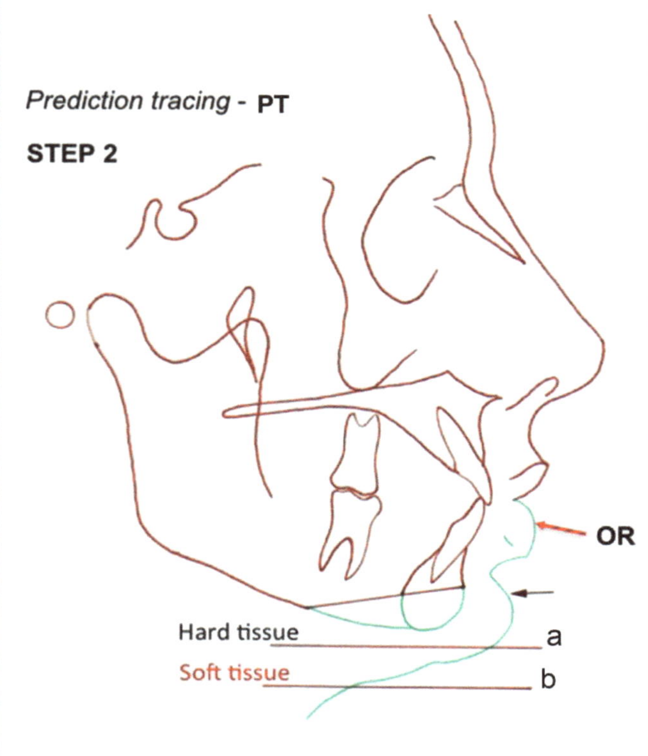

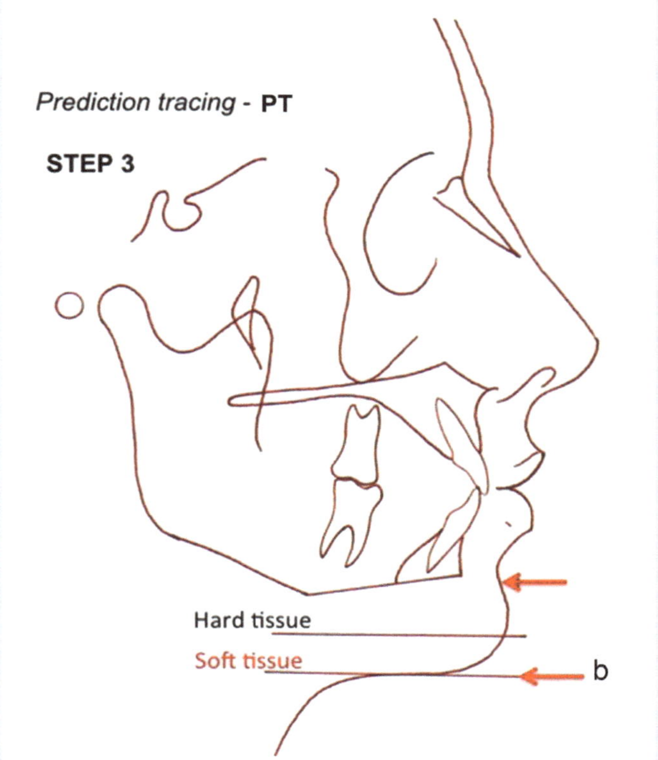

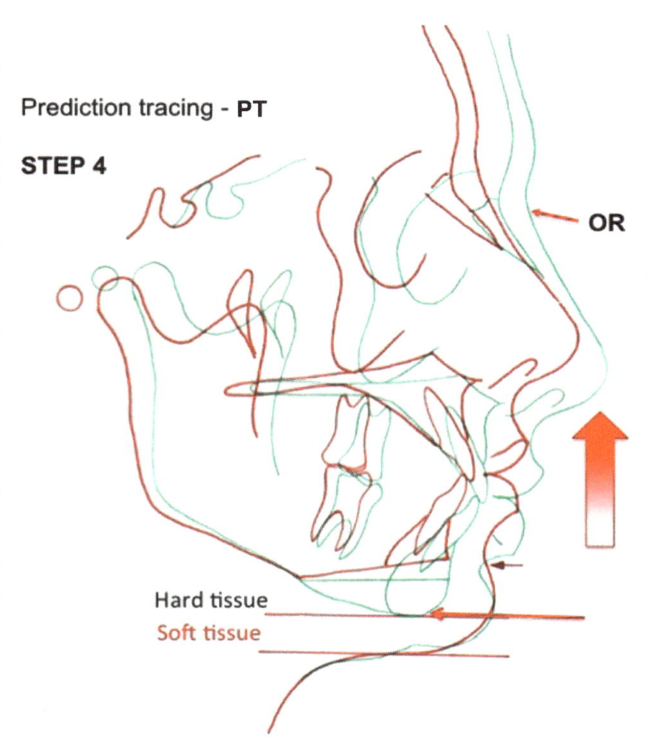

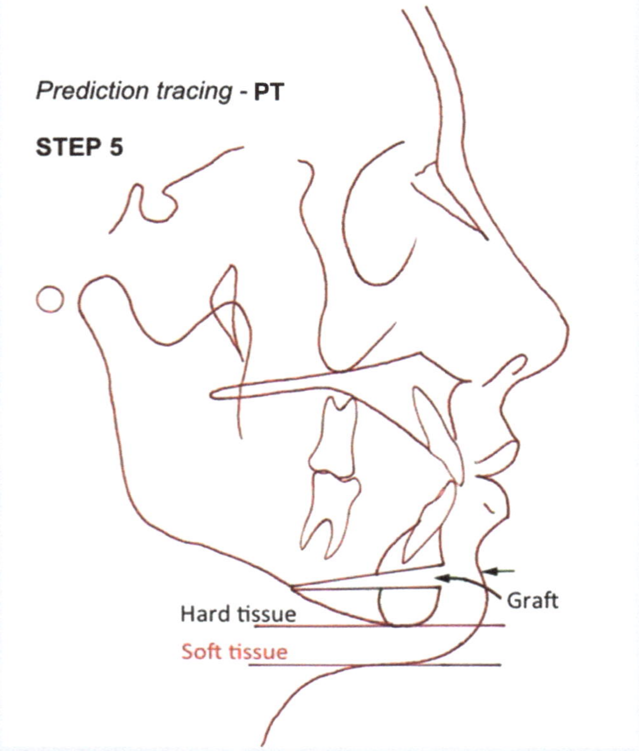

Figure 3.15 *The final tracing indicate the hard and soft tissue changes as well as the expected bone defect that may have to be grafted.*

Soft Tissue Changes Associated With Vertical Augmentation

Chin(V)	1:1	Me':Me Interpositional	Wessberg (1980)[17]
Chin(V)	9.6:1	Me':Me Interpositional	Reyneke (2000) unpubl

TABLE 3.

Prediction Tracing For Vertical Chin Reduction

STEP 1. Prepare an OT as previously dicussed *(Fig 3.16)*. Vertical cephalometric guidelines to assist in planning the ideal height of the chin should be drawn on the OT and include:

Vertical Relation Between Middle and Lower Facial Third = 1:1

Stms-Labial Fold:Labial Fold-Menton = 1:2

Sn-Li:L –Me' =1:1

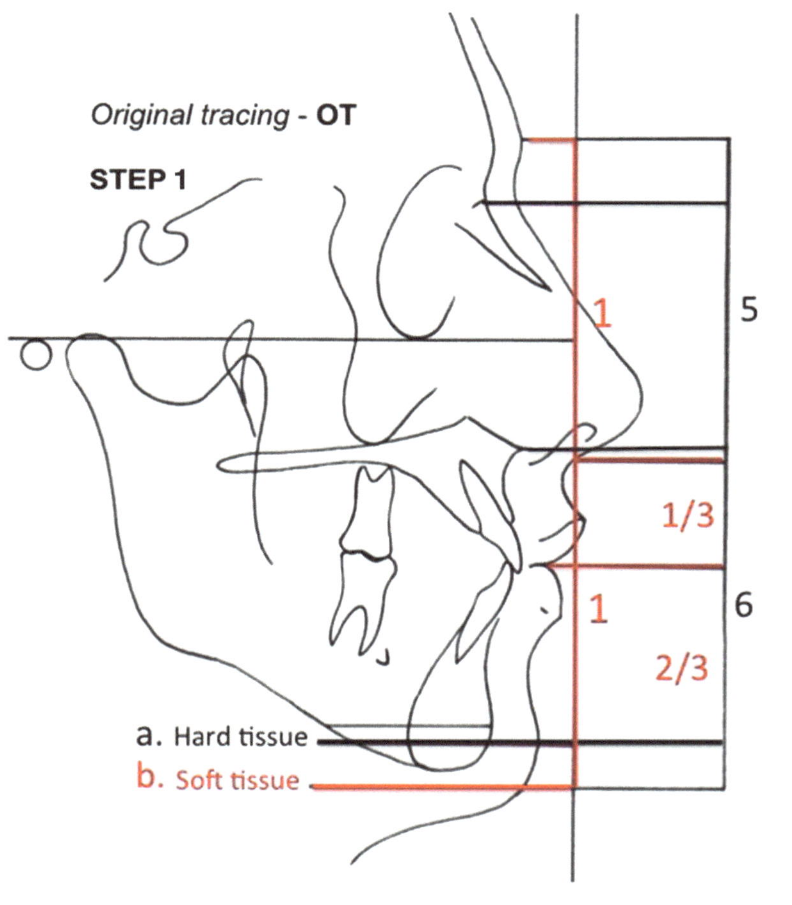

Figure 3.16 - STEP 1 *Prediction tracing for vertical reduction genioplasty. An original tracing (OT) is created and the ideal hard* **(a)** *and soft tissue* **(b)** *heights are indicated by constructing two horizontal lines as described in the text.*

When planning the height of the horizontal osteotomy, keep in mind that the chin will be vertically reduced. The first horizontal osteotomy should therefore be placed low on the chin. This will facilitate a safe ostectomy below the mental foramen and the apexes of the incisor teeth.

STEP 2. A PT is traced. Trace all hard tissue structures above the osteotomy line and all soft tissue structures above the lower lip (Stms) *(Fig 3.17)*.

STEP 3. The ideal chin shape with reduced height is drawn on the PT *(Fig 3.18)*.

STEP 4. Move the PT inferiorly over the OT until the soft tissue of the PT and OT coincide *(Fig 3.19)*. The soft tissue change in relation to hard tissue repositioning is not as predictable as horizontal and vertical augmentation *(Table 4)*. The soft tissue of the chin tends to advance slightly as the chin height is reduced due to bunching of the soft tissue. Slight advancement of the chin should also be considered to achieve an esthetically pleasing labiomental fold *(Fig 3.19, Arrow 1)*.

Figure 3.20 illustrates the completed PT indicating the amount of hard tissue reduction and expected soft tissue result *(Fig 3.20, Arrow 2)*.

Figure 3.17 - STEP 2 *The prediction tracing (PT). Trace all the structures that will not be influenced by the surgery on a clean piece of tracing paper in red. Also ad the constructed horizontal lines* **(a)** *and* **(b)**.

Figure 3.18 - STEP 3 *Draw the desired soft tissue of the chin in red (arrows). Use the horizontal line indicating the desired soft tissue height of the chin as a guide.*

Figure 3.19 - STEP 4 *Slide the PT inferior (arrow) over the OT until the soft tissue of the PT is slightly below the soft tissue line (red). The relative soft tissue change to hard tissue repositioning is about 0,26:1 (Refer to Table 4). The chin on the OT will effectively move superior relative to the PT.*

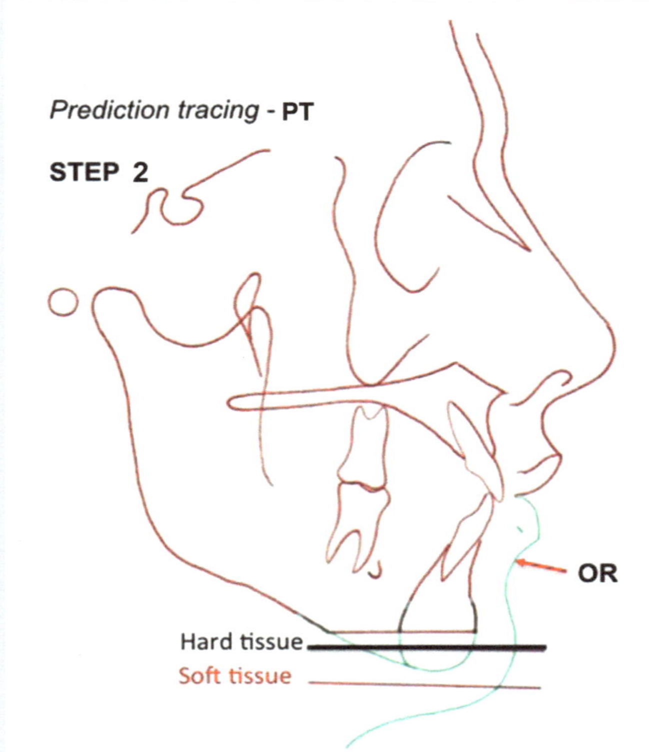

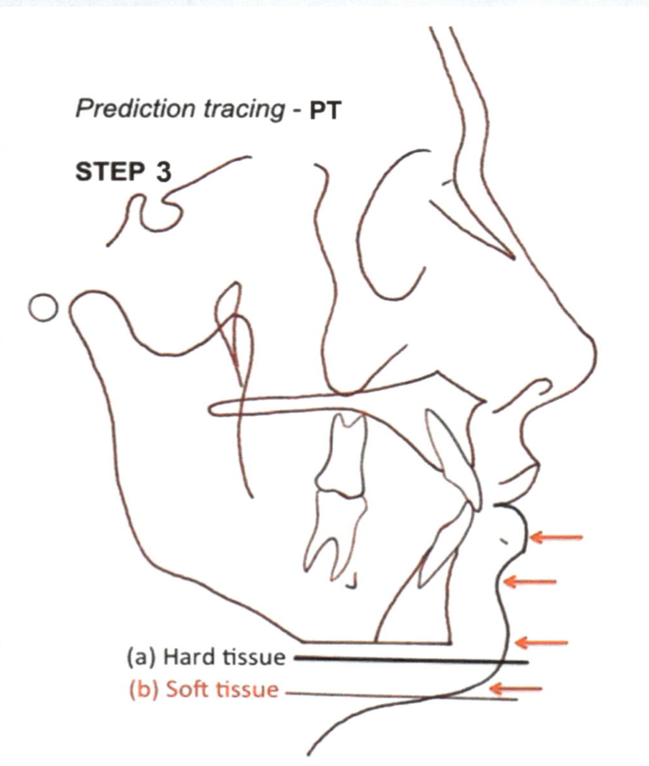

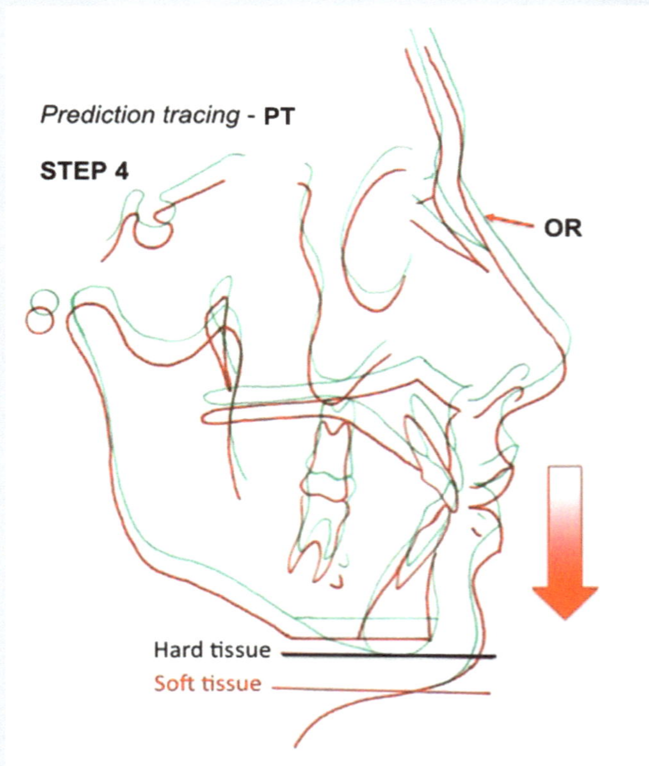

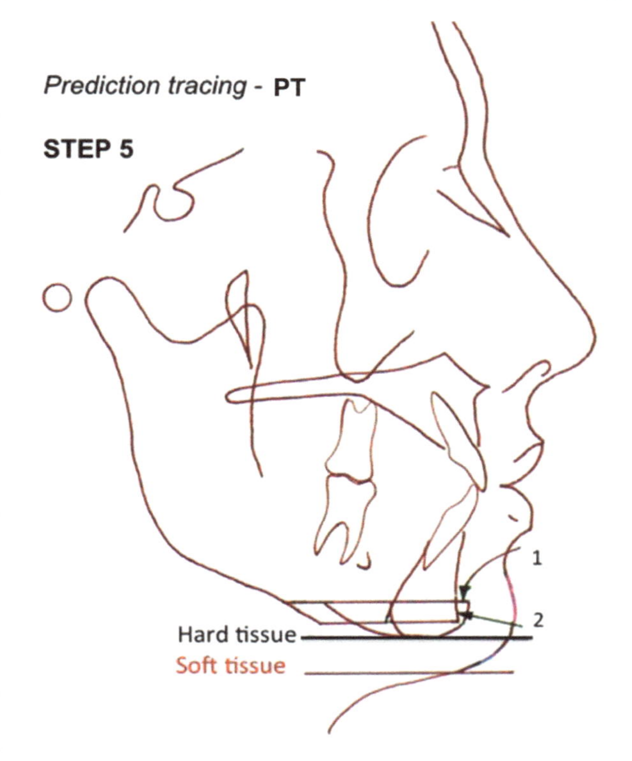

Figure 3.20 - STEP 5 Trace the hard tissue chin in red. The chin is advanced slightly to improve the labiomental fold contour (1). The required hard tissue reduction is indicated by the arrow (2).

Soft Tissue Changes Associated With Vertical Reduction Genioplasty

Chin(V)	-0.25:1	Me':Me Inf. Border Ostectomy Degloving	Hohl, Epker (1976)[16]
Chin(V)	-0.26:1	Pog':Pog Horizontal With Broad Pedicle	Park, Ellis (1989)[14]

TABLE 4.

Chapter 4 - Surgical Technique

Over the last 35 years, the versatility of an osteotomy of the anterior part of the inferior border of the mandible has enabled surgeons to modify the genial area in all three dimensions.[1–9] The chin is one of the most noticeable facial structures and it is essential that surgeons develop an artistic application and equity in the execution of the surgical technique.

Step 1: Infiltration of the Soft Tissue with a Vasoconstrictor.

Infiltrate the area of dissection with 2 ml of local anesthetic containing a vasoconstrictor (1:100,000 adrenaline) 10 minutes before surgery *(Fig 4.1)*. Do not inject more than 2 ml of local anesthetic, as a large volume of local anesthetic in the tissue will distort the soft tissue shape of the chin and render intraoperative clinical assessment of the esthetics difficult. Avoid injecting into the mental neurovascular bundle.

Step 2: Mucosal Incision.

Make the first soft tissue incision only through the labial mucosal layer from just distal to the canine to a similar point on the contralateral side *(Fig 4.2)*. Branches of the mental nerve can often be identified in the submucosal tissue laterally and should be avoided. Leave at least 5 mm of non-keratinized mucosa superiorly for ease of suturing the mentalis muscle, submucosal layer, and mucosa later *(Fig 4.2)*.

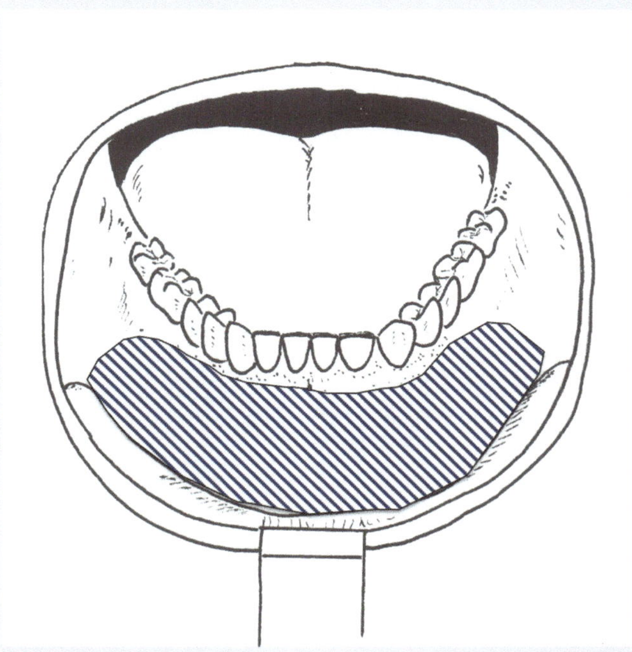

Figure 4.1 - STEP 1:
Infiltration of soft tissue with a vasoconstrictor.

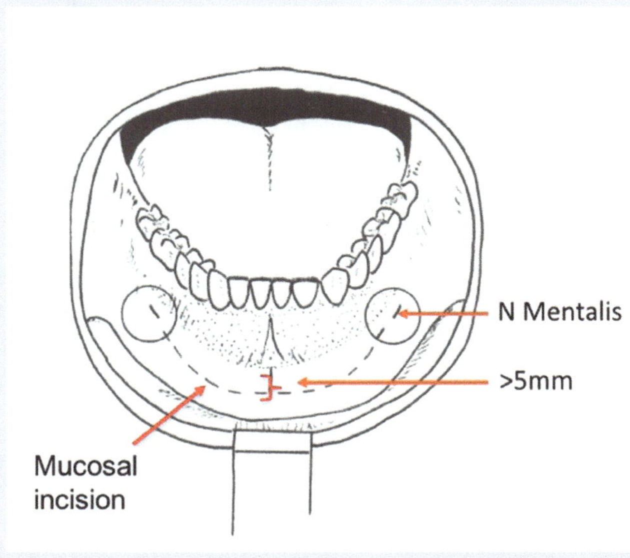

Figure 4.2 - STEP 2:
Mucosal incision.

Step 3: Submucosal Incision.

The second incision is performed through the submucosal tissue, mentalis muscle, and periosteum onto the bone while taking care not to damage the terminal branches of the mental nerve at the lateral aspects of the incision. This incision is angled at 45° to the bone so that more submucosal tissue, muscle, and periosteum is left at the superior aspect for ease of re-approximation later *(Fig 4.3).*

Step 4: Mucoperiosteal Dissection.

Start the mucoperiosteal dissection from the center and dissect laterally and inferiorly. Identify the mental nerves bilaterally. The neurovascular bundle should not be deliberately dissected free, but rather left attached to the periosteum and simply visually located to facilitate protection of the nerve *(Fig 4.4).* Elevate the mucoperiosteum at the superior aspect of the incision to facilitate suturing later.

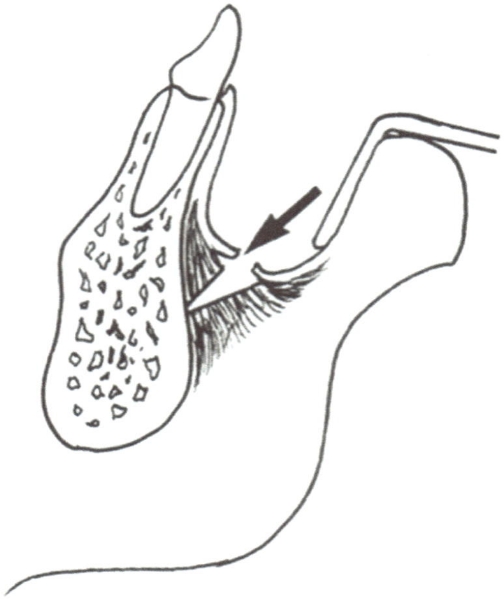

Figure 4.3 - STEP 3:
Submucosal incision.

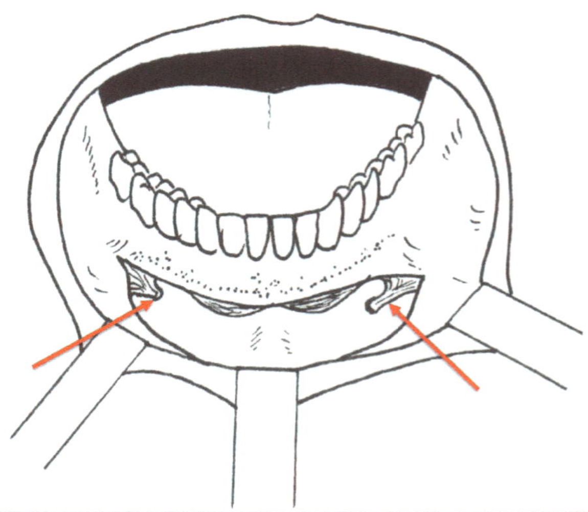

Figure 4.4 - STEP 4:
Mucoperiosteal dissection.

Step 5: Reference Marks

Mark the dental midline on the bone superiorly and inferiorly to the planned osteotomy line using a 701 bur. Make small, shallow holes, avoiding the roots of the incisor teeth, and score a line into the cortex to connect the holes *(Fig 4.5a)*. The inferior hole is deepened by angling the bur superiorly and extending the hole well through the cortex *(Fig 4.5b, arrow)*. This hole is intended for the placement of a positioning wire to control the segment during final repositioning of the chin. Place the hole in thick bone to ensure that the wire does not pull through *(Fig 4.5b)*. To guarantee accurate repositioning of the chin, place reference marks ±10 mm lateral to the midline as well.

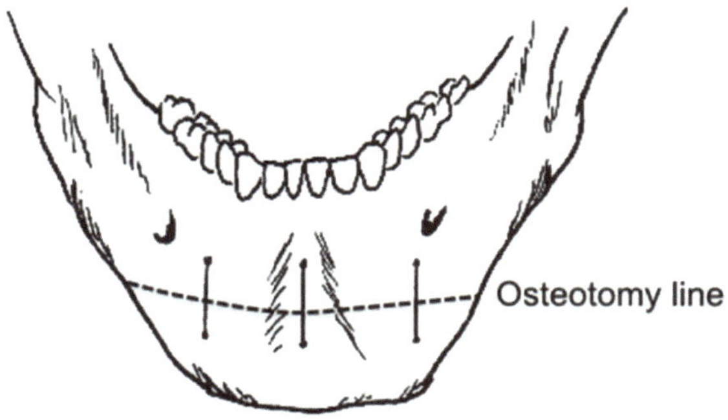

Figure 4.5a - STEP 5:
Reference marks.

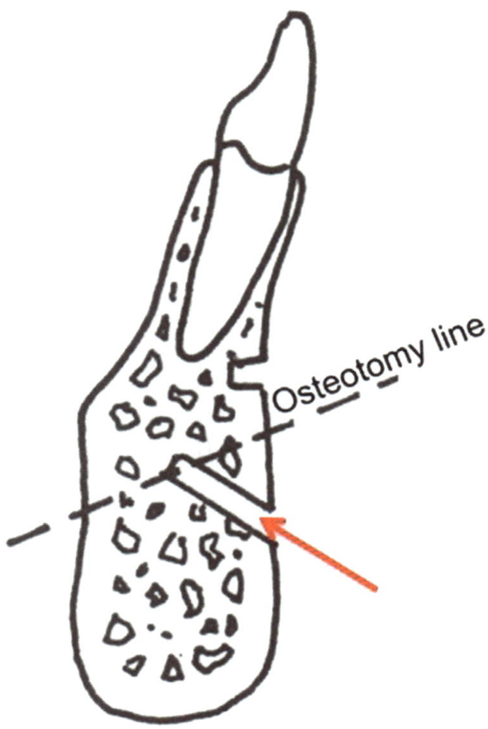

Figure 4.5b - STEP 5:
Placement of holding wire purchase hole.

Step 6: Design the Osteotomy.

The following text will discuss the basic technique for advancing the chin using tricortical screw or boneplate fixation. The techniques for anteroposterior reduction, vertical change, correction of asymmetry, and change in width of the chin are discussed from Steps 16 through 20.

The osteotomy should be performed at least 5 mm below the roots of the incisor and canine teeth and 5 mm below the mental foramen *(Fig 4.6a).* Visualize and mark the angle of the osteotomy on the bone surface guided by the surgical visual treatment objective.

Most genioplasty procedures are performed to augment the chin. Consideration must be given to the angulation of the osteotomy, as variations in the angle will lead to changes in the vertical dimension of the chin, with obvious esthetic consequences. The angle of the osteotomy will create a plane along which the bony segment will slide as it is advanced *(Fig 4.6b).* The steepness of the angle of the osteotomy will be influenced by three factors: the aesthetic requirements, the roots of the incisor and canine teeth, and the position of the mental foramina. Keep in mind that the course of the mental nerve prior to its exit through the mental foramen is ±5 mm inferior and anterior to the foramen *(Fig 4.6a).*

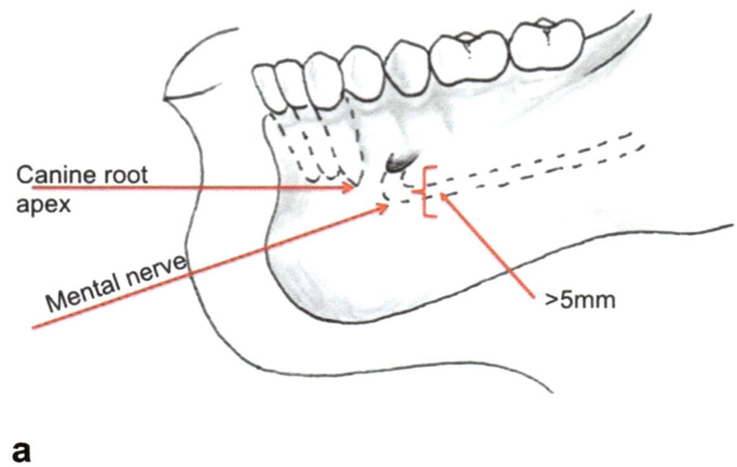

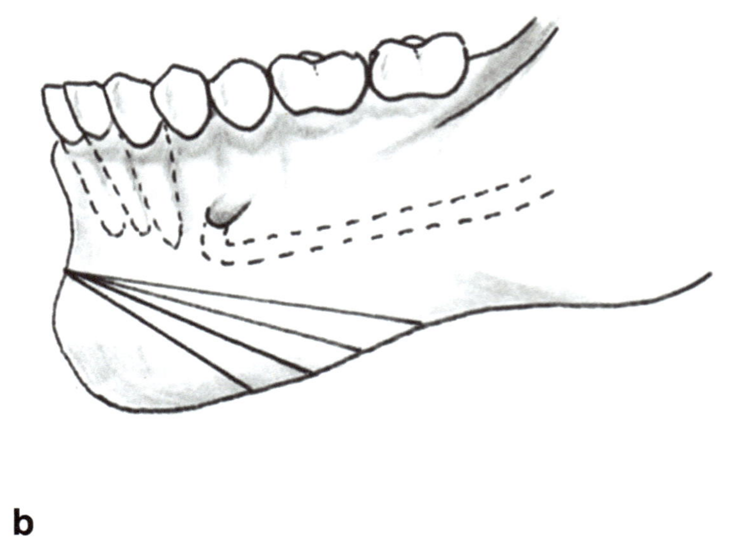

Figure 4.6 - STEP 6:
a. *Osteotomy design.* **b.** *Osteotomy angulation.*

Figure 4.6c illustrates the difference in vertical change after advancing the chin along two different planes. Care should be taken not to angle the osteotomy too steep. A vertically angled osteotomy will exit the inferior border posteriorly in the parasymphyseal area, which may create a disruption in the smooth lower border of the mandible. This step in the bone may be visible in individuals with thin skins. By altering the height of the osteotomy, the height of the labiomental fold and the shape of the chin button can be controlled *(Fig.4.6d)*.

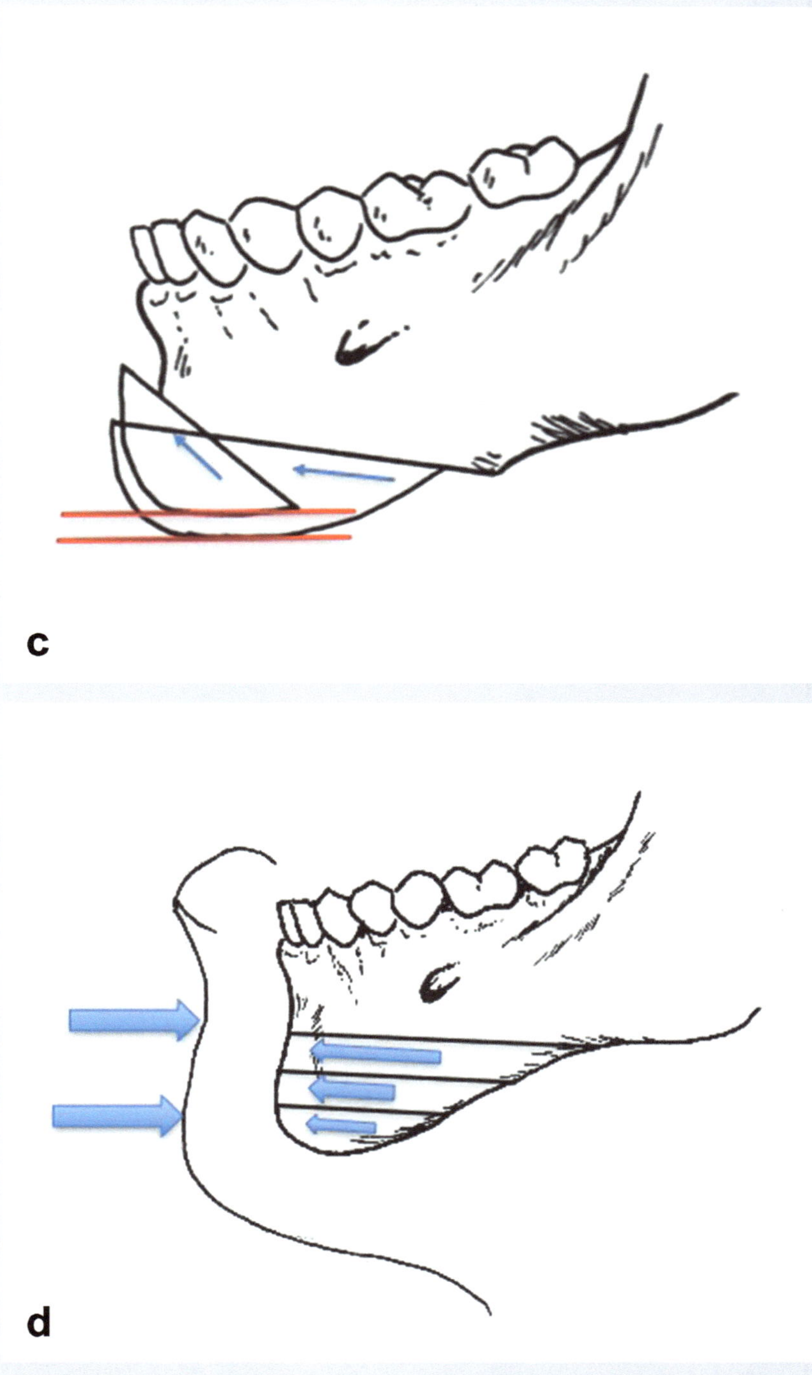

c

d

Figure 4.6 - STEP 6:
c. *Vertical control.* **d.** *Control of the labiomental fold.*

Step 7: Osteotomy of the Chin.

The osteotomy is performed using an oscillating saw. Start in the center and carry the osteotomy laterally *(Fig 4.7a)*. Ensure that the osteotomies are completed and include the lower border and lingual cortex of the mandible at the posterior end of the osteotomy *(Fig 4.7b)*. Failure to complete the osteotomy may lead to an unfavorable fracture, making accurate positioning of the segment difficult *(Fig 4.7c)*.

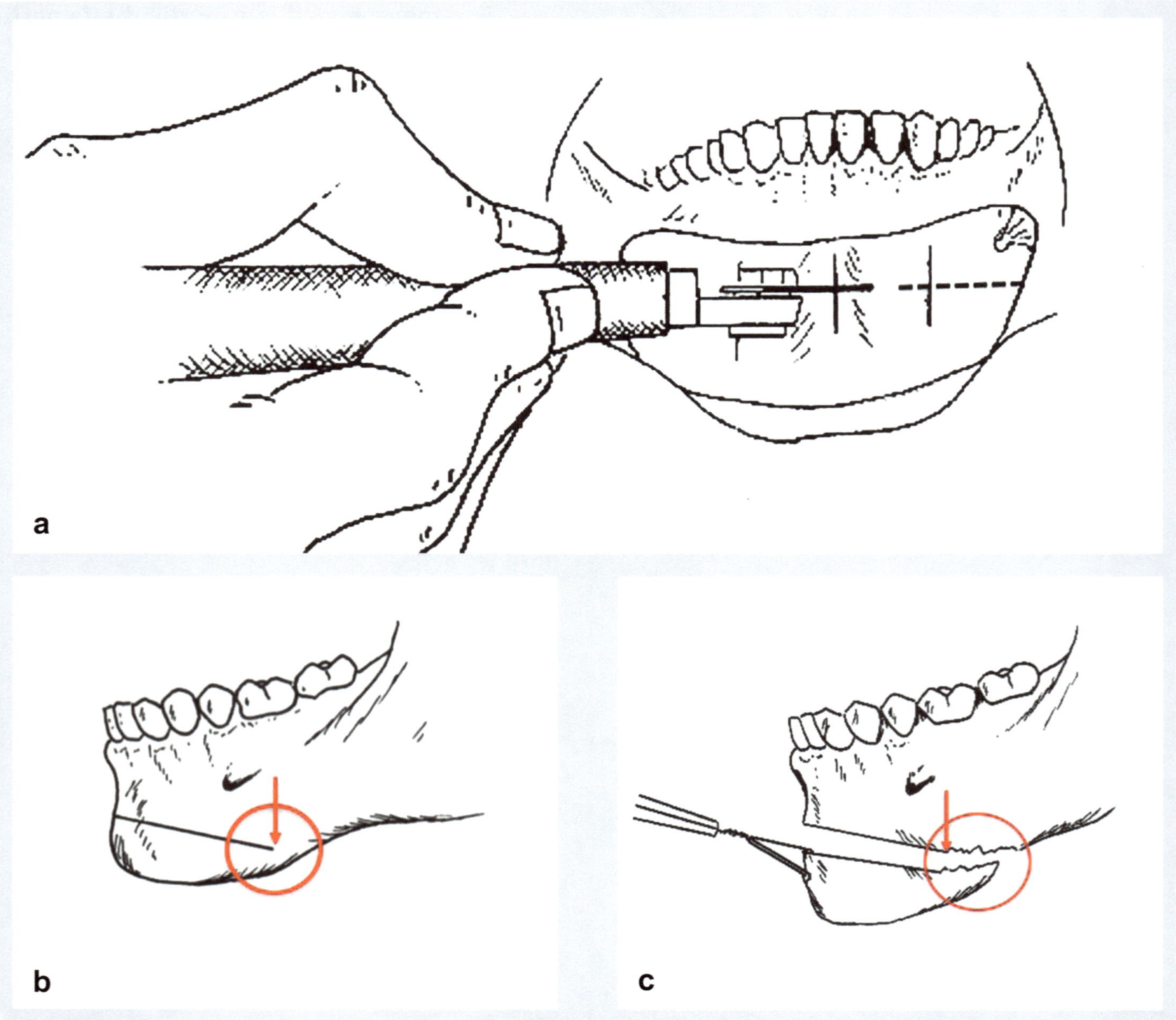

Figure 4.7 - STEP 7: a. *The horizontal genioplasty osteotomy.* **b.** *incomplete (arrow) the lower border osteotomy.* **c.** *Unfavorable lower border fracture (circle).*

Step 8: Mobilization of the Chin.

After completing the osteotomy, the chin segment should be mobile. It may, however, be necessary to carefully complete the osteotomy using a small osteotome in the osteotomy line *(Fig 4.8)*.

In cases where a genioplasty is combined with a bilateral sagittal split mandibular ramus osteotomy, the author prefers to perform the genioplasty after completing the sagittal split osteotomy. Once the mandible has been repositioned and the teeth are still held in occlusion by inter-maxillary fixation, surgeons have an opportunity to evaluate the esthetics by visualizing the soft tissue changes to the chin directly. Maintaining the teeth in occlusion while performing the genioplasty provides the added advantage of support to the mandible and reduction of the forces on the recently placed fixation. However, care should be taken not to apply too much force to the mandible while performing the genioplasty, as this may dislodge the orthodontic brackets or cause fixation failure at the sagittal split osteotomy site. An alternative method is to perform the genioplasty before the sagittal split osteotomy.

Step 9: Engage Positioning Wire.

Place an "018" wire through the hole drilled in the osteotomised segment during placement of the reference marks *(Fig 4.5, Step 5)* and attach a wire twister to it *(Fig 4.9)*. This wire will assist during the final mobilization phase *(Fig, 4.10, Step 10)* and also be of great help when repositioning the chin segment.

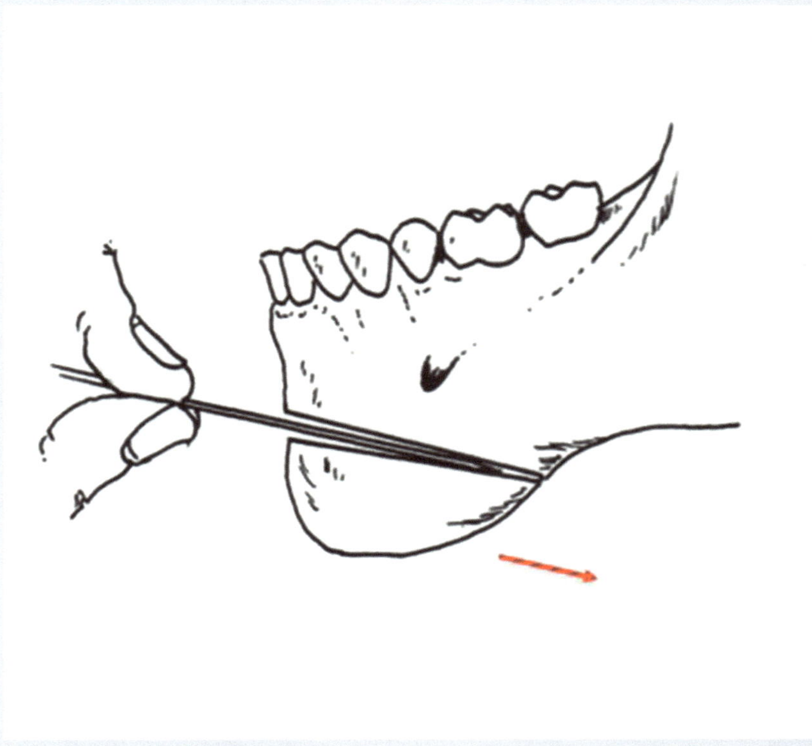

Figure 4.8 - STEP 8:
Mobilization of the chin segment.

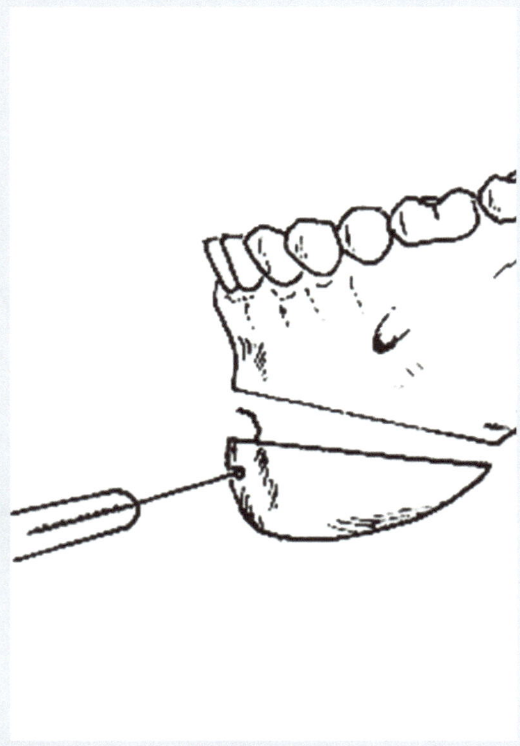

Figure 4.9 - STEP 9:
Positioning wire.

Step 10: Final Mobilization of the Chin Segment.

Place a Howarth elevator behind the lingual cortex and pull the chin forward by stretching the soft tissue made up of the suprahyoid muscles and periosteum *(Fig 4.10)*. Adequate mobilization of the segment will allow easy and accurate repositioning of the chin.

Step 11: Refinement of the Osteotomy.

Interference's are often found at the posterolingual area of the mobilized segment. *(Refer to Fig 4.7c)* Failure to remove any irregularities on the sliding surface of the chin will prevent accurate repositioning. Remove the bony interferences using a large round vulcanite bur while protecting the soft tissues, e.g., sublingual salivary gland, facial artery, mentalis nerve, and geniohyoid muscles *(Fig 4.11)*.

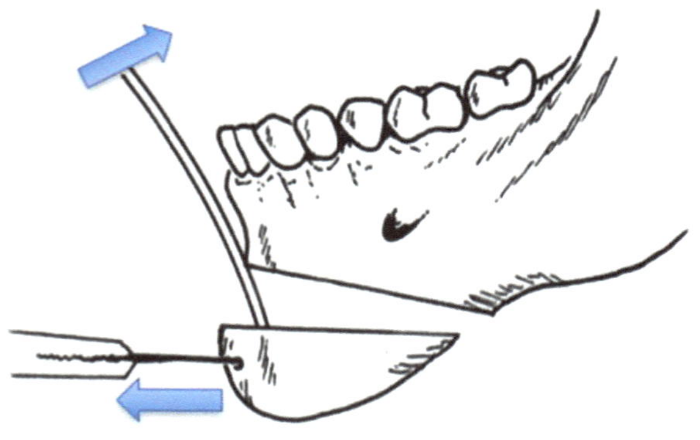

Figure 4.10 - STEP 10:
Final mobilization of the chin segment.

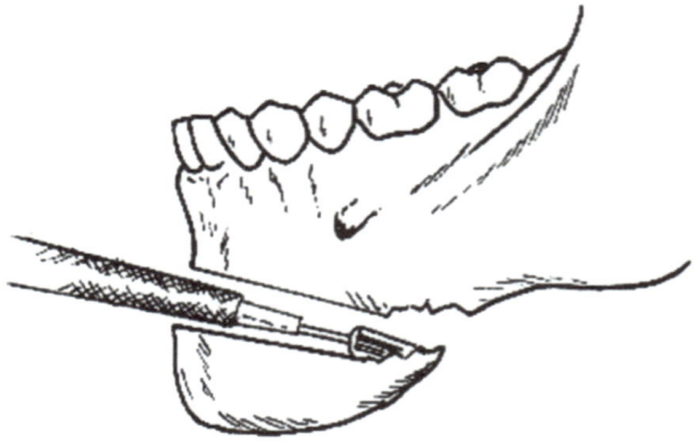

Figure 4.11 - STEP 11:
Refinement of the osteotomy.

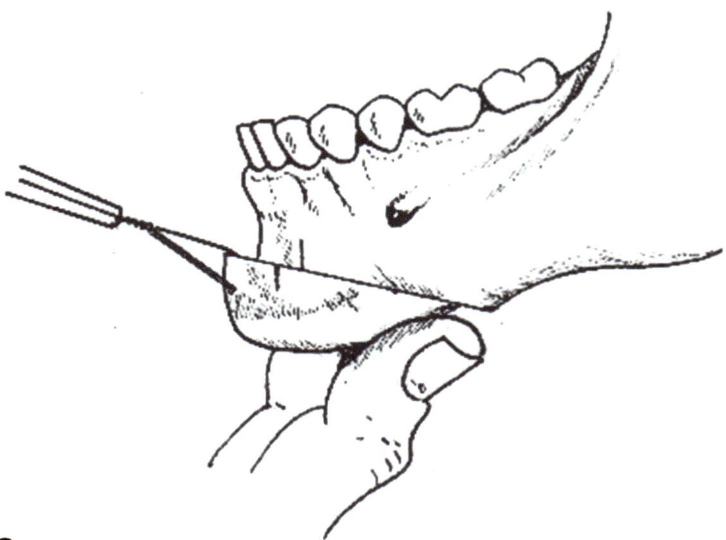

a

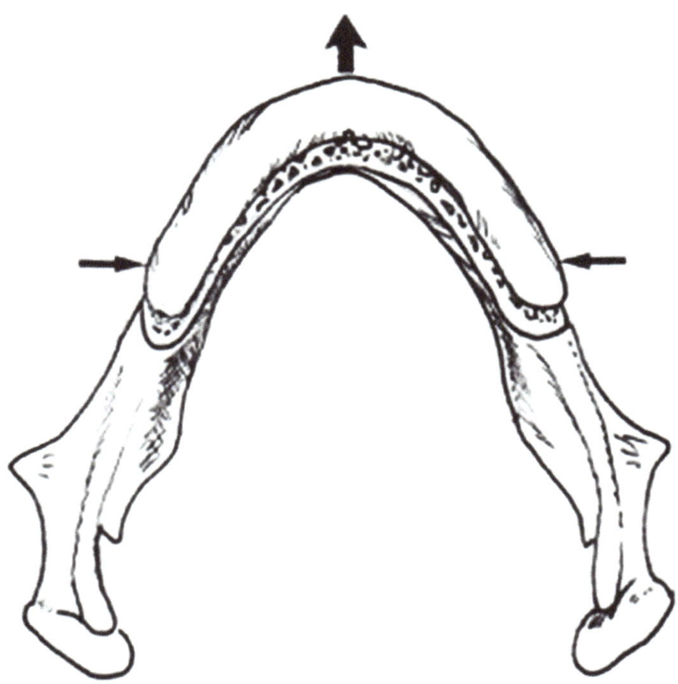

b

Figure 4.12- STEP 12:
a. *Repositioning of the chin segment.*
b. *Checking lower border contour.*

Step 12: Repositioning of the Chin.

Utilize the positioning wire and extra-oral digital pressure to accurately reposition the chin according to the treatment plan (*Fig 4.12a*).

The extent of chin repositioning is decided upon after clinical examination, diagnosis, and development of a cephalometric prediction. A golden rule in orthognathic surgery is "never change your treatment plan on the operating table." The genioplasty procedure, however, may be an exception to the rule when the clinical judgement of the surgeon at the time of surgery may change the repositioning of the chin slightly. As the chin is advanced, some lateral augmentation takes place as the posterior ends of the segment become relatively wider than the lower border of the mandible (*Fig 4.12b arrows*).

Step 13: Drill Holes for the Placement of Two Screws.[10]

Countersink two holes in the buccal cortex ±8 mm on either side of the midline reference on the osteotomised segment. Position the countersink holes at least 5 mm from the superior edge of the segment and direct the hole upward to accommodate the head of the screw. The assistant holds the chin firmly in position using the positioning wire while the holes are drilled and bone screws are placed by the surgeon. Drill the holes into the center of the countersink hole using a trochar to protect the soft tissue *(Fig 4.13 (arrow)*. The drill is angled appropriately to engage all three cortices. Ensure that the screw is long enough to engage all three cortices.

Step 14: Placement of the Tricortical Screws [10,11]

The appropriate screw length is selected and the genial segment fixated with two screws, one on each side of the midline *(Fig 4.14a)*.

In cases where the labiomental fold needs to be enhanced, the anterior acute edge of the chin segment should be contoured. Contouring is, however, not routinely indicated, as the bone in this area will re-contour by resorbtion at the anterior edge, and new bone deposition on the mandible, superior to the segment, will take place – the so called "bow tie" effect *(Fig 4.14b)*.[12]

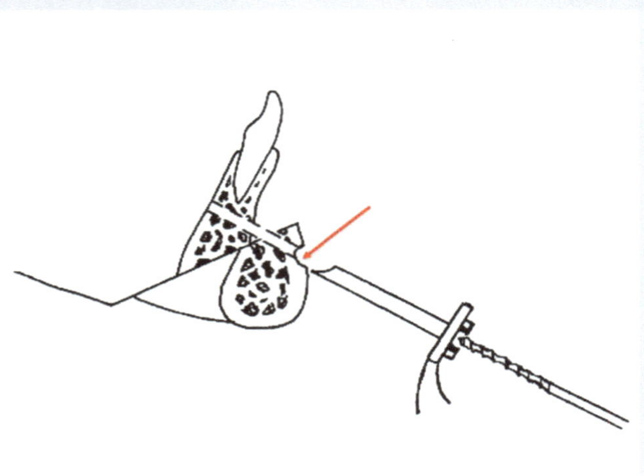

Figure 4.13 - STEP 13:
Drill the holes for placement of two screws.

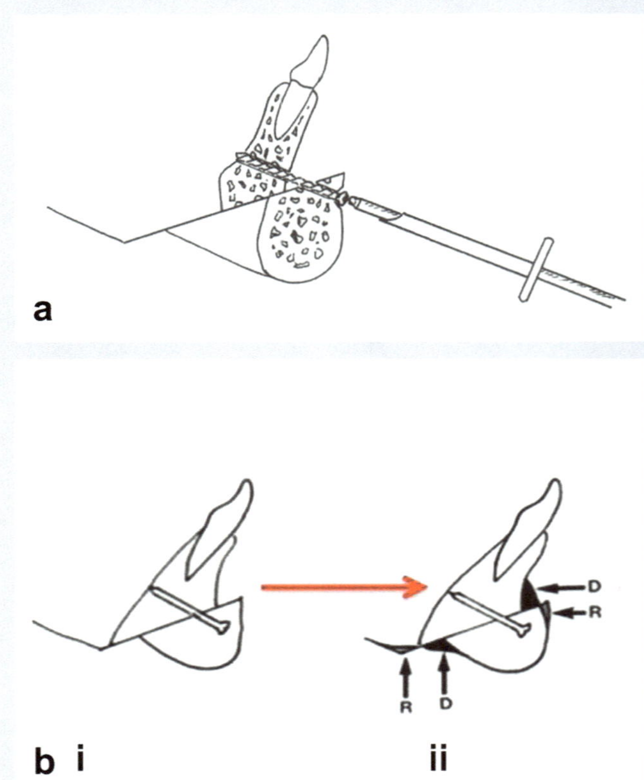

Figure 4.14 - STEP 14:
a. *Placement of tri-cortical screws.* **b.** *The "bow tie" effect.*

Step 15: Bone Plate Fixation as an Alternative to Screw Fixation.

Use an X-shaped, H-shaped, two straight boneplates, or a pre-bent plate with two screws on either side of the osteotomy. The positioning wire and digital pressure are used to help stabilize the chin segment in its planned position *(Fig 4.15a)* while the bone plates are bent to fit accurately and passively. Make sure not to damage the roots of the incisor teeth with the screws. It is recommended that fixation is placed on each side of the midline *(Fig 4.15b)*.[8]

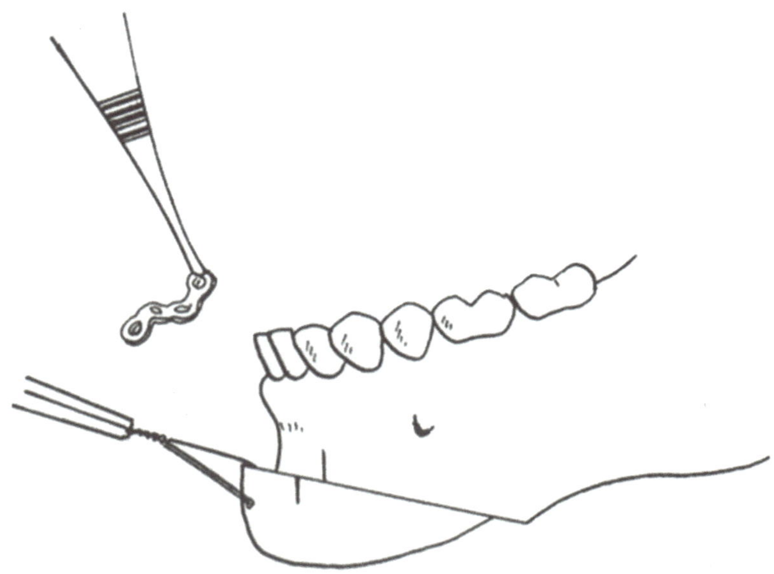

a

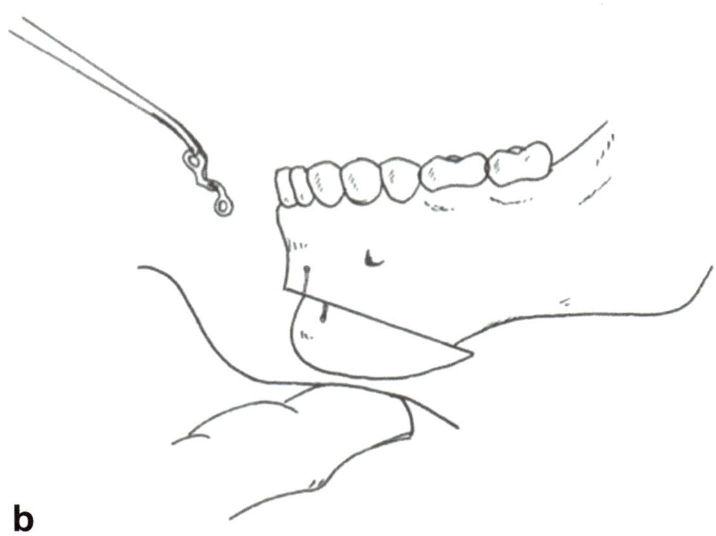

b

Figure 4.15 - STEP 15:

a. *Bone plate fixation using potioning wire.*

b. *Digital pressure may assist bone plate fixation.*

Step 16: Anteroposterior Reduction of the Chin.

Position the chin by means of extra-oral digital pressure, check the position of the bone against the reference marks using calipers, and then bend the appropriate plate to fit accurately and passively. Use an X-, H-shaped, two straight plates, or a prebent plate). When the chin is set back, the posterolingual area of the chin segment often results in a palpable step defect on the inferior border of the mandible *(Fig 4.16a, arrows)*. To contour this area, the osteotomized segment is pulled downward and forward and the posterolingual aspect of the chin segment is then contoured. It is, however, possible and often indicated to widen the posterior area of the segment. This is achieved by performing a midline osteotomy of the chin segment *(Fig 4.16b)*. Take special care to protect the soft tissue during this step.

Anteroposterior reduction of the chin may result in flattening of the labiomental fold. The sharp anterior edge on the superior aspect may be contoured to counter this effect and enhance the depth of the labiomental fold and chin shape *(Fig 4.16c, see arrow)*.

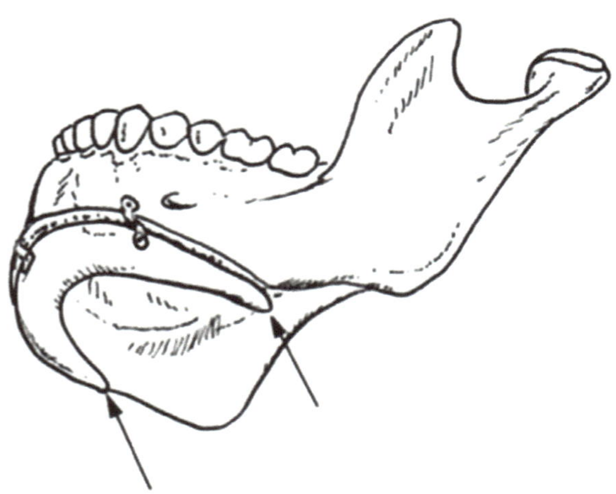

a

Figure 4.16 - STEP 16: **a.** *Checking the lower border contour.*

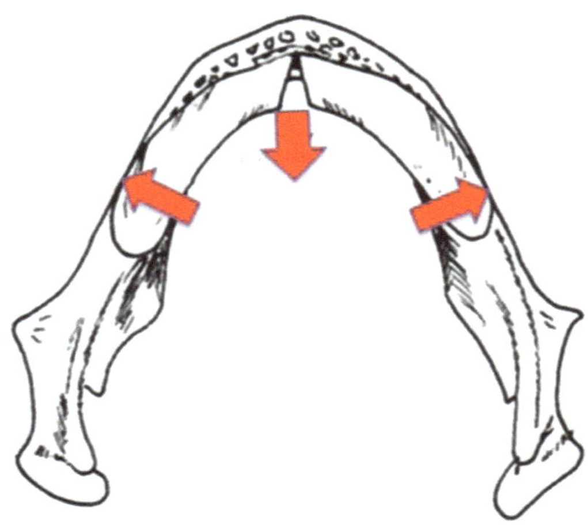

b

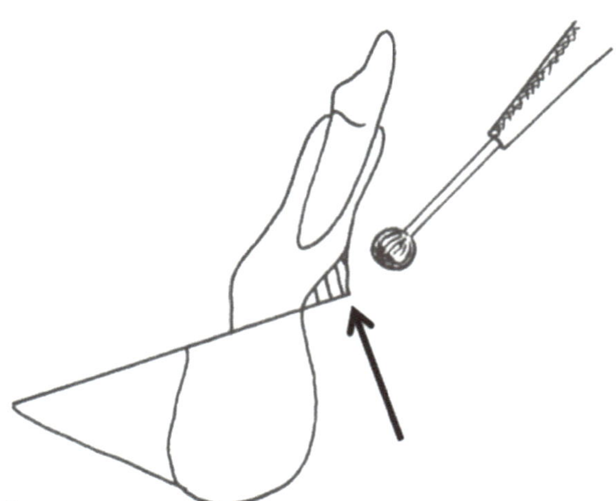

c

Figure 4.16 - STEP 16: **b.** *Correcting lower border defects.* **c.** *Control of the labiomental fold.*

Step 17: Vertical Increase of Chin.

Drill reference marks to record the vertical dimensions of the chin *(Fig 4.17a)*. Once the chin segment has been mobilized, fix two boneplates of appropriate length to the inferior segment. While the assistant maintains the required space between the bone segments, using the positioning wire and an instrument wedged between the segments, fix the screws through the plates onto the bone superiorly *(Fig 4.17b)*. At least two screws should be placed superiorly and inferiorly to the osteotomy using an H-shaped, X-shaped or two straight plates to secure the segment and maintain the height. It is recommended that a bone graft be placed in the defect. The esthetic requirements will dictate the shape of the bone graft. Make sure not to force the bone graft into the defect as it may displace or mobilize the chin segment. Freeze-dried bone or hydroxyapatite may be used as a grafting material.

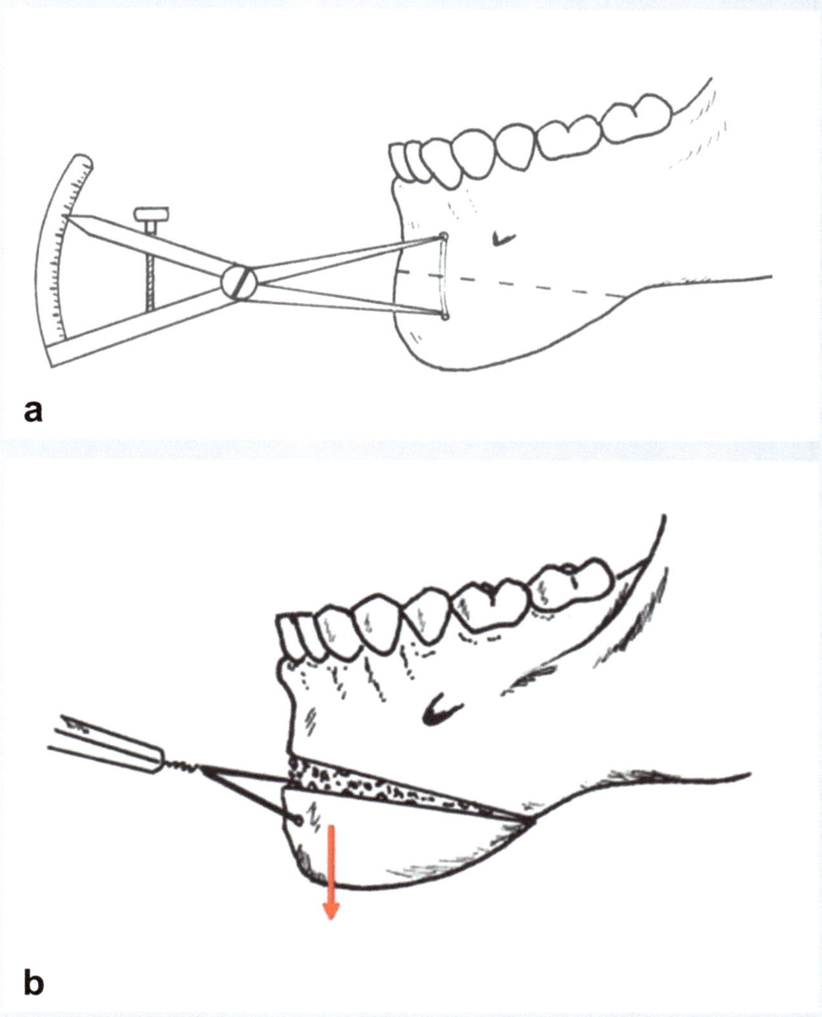

Figure 4.17 - STEP 17:
a. *Increase of the anterior chin height.*
b. *Positioning, grafting and fixation of the chin segment.*

Step 18: Vertical Reduction of Chin.

The reference marks are used to record the vertical dimensions of the chin. To maintain symmetry of the chin, the marks are placed in the midline and ±10 mm lateral to the midline. The vertical distances between them are recorded to assist with accurate vertical repositioning. Perform the first osteotomy low enough to facilitate the second osteotomy from the superior aspect *(Fig 4.18a)*. The lower osteotomy is completed and the chin segment is mobilized. Mark the amount and shape of bone to be removed and then complete the superior osteotomy. The shape of the ostectomized bone will influence the final anteroposterior position of the tip of the chin, i.e., if the ostectomy is wider on the anterior aspect, the chin will rotate anteriorly, *(Fig 4.18b, arrows)*, whereas a wider ostectomy posterior will rotate the chin posteriorly *(Fig 4.18c, arrows)*. Maintain as much soft tissue attachment to the chin as possible to ensure good blood supply to the repositioned bone and to reduce dead space. A large soft tissue pedicle will also reduce postoperative bone resorbtion and enhance predictable esthetic results.

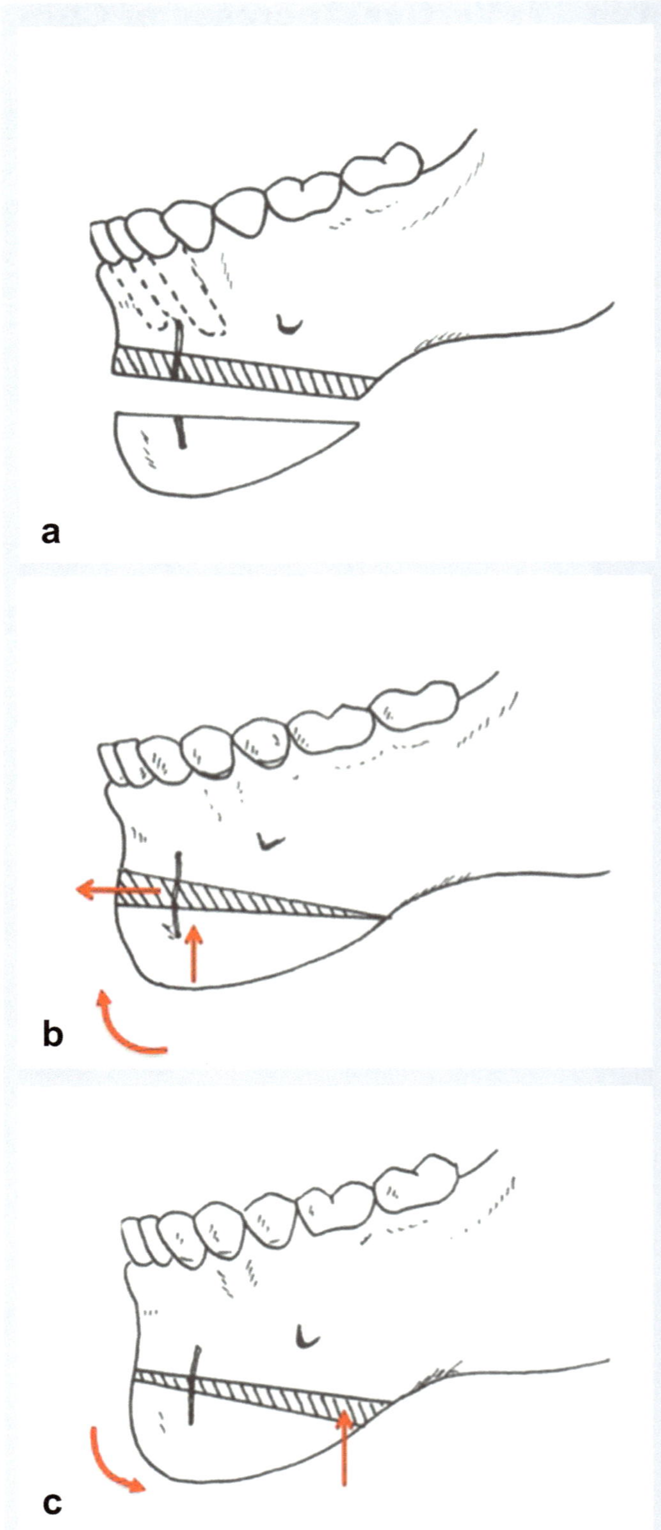

Figure 4.18 - STEP 18: **a.** *Vertical reduction of the chin.* **b & c.** *Anteroposterior control of the chin during vertical reduction.*

Step 19: Correction of Asymmetry of the Chin.

Drill reference marks to record the transverse and vertical dimensional changes of the chin. For lateral movement of the chin, the dental midline is marked as well the midline of the chin. The asymmetry is corrected by sliding the segment laterally until the dental midline (facial midline) mark and chin midline mark coincide *(Fig 4.19a)*. However, when correction of the asymmetry requires correction of a cant of the lower border, marks are placed lateral to the midline to record vertical dimensions on both the left and right sides. Depending on the height of the chin, the cant is corrected by increasing the height on one side (by downgrafting) *(Fig 4.19b)*, reducing the height on the contralateral side (by ostectomy) *(Fig 4.19c)* or a combination of the above *(Fig 4.19d & e)*.

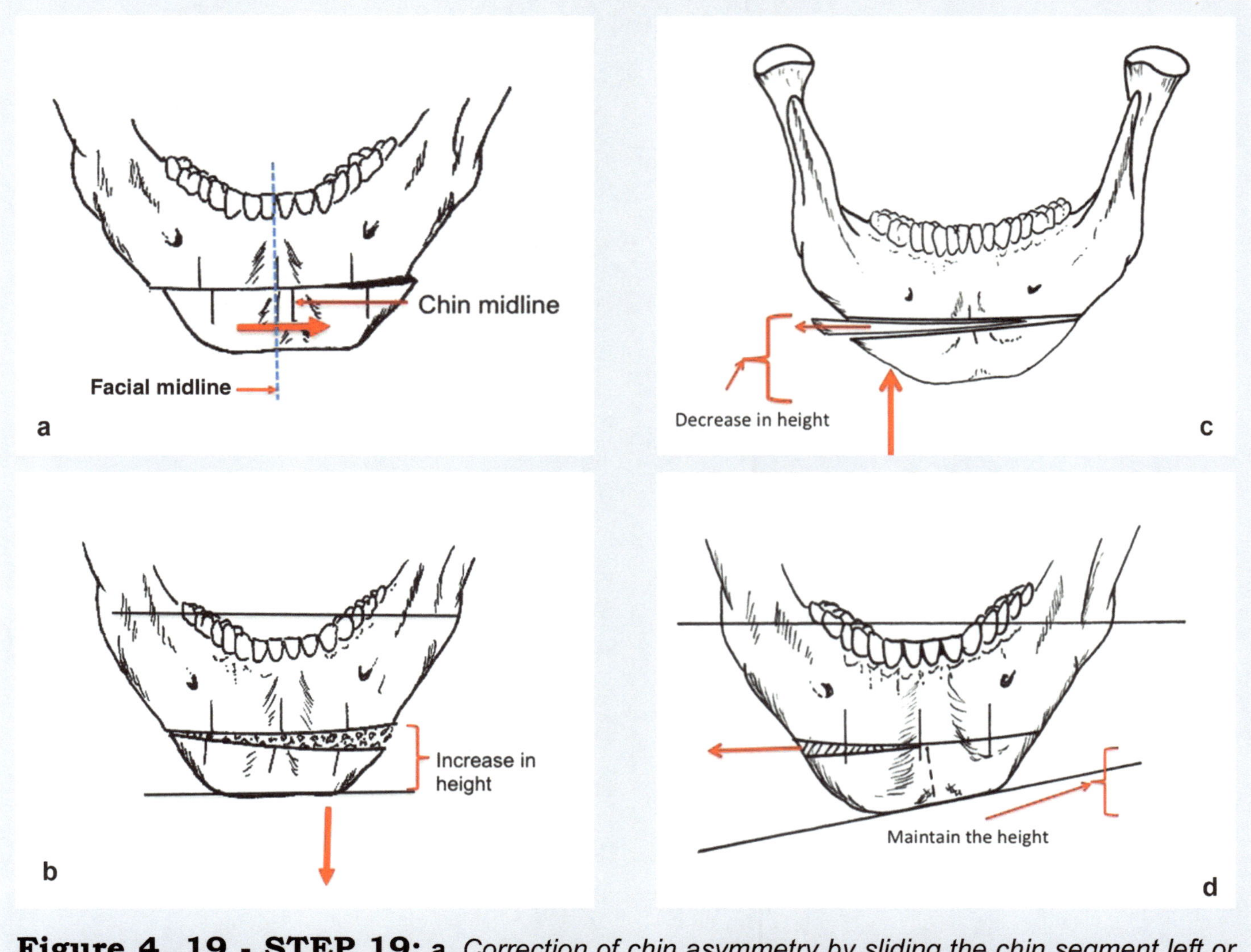

Figure 4. 19 - STEP 19: **a.** *Correction of chin asymmetry by sliding the chin segment left or right.* **b.** *Correction of chin asymmetry and simultaneous vertical increase.* **c.** *Correction of chin asymmetry and simultaneous vertical reduction.* **d.** *Correction of chin asymmetry maintaining the height.*

Large cants of the chin contour, i.e., unilateral condylar hyperplasia or hypoplasia, may have to be corrected by a propeller osteotomy. In this case, the first osteotomy is performed superiorly and parallel to the occlusal plane or interpupillary plane. A second osteotomy is performed parallel to the lower border of the chin *(Fig 4.19f)*. The small triangular-shaped segment is now rotated by 180° while maintaining its muscle attachment *(Fig 4.19g)*. The inferior segment can now be secured by means of rigid fixation *(Fig 4.19h)*.

Anteroposterior asymmetries are corrected by advancing one side of the chin segment more than the other or vice versa, setting one side further back than the other.

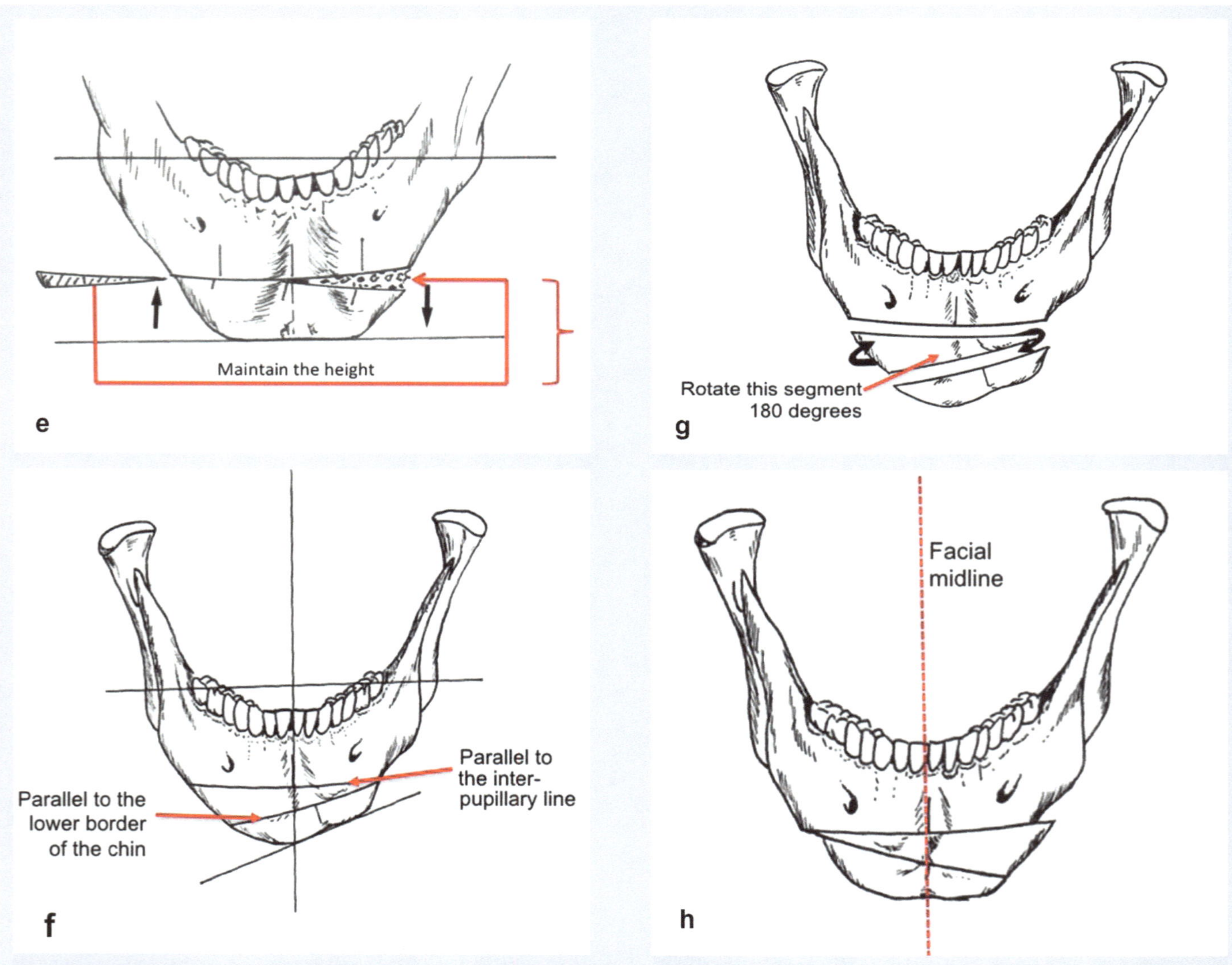

Figure 4.19 - STEP 19: **e.** *Maintaining the anterior chin height.* **f, g, h.** *The steps in the propeller osteotomy.*

Step 20: Altering Width of Chin.[10]

Place reference marks, recording the presurgical chin dimension with a fissure 701 bur.

Widen or reduce the chin width by altering the posterior dimension of the chin. Before the chin is mobilized, place a straight fixation plate (4-hole) horizontally across the midline below the planned osteotomy line to the labial cortex of the chin *(Fig 4.20a).*

Widening the Chin.

Perform a midline osteotomy through the buccal and
lingual cortexes of the mobilized chin segment and complete the osteotomy with a small osteotome. The chin can now be widened by using the boneplate as a hinge *(Fig 4.20b).* A small triangular bone graft may be placed in the lingual bone defect.

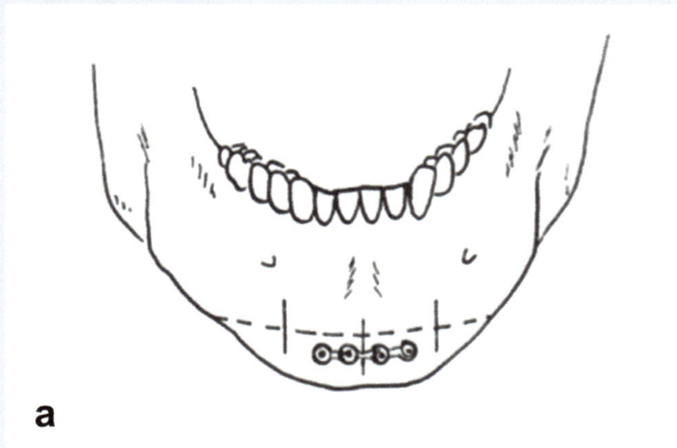

Figure 4.20 - STEP 20:
a. *Altering the transverse chin dimension. Note: the four hole plate is placed before the osteotomy is performed.*
b. *Widening the posterior chin.*

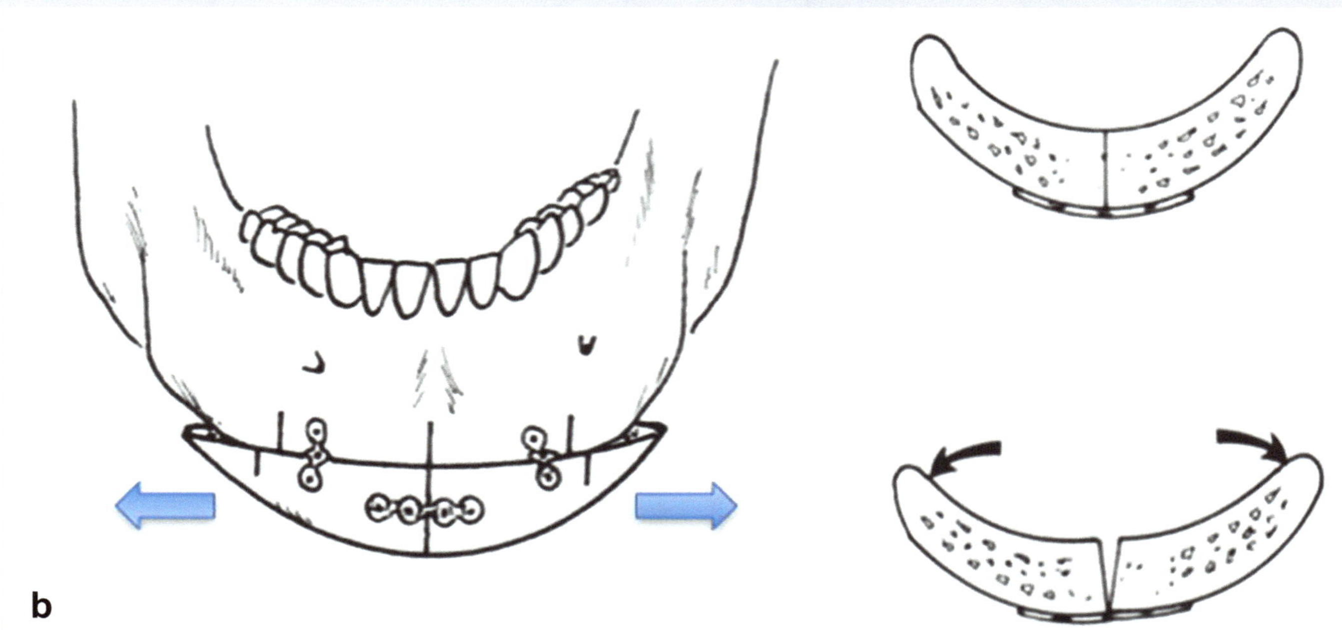

Narrowing the Chin.

Perform a triangular midline ostectomy on the lingual aspect of the mobilized chin segment and narrow the chin by using the boneplate as a hinge. The lower border of the mandible posterior to the chin may be contoured where indicated *(Fig 4.20c).* Once the desired shape of the chin has been achieved, further fixation can be placed. Fixation should be placed on both sides of the midline osteotomy.

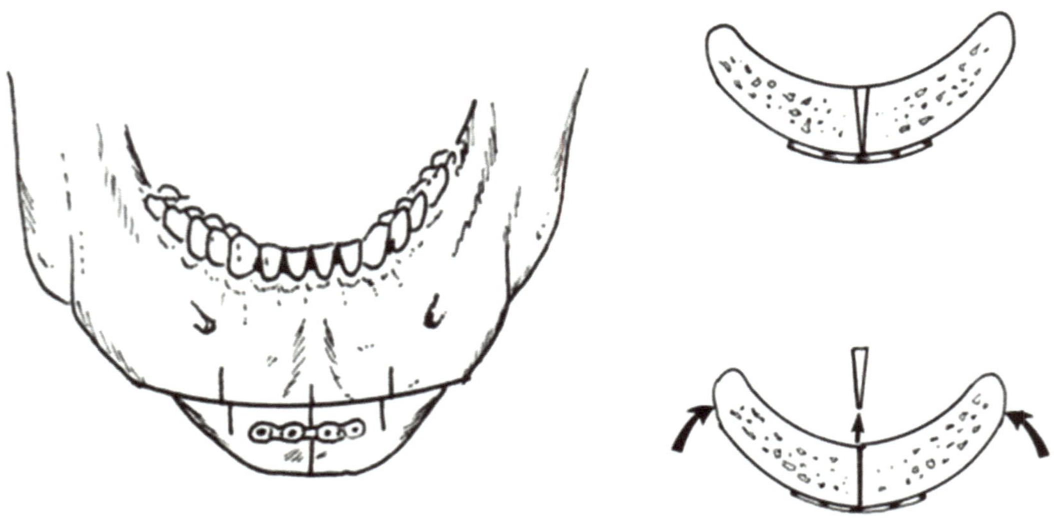

Figure 4.20 - STEP 20:
c. *Narrowing the posterior chin.*

Widening or Narrowing the Chin by Altering the Anterior Dimension of the Chin.

Narrowing the Chin.

A predetermined amount of bone is ostectomized from the center of the mobilized segment to narrow the chin. Complete all the osteotomies before mobilizing the segments to simplify the removal of the ostectomized bone *(Fig 4.20, d & e)*. The lower border of the mandible posterior to the segment may be contoured when required.

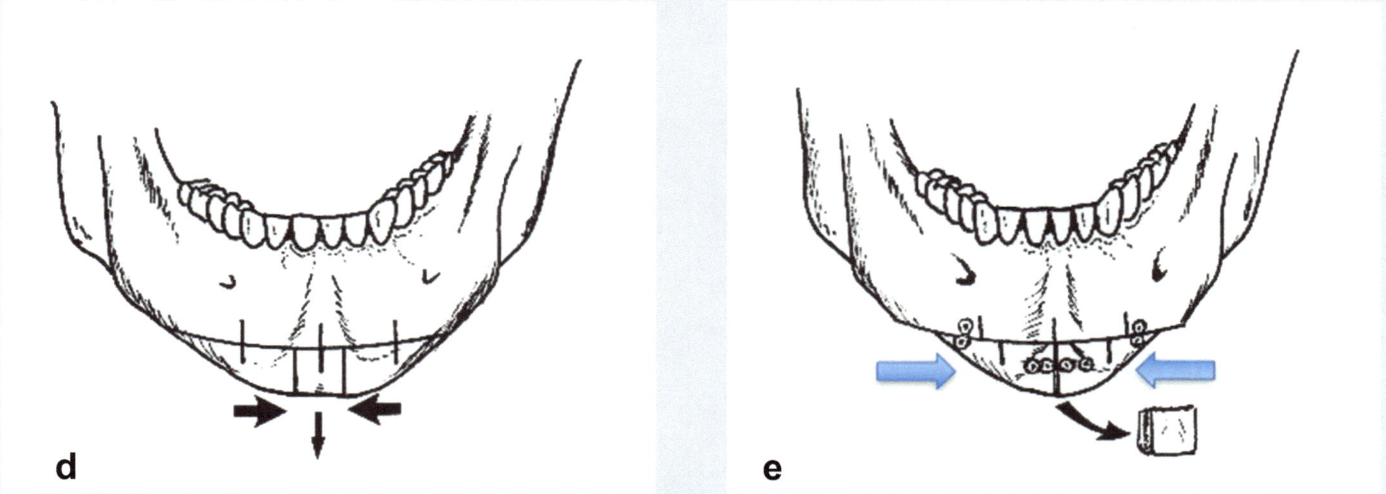

Figure 4.20 - STEP 20: **d & e.** *Narrowing the anterior chin.*

Widening of the Chin.

The anterior width can be increased and squareness of the chin enhanced by a midline osteotomy that moves the segments laterally *(Fig 4.20f)*. A bone graft is then secured between the segments *(Fig 4.20g)*.

Step 21: Suture the Submucosal Tissue

Care should be taken to meticulously reapproximate the mentalis muscle, periosteum, and mucosa. Place an interrupted midline suture first to accurately re-establish midline soft tissue alignment. A 3/0 chromic suture is then used in a continuous fashion to reapproximate the periosteum and muscle.

Step 22: Suture the Mucosa

Place a single midline 4/0 chromic suture to re-establish lip symmetry. A continuous suture is then used to secure the rest of the mucosa.

Step 23: Dress the Wound

Apply a pressure dressing. The pressure dressing should remain on the chin for 48 hours postoperatively.

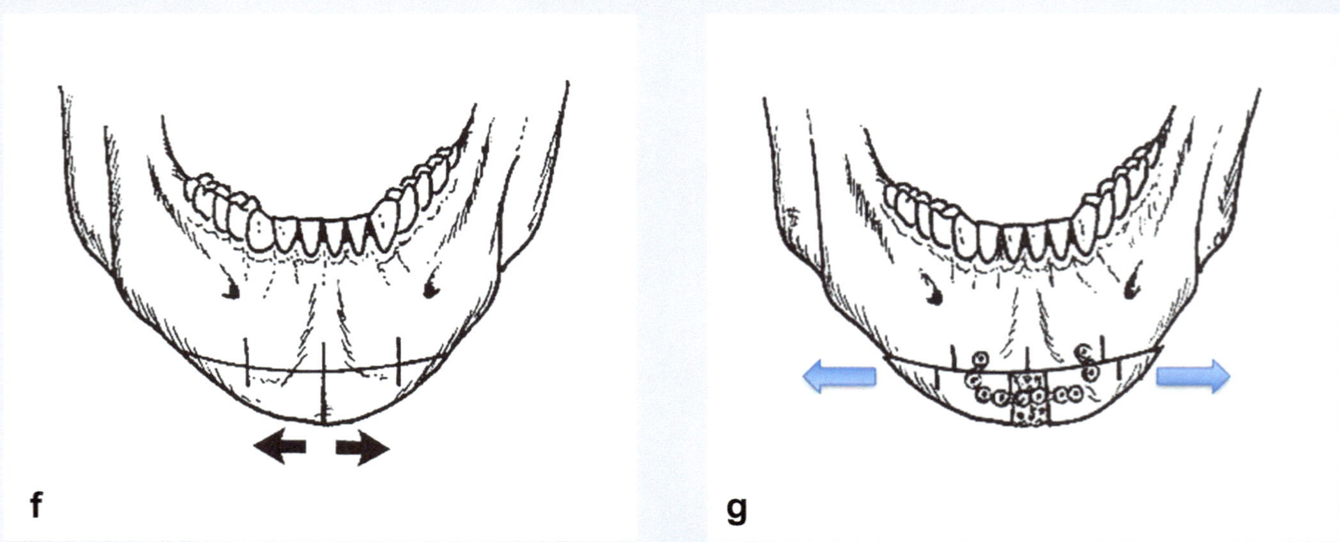

Figure 4.20 - STEP 20: **f, g.** *Widening the anterior chin.*

Chapter 5 - Clinical Treatment

Anteroposterior Deficiency – Microgenia

Anteroposterior augmentation by horizontal sliding osteotomy is the most common operation to correct an anteroposterior-deficient chin.[1–4] This procedure provides surgeons with versatility to correct chin deformities in all three dimensions of space, especially where concomitant vertical and transverse corrections are required.

The sliding genioplasty for anteroposterior chin augmentation has distinct advantages above the use of alloplastic materials for chin augmentation. Some unwanted sequelae associated with the use of alloplastic materials as chin implants are poor chin contour esthetics, resorbtion of bone, resorbtion of the incisor tooth roots under the implant, mobility to palpation, limited dimensional correction, both early and late infections, inability to change vertical chin dimensions, non-infectious inflammatory responses, and unpredictable soft tissue response.[5–10]

Typical Clinical Characteristics of Anteroposterior Deficiency

Frontal view:

- The chin appears weak and is often narrow.
- Soft tissue "marionette groves" often exist in adults.
- Poor chin–neck definition with a double chin appearance.

Profile view:

- Retruded weak chin.
- Increased lip–chin–submental angle.
- Decreased chin–neck length.
- Increased submental–neck angle.
- Poor lower border definition.
- Deep labiomental fold.

Treatment

Treatment for an anteroposterior-deficient chin is anteroposterior augmentation by horizontal sliding genioplasty. The anteroposterior chin position is determined by an integration of the clinical evaluation, cephalometric analysis, and the development of a surgical visual treatment objective. Various cephalometric indices may be used as indicators of "ideal" hard and soft tissue chin position in relation to other facial structures. The cephalometric parameters are discussed in Chapter 2 and development of the visual treatment objective are discussed in Chapter 3.

Esthetic Objectives

- **To maintain an existing smooth lower border or establish a smooth line.** Care should be taken when performing the horizontal osteotomy not to angle the osteotomy too vertical or "steep." This will not only decrease the chin height as the chin is advanced but may also create a step on the lower border, disrupting the well-defined lower border of the mandible. This disruption will be especially visible in individuals with thin skin.
- **To enhance the chin shape anteroposterior and transversely.**
- **Chin projection.** Make sure to achieve adequate chin projection while establishing a harmonious, smooth line from the lower lip, labiomental fold, and the chin button.
- **Transversely.** The width of the chin should be balanced with other facial features, especially the bizygomatic and bigonial facial widths. The head and facial shape, age, and gender of the patient will influence the final width of the chin. Patients with deficient chins often have leptoprosopic facial structures with "pointed chins." Simultaneous widening and advancing of the chin will reduce parasymphyseal depressions or groves.
- **Mandibular height.** The anterior mandibular height (excess or deficiency) should be corrected at the same time. Bear in mind that the angle at which the osteotomy is performed will influence the height as the chin is advanced. A "steep" angle will reduce the height as the chin slides anteriorly and superiorly.
- **Labiomental fold.** The magnitude of advancement, the height of the horizontal osteotomy, as well as the angle at which it is performed will also determine the height of the labiomental fold. Unless the depth of the labiomental fold needs to be enhanced, the acute anterior edge of the advanced chin segment is not contoured. The bone will contour by resorbtion of the edge and new bone deposition on the anterior surface of the mandible just superior of the advanced segment in the so-called "bow tie" effect.

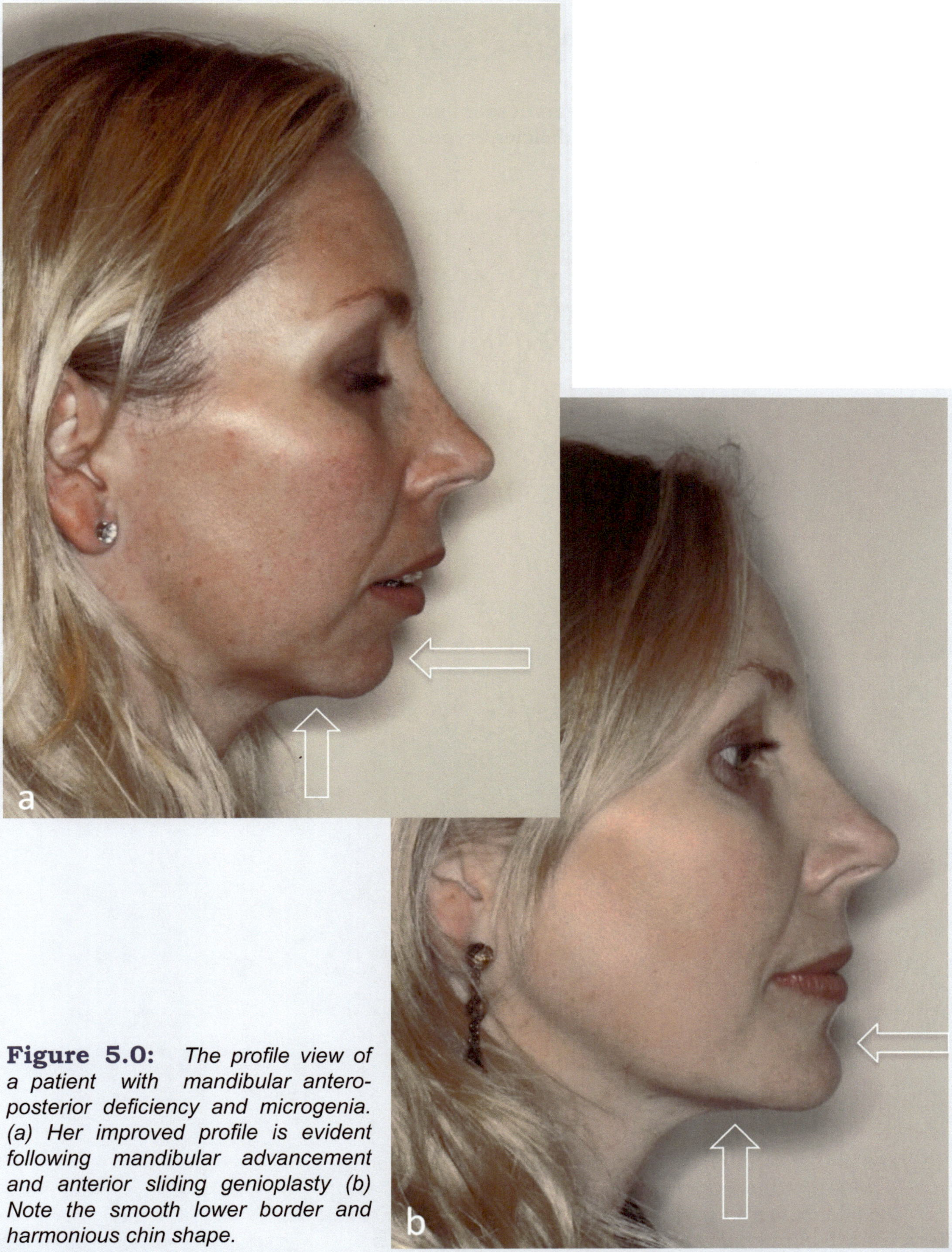

Figure 5.0: *The profile view of a patient with mandibular antero-posterior deficiency and microgenia. (a) Her improved profile is evident following mandibular advancement and anterior sliding genioplasty (b) Note the smooth lower border and harmonious chin shape.*

Anteroposterior Chin Augmentation

CASE 1: This 17-year-old male of Asian descent was referred to the orthodontist for correction of bimaxillary protrusion and a deficient chin.

Main complaint:
The patient complained that his chin appeared too small.

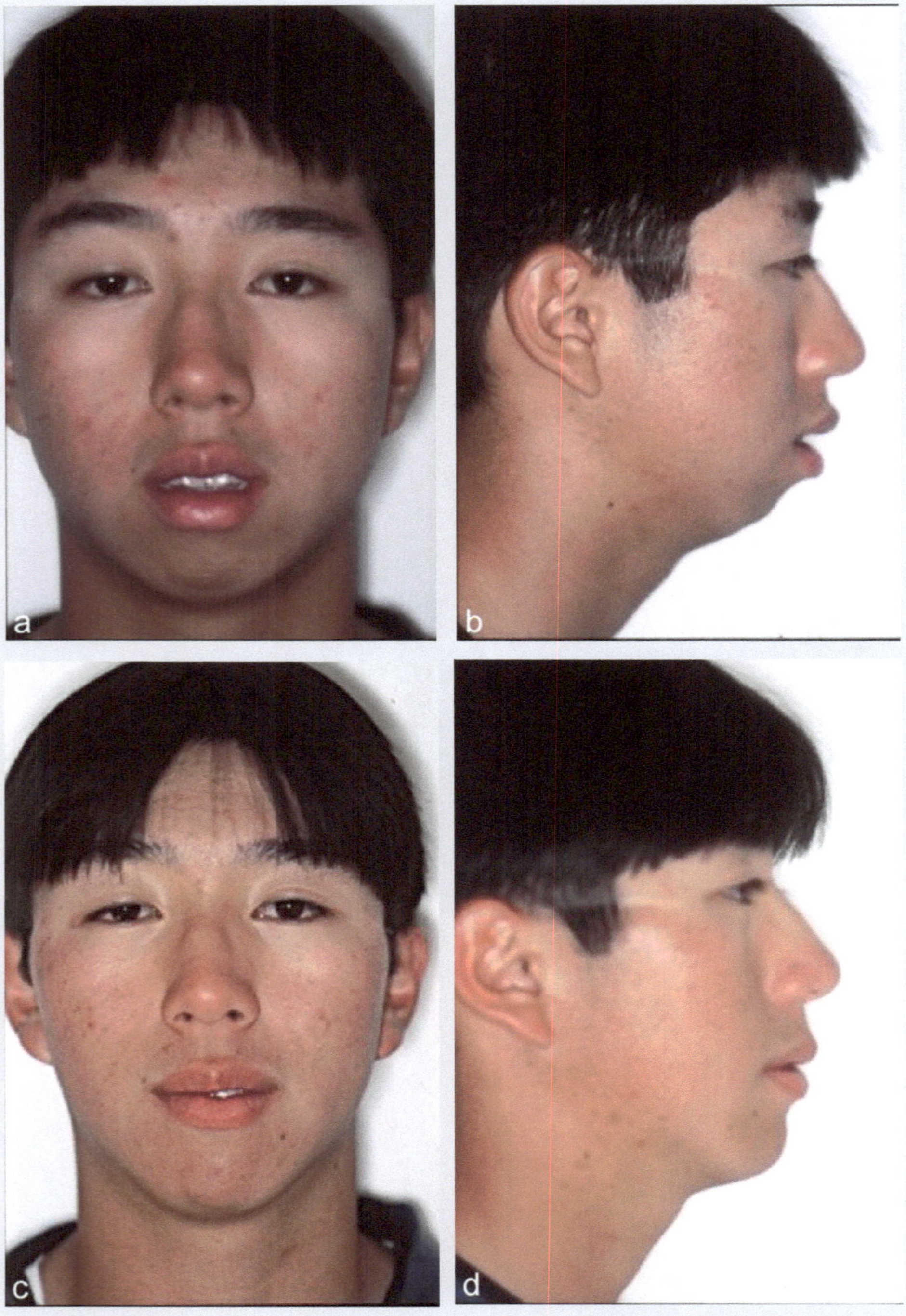

Figure 5.1 - CASE 1: *The pre-treatment frontal (a) and profile (b) and post-treatment frontal view (c) and profile view (d). The treatment plan consisted of orthodontic correction of the bimaxillary protrusion and surgical advancement of the chin.*

Diagnosis:

1. Dental: Class I bimaxillary protrusion.
2. Skeletal: Microgenia.
3. Soft tissue:
   - Anteroposterior deficient chin.
   - Full, protrusive lips.
   - Increased lip–chin–submental angle.
   - Short chin–neck length.
   - Flat labiomental fold.

Treatment:

1. Orthodontic correction of bimaxillary protrusion.
2. Advancement genioplasty.

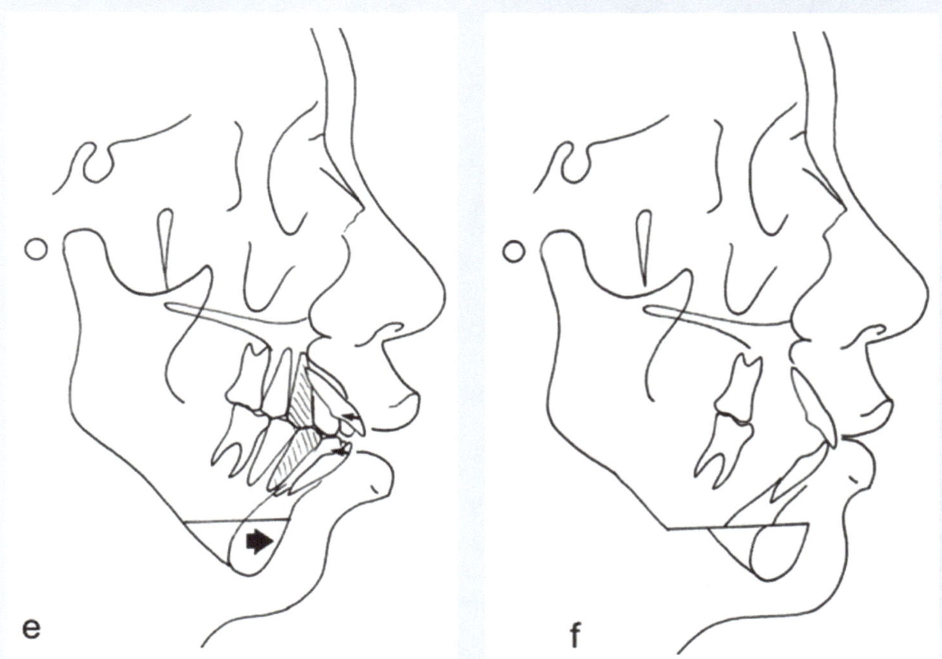

Figure 5.1 - CASE 1: *The pretreatment cephalometric tracing and treatment plan (e) and predicted postoperative cephalometric tracing (f).*

Anteroposterior Chin Augmentation Combined With Mandibular Advancement

CASE 2: A 16-year-old female patient consulted the orthodontist regarding treatment for her increased overjet.

Main complaint:
The patient felt that her bite was uncomfortable, her overjet was increased, and her upper incisors were too prominent.

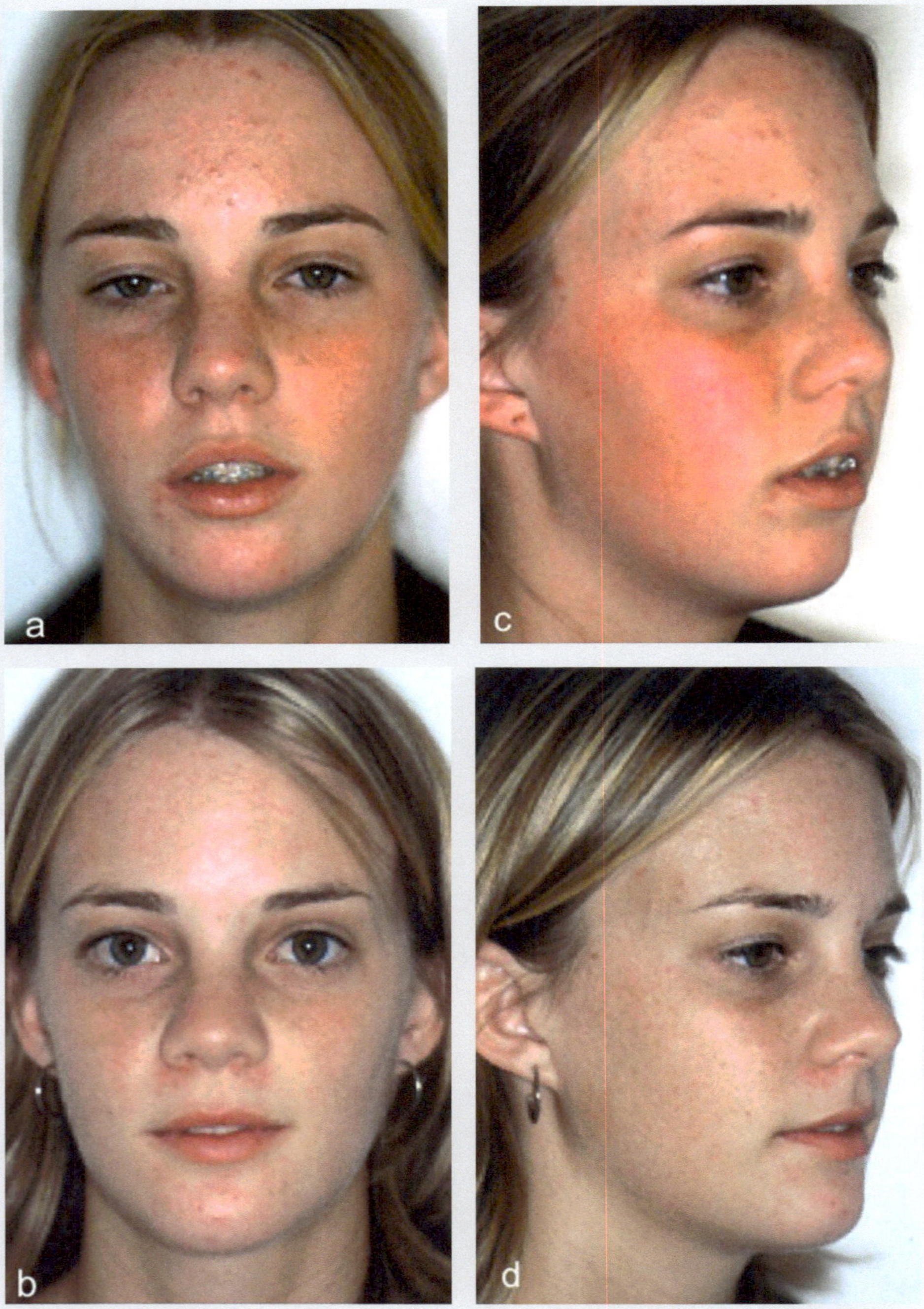

Figure 5.2 - CASE 2. *The vertical maxillary excess, mandibular anteroposterior deficiency and microgenia of the patient are evident in the frontal view (a) and three-quarter view (c). The improved esthetic results are demonstrated in (b) and (d).*

Diagnosis:

1. Dental: Class II dental relation.
2. Skeletal:
   - Vertical maxillary excess.
   - Mandibular anteroposterior deficiency.
   - Microgenia.
3. Soft tissue:
   - Convex profile.
   - Anteroposterior chin deficiency.
   - Deep labiomental fold.
   - Increased lip–chin–submental angle.
   - Increased submental–neck angle.
   - Short chin–neck length.
   - Increased interlabial gap.

Treatment:

1. Preoperative orthodontic alignment to facilitate a Class I occlusion after mandibular advancement.
2. Le Fort I maxillary osteotomy with superior repositioning of the maxilla.
3. Bilateral sagittal split ramus osteotomy, advancing the mandible.
4. Genioplasty, advancing the chin.

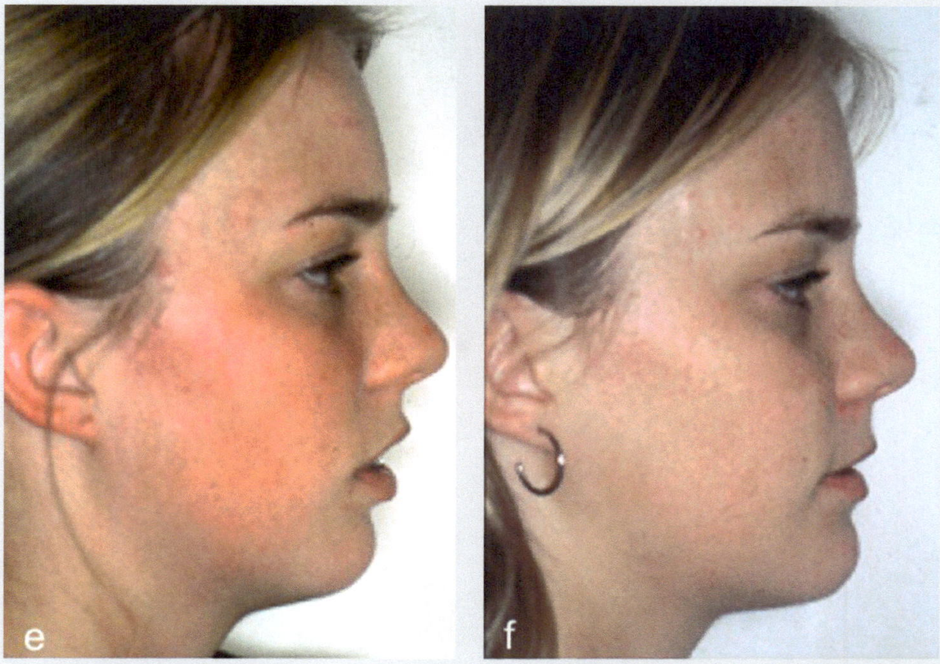

Figure 5.2 - CASE 2. *The vertical maxillary excess, mandibular anteroposterior deficiency and microgenia of the patient are evident in the profile view (e). Treatment plan: A le Fort superior repositioning of her maxilla, a bilateral sagittal split mandibular advancement and advancement sliding genioplasty. The improved esthetic results are demonstrated in (f).*

Anteroposterior Chin Augmentation Combined With Mandibular Setback

CASE 3: This 19-year-old male patient received orthodontic treatment for a skeletal Class III occlusion and was referred to the surgeon for surgical correction.

Main complaint:
The patient was concerned about the prominent appearance of his lower lip.

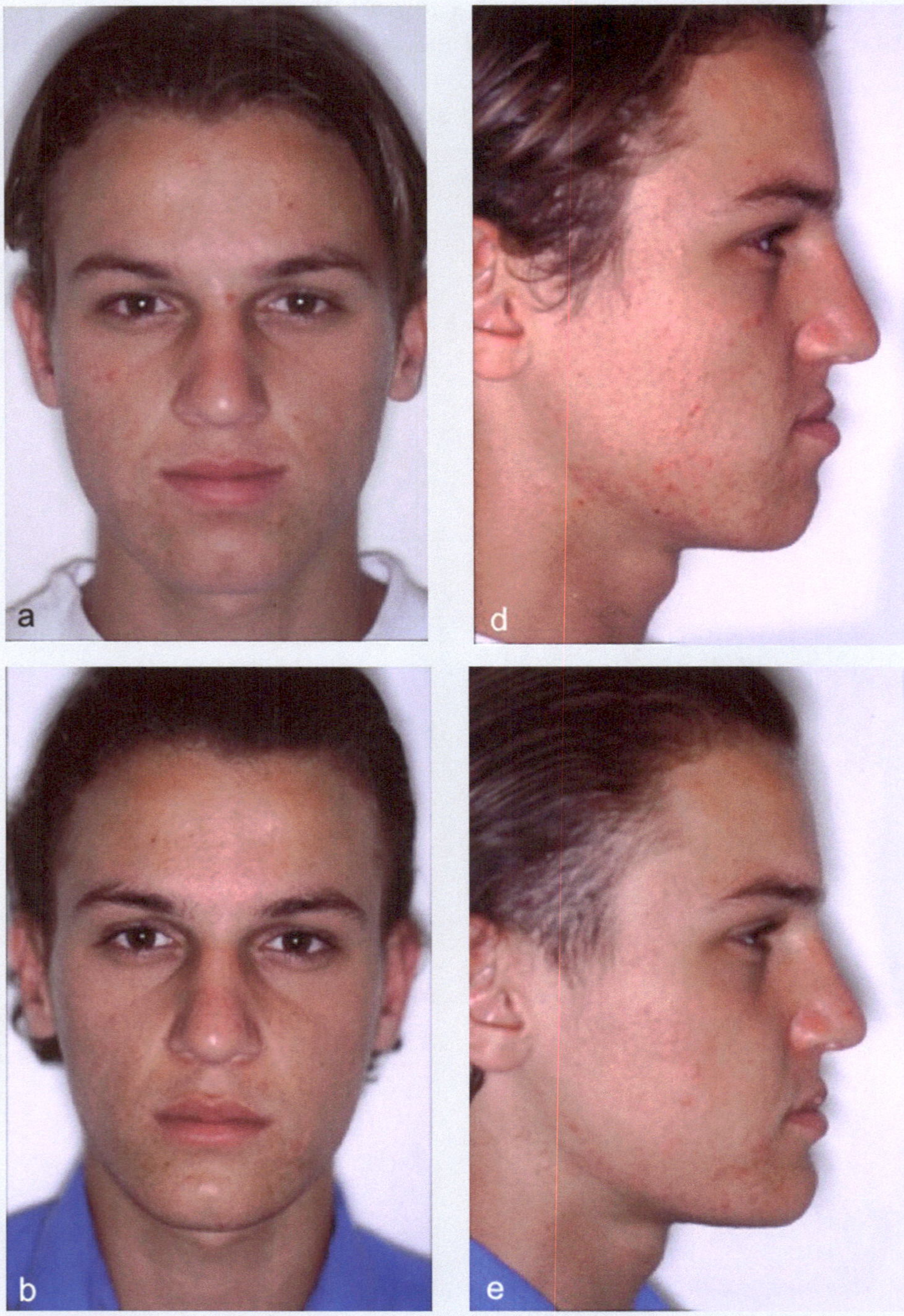

Figure 5.3 - CASE 3. *A patient with a Class III occlusion as a result of maxillary anteroposterior deficiency. The chin is rounded and ill-defined with the lower lip everted and ahead of the chin. Frontal view (a), profile (d). After a le Fort I maxillary downsliding osteotomy and advancement genioplasty (b) and (e).*

Diagnosis:

1. Dental: Class III dental relationship.
2. Skeletal:
   - Maxillary anteroposterior deficiency.
   - Maxillary vertical deficiency.
   - Anteroposterior chin deficiency.
3. Soft tissue:
   - Flat paranasal areas.
   - Concave profile.
   - Ill-defined, rounded chin.
   - Everted lower lip.

Treatment:

1. At the time of surgical consultation, the orthodontic preparation for surgery was completed.
2. Advance and downsliding le Fort I maxillary osteotomy.
3. Advancement genioplasty.

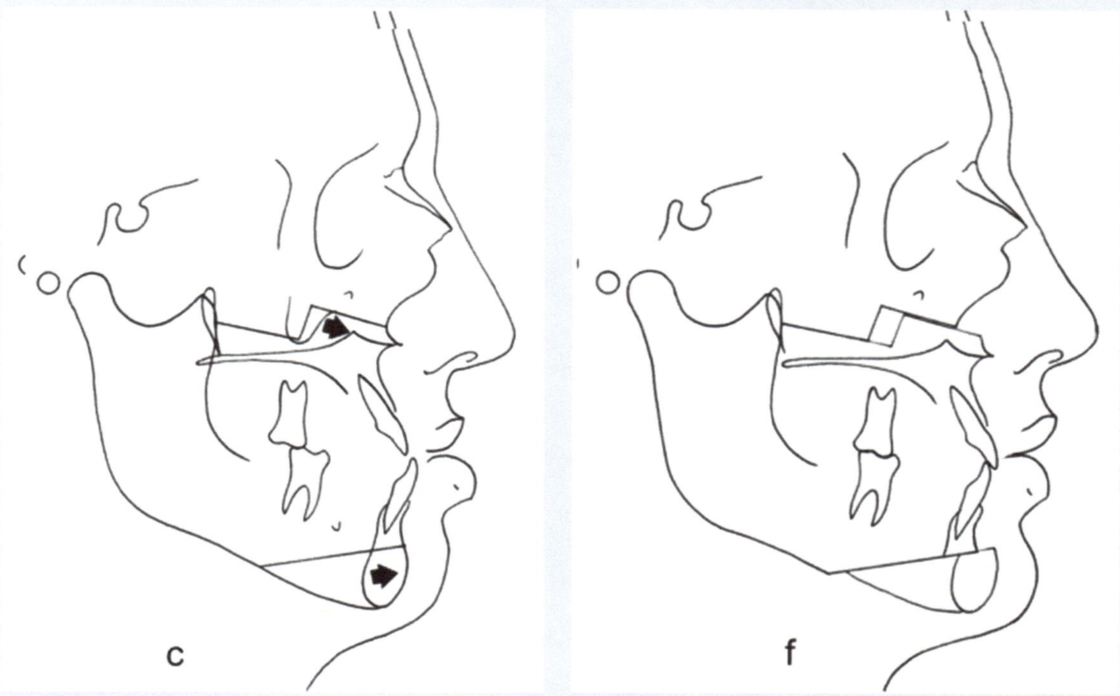

Figure 5.3 - CASE 3. *A patient with a Class III occlusion, as a result of maxillary anteroposterior deficiency, cephalometric tracing with treatment plan (c) for a le Fort I maxillary downsliding osteotomy and advancement genioplasty is illustrated in (f).*

Anteroposterior Chin Augmentation With Superior Repositioning of Maxilla and Advancement of Mandible

CASE 4: The dentist referred this 16-year-old male patient to the surgeon for orthognathic surgical correction of a skeletal Class II relation.

Main complaint:
The inability to close his lips.

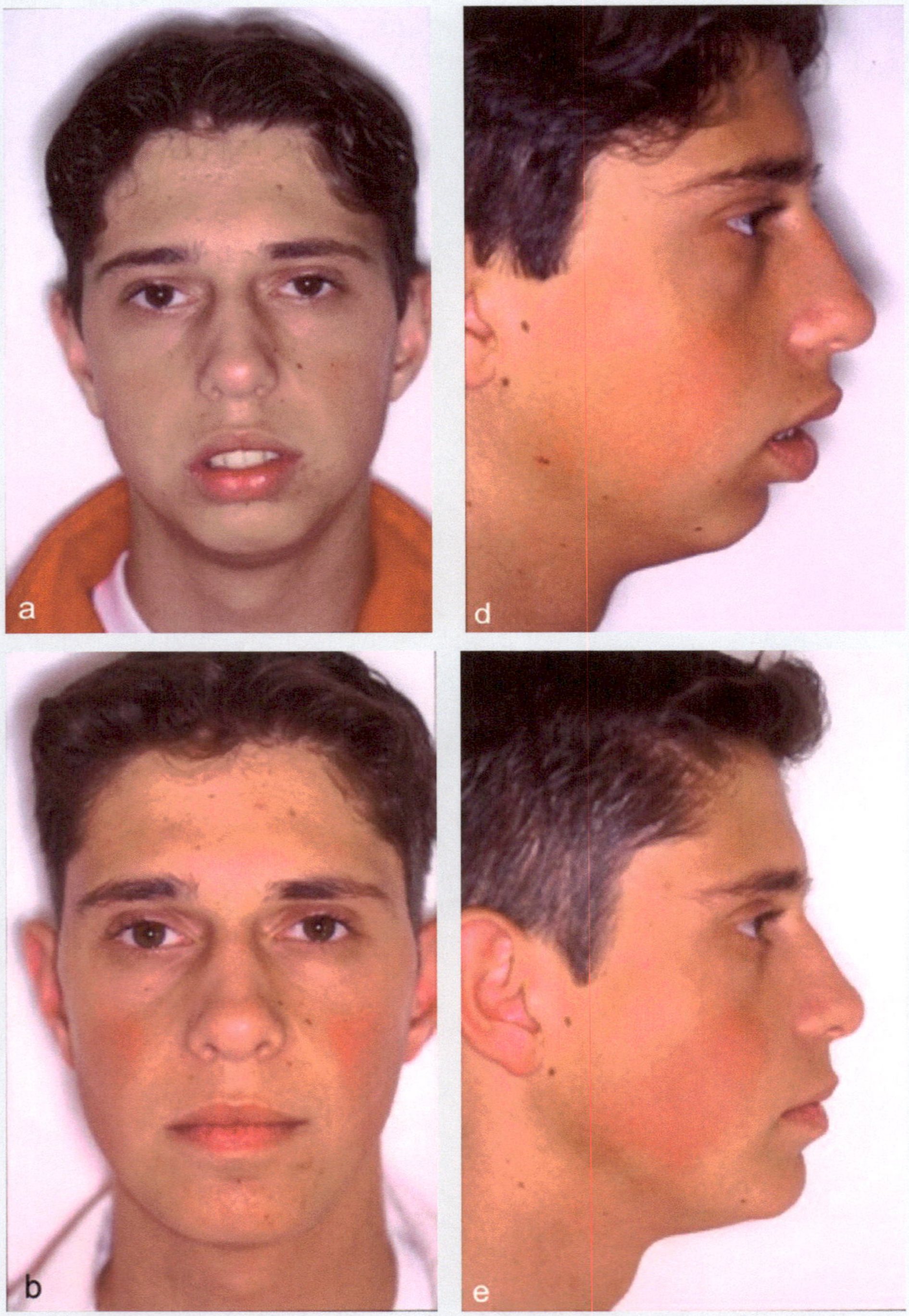

Figure 5.4 - CASE 4. *A patient with vertical maxillary excess, mandibular anteroposterior deficiency, microgenia and a Class II malocclusion (a) and (d). The post treatment results (b) and (e).*

Diagnosis:

1. Dental: Class II dental relation.
2. Skeletal:
   - Vertical maxillary excess.
   - Mandibular anteroposterior excess.
   - Microgenia.
3. Soft tissue:
   - Convex profile.
   - Incompetent lips.
   - Everted lower lip.
   - Anteroposterior-deficient chin.
   - Deep labiomental fold.
   - Increased lip–chin–submental angle.
   - Increased interlabial distance.

Treatment:

1. Orthodontic leveling and alignment of the dental arches.
2. Le Fort I maxillary osteotomy with superior repositioning of the maxilla.
3. Bilateral sagittal split ramus osteotomy, advancing the mandible.
4. Advancement genioplasty.

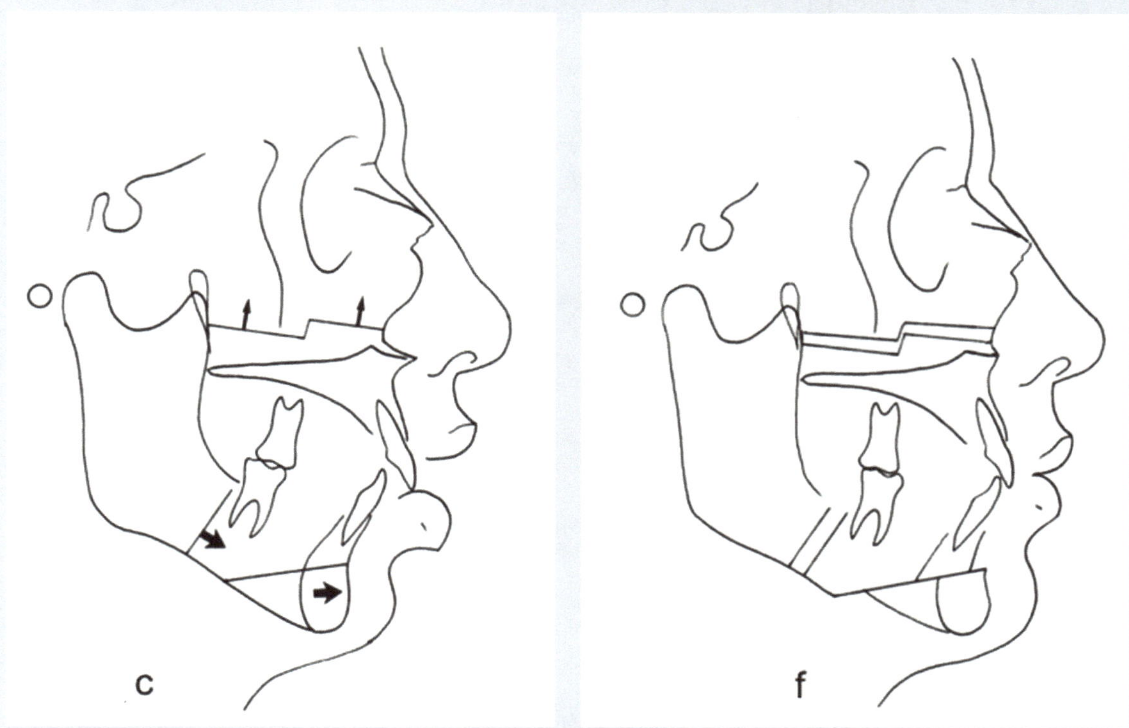

Figure 5.4 - CASE 4. *The cephalometric tracing of a patient with vertical maxillary excess, mandibular anteroposterior deficiency, microgenia and a Class II malocclusion with treatment plan (c) and post treatment results (f).*

Anteroposterior Chin Augmentation with Superior Repositioning of Maxilla, Advancement of Mandible, Advancement Genioplasty, and Bone Graft to the Chin

CASE 5: This patient was seen by the orthodontist from an early age regarding a severe Class II open bite malocclusion. Preoperative orthodontic dental alignment commenced at the age of 13 years *(Fig 5.5, a–d)* and surgery performed when the patient was 16 years old.

Main complaint:
The patient was unable to chew his food and his severely deficient lower jaw concerned him most.

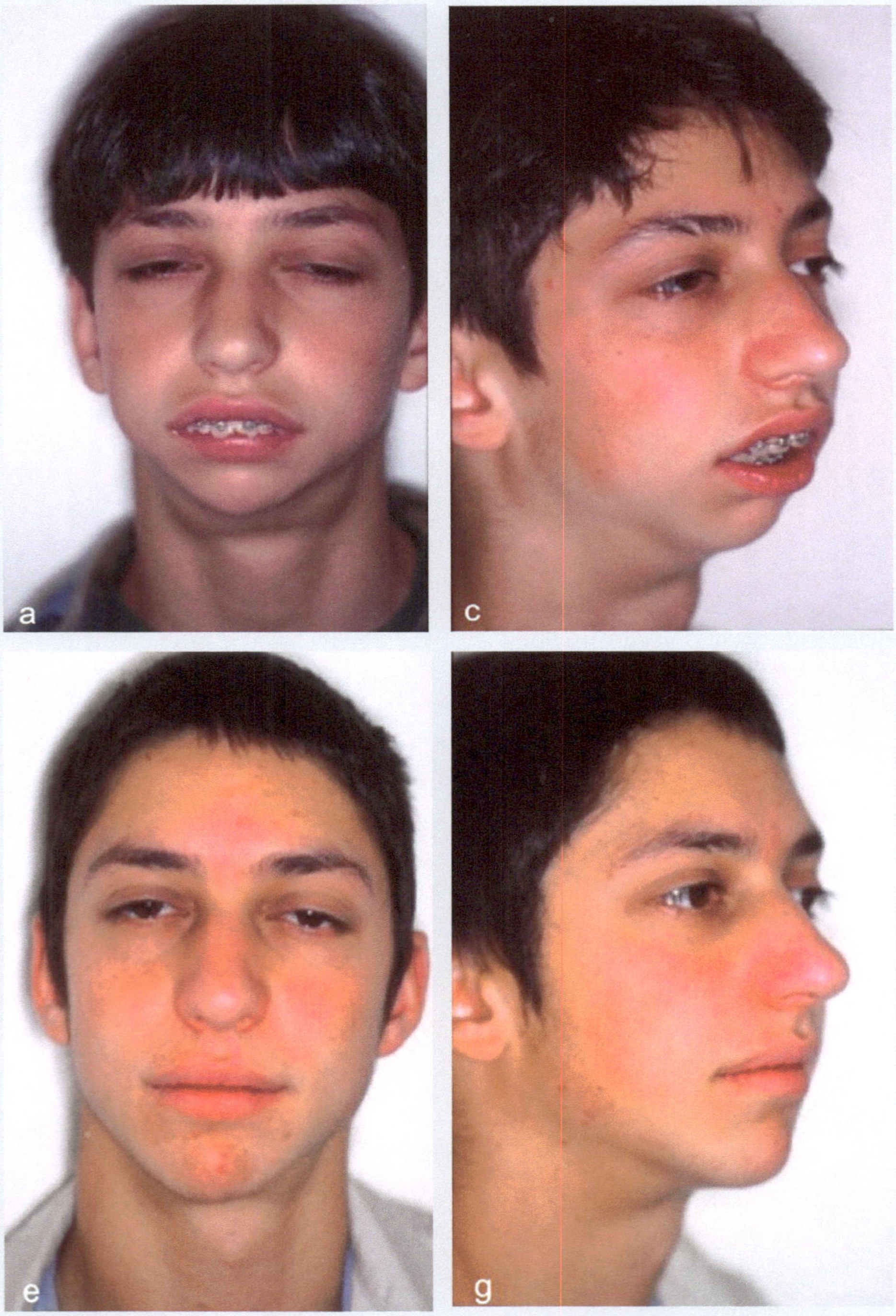

Figure 5.5 - CASE 5. *The preoperative frontal (a) and ¾ view (c) of a 13 year old patient demonstrating the severe convex facial profile. The 16 year olds postoperative results (e) and (g).*

Diagnosis:
1. Dental: Class II anterior open bite.
2. Skeletal:
   - Vertical maxillary excess.
   - Mandibular anteroposterior deficiency.
   - Microgenia.
3. Soft tissue:
   - Convex profile.
   - Lip incompetence.
   - Mandibular anteroposterior deficiency.
   - Anteroposterior chin deficiency.
   - Increased lip–chin–submental angle.
   - Increased submental–neck angle.
   - Decreased chin–neck length.
   - Everted lower lip.

Treatment:
1. Orthodontic alignment of the dental arches.
2. Le Fort I maxillary osteotomy superior repositioning of the maxilla.
3. Bilateral sagittal split ramus osteotomy, advancing the mandible.
4. Large advancement genioplasty.
5. Bone graft to the triangular bone defect superior to the advanced chin segment.

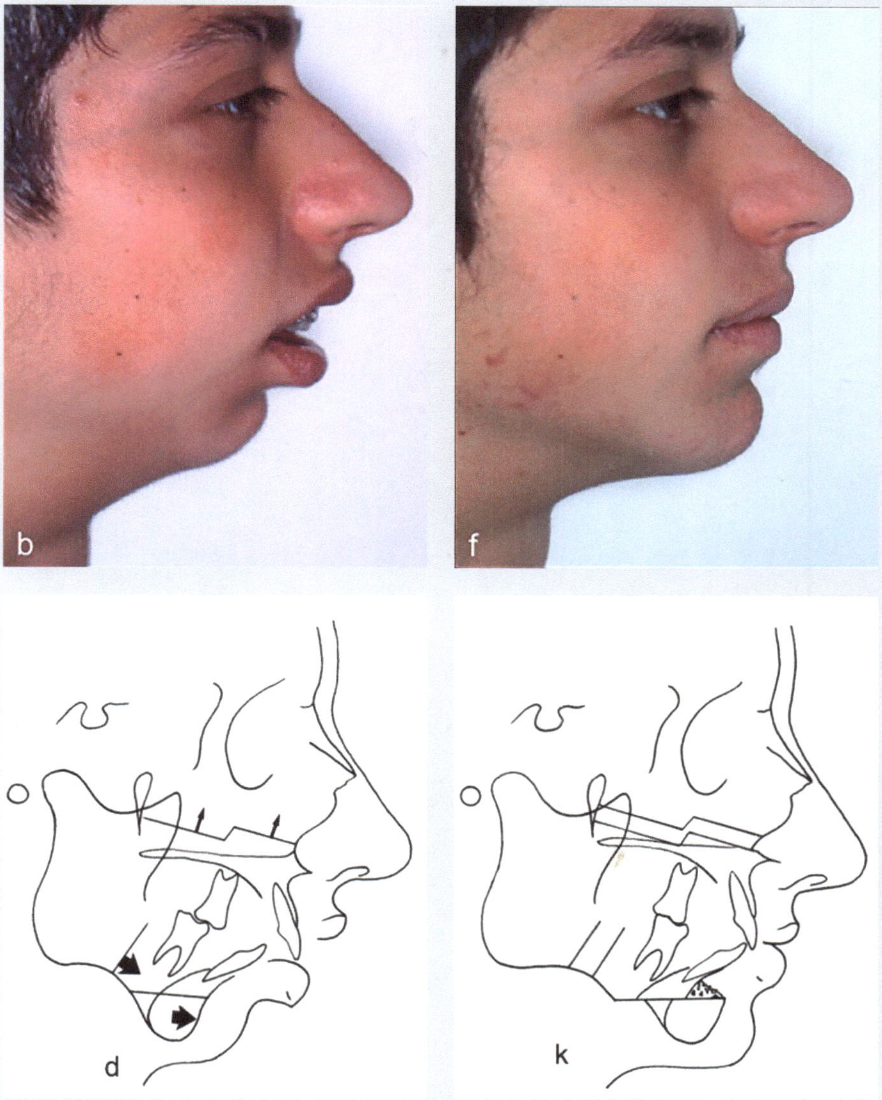

Figure 5.5 - CASE 5. *The preoperative profile view of a patient at age thirteen with a severe convex facial profile. The postoperative profile (f). The soft tissue, dental and skeletal relationship (d). Note the bone grafted superior to the chin segment to enhance the chin shape (k).*

Mandibular Advancement and Advancement Genioplasty

CASE 6: A patient with mandibular anteroposterior deficiency, and microgenia. The treatment results are illustrated following advancement of her mandible, and advancement of her chin.

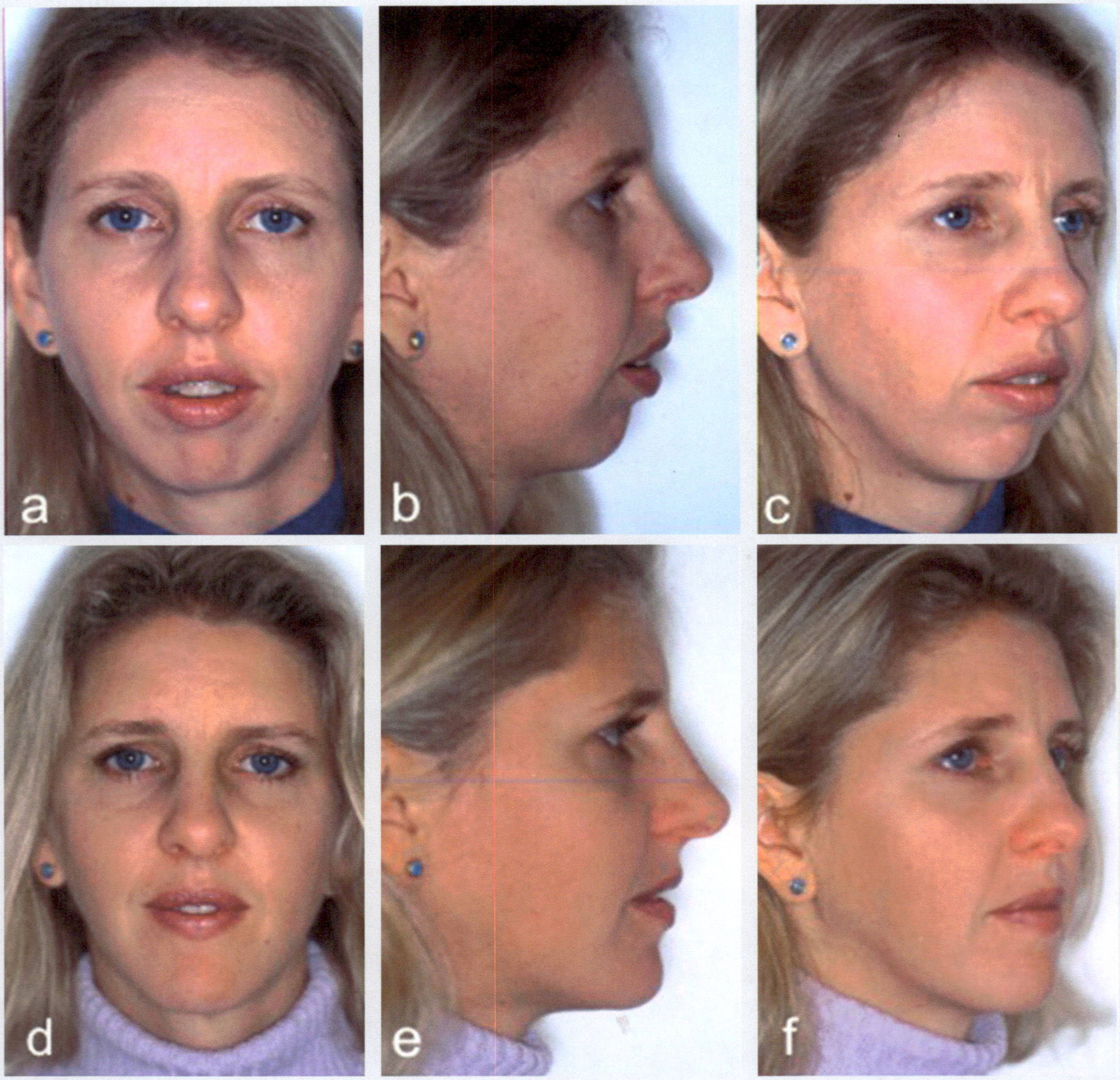

Figure 5.6 - CASE 6. *Note the convex profile due to mandibular anteroposterior deficiency and microgenia. The patient has a short chin-throat length, obtuse lip-chin-submental angle, an everted lower lip and a strong mentalis muscle action (a, b and c). The esthetic improvement is evident following mandibular advancement and advancement genioplasty (d, e and f).*

Superior Repositioning of the Maxilla and Advancement of the Chin

Case 7: The lower facial third of the patient is increased due to vertical maxillary excess. Her chin is anteroposteriorly deficient with an everted lower lip. Her maxilla was superiorly repositioned and her chin advanced. Photos illustrate the pre-treatment (a-d), and the post-treatment (e-h) features. Note the straighter profile, improved lip competence, improved chin projection, and more attractive smile.

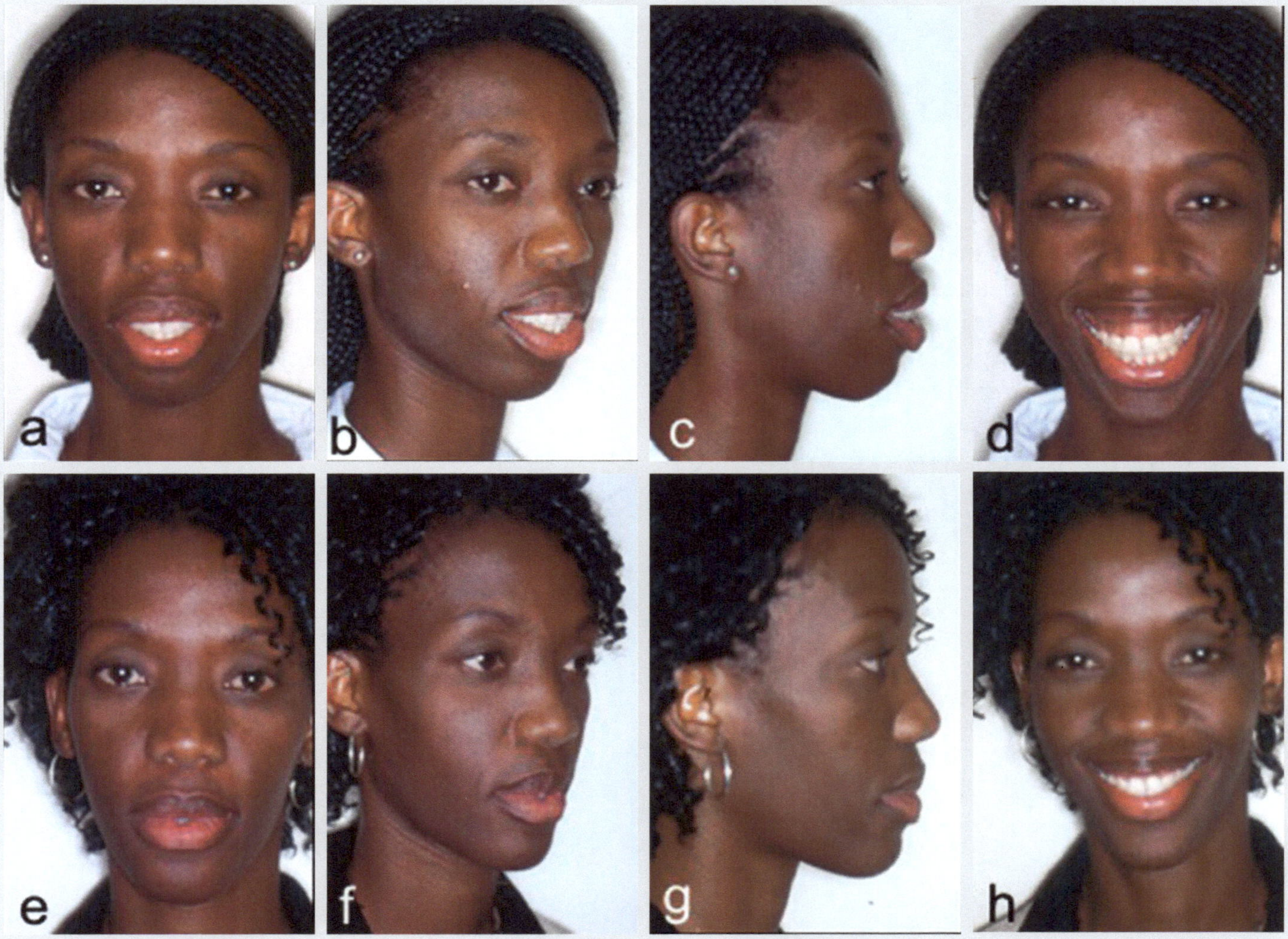

Figure 5.7 - CASE 7. *The patient's main complaint was her gummy smile. She also presented with a poorly shaped and deficient chin (top row). Her maxilla was superiorly repositioned allowing the mandible to auto rotate. Her chin was advanced by means of a sliding genioplasty (bottom row).*

Anteroposterior Excess – Macrogenia

This chin deformity is mostly caused by skeletal prominence of the symphysis of the chin, however, excessive soft tissue thickness may also lead to poor esthetic chin projection.[11,12]

Macrogenia may occur in patients with a Class I, II, or III occlusions. In patients with Class III malocclusions, the chin will be accentuated by dental compensation (retroclination of the lower incisor teeth), flattening the labiomental fold and resulting in a more prominent chin. Likewise, in patients with Class II occlusions, the excessive chin will be accentuated by a deep labiomental fold, resulting in a more "knobby chin." Without orthodontic correction of the malocclusion, reduction genioplasty is contraindicated in the above two instances.[13]

Typical Clinical Characteristics of Anteroposterior Excess

Frontal view:
- The chin is prominent and "knobby."
- Deep labiomental fold (often in patients with a Class II division 1 malocclusion). When dental compensation for a class III occlusion is present, the labiomental fold may be obtuse.
- The chin often "separates" from the rest of the mandible.

Profile view:
- Increased chin projection.
- Deep labiomental fold.
- Decreased lip–chin–submental angle.
- Increased chin–neck length.
- Pogonion ahead of the lower lip.

Treatment

The chin prominence is reduced by a posterior sliding genioplasty. Careful preoperative appraisal of the patient's esthetic features and treatment planning for esthetic anteroposterior chin reduction are critical. Poor planning, without taking all esthetic aspects into consideration, may make the esthetics worse.

Esthetic Objectives

Although the primary goal of the procedure is to position the chin in its ideal anteroposterior relation to other facial structures, the basic planning for this procedure must take the following important aspects into account:

- **The depth of the labiomental fold.** Anteroposterior reduction of the chin will reduce the depth of the labiomental fold. A flattened labiomental fold is esthetically unsatisfactory.
- **The final position of the bony chin** should be in proper relationship to the lower incisors as determined by cephalometric parameters, e.g., NB:Pog', A:Pog', and subnasale perpendiculars.
- **The smooth lower border of the mandible** will be affected by the retropositioned chin. The posterior aspects of the chin segment will create unesthetic irregularities on the inferior border of the mandible with loss of the smooth continuous line. This can be prevented by reduction of the posteromedial aspect of the chin segment. *(See Chapter 4, Surgical Technique.)*
- Bear in mind that the **angle of the horizontal osteotomy** will influence the final vertical dimension of the chin. A "steep" osteotomy will increase the height as the chin slides backward and downward.
- **The transverse dimension of the chin** should be carefully considered because as the chin segment is moved posteriorly, the posterior aspect will become relatively narrow. To maintain the width, squareness, and contour of the lower border, it may be required to widen the posterior aspect of the chin by means of a two-piece genioplasty. *(See Chapter 4, Surgical Technique.)*

Anteroposterior Chin Reduction

Case 8: This 16-year-old female patient was referred to the surgeon after orthodontic alignment of her teeth and establishment of a Class I occlusion.

Main complaint:
The patient was unhappy about her large chin.

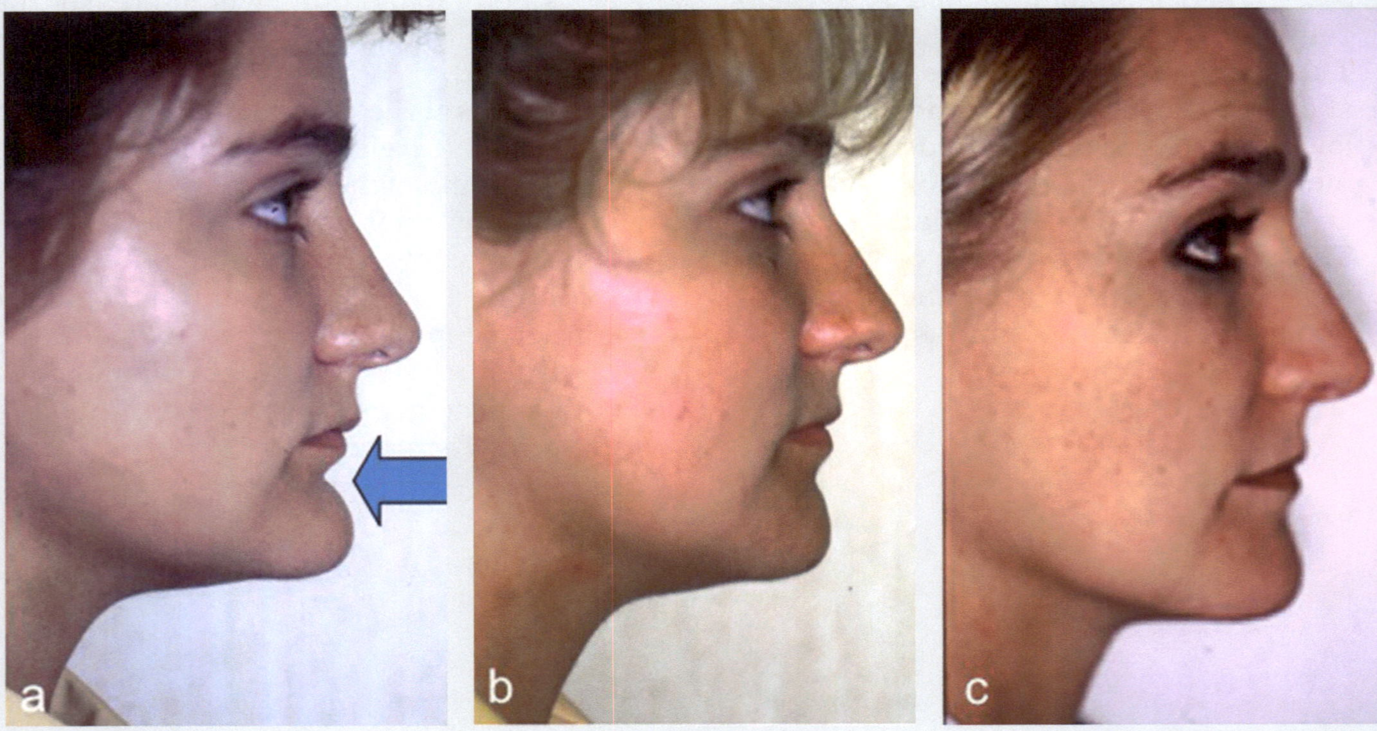

Figure 5.8 - CASE 8. *A patient with macrogenia. Note the prominent chin and deep labio-mental fold (arrow) in the pretreatment profile view (a). The post treatment result after 1 year in figure (b) and 10 years after treatment (c).*

Diagnosis:

1. Dental: Class I.
2. Skeletal: Macrogenia.
3. Soft tissue:
   - Chin anteroposteriorly excessive.
   - Deep labiomental fold.
   - Increased chin–neck length.
   - Acute lip–chin–submental angle.

Treatment:

Reduction sliding genioplasty.

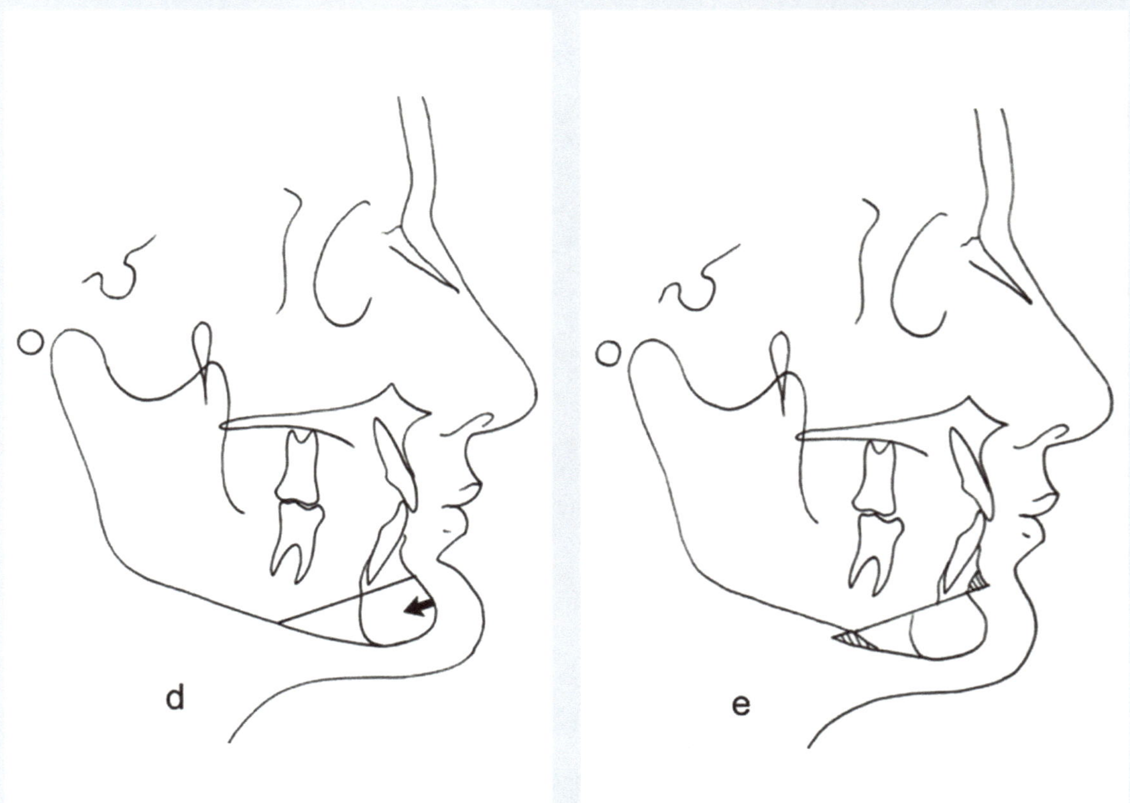

Figure 5.8 - CASE 8. *A patient with macrogenia. Note the prominent chin and deep labiomental fold (arrow) in the cephalometric tracing (d). The long term soft and hard tissue changes post treatment are demonstrated in (e).*

Anteroposterior Chin Reduction Combined with Mandibular Advancement

Case 10: This 15-year-old male was referred to the orthodontist for treatment of a Class II occlusion. The treatment plan consisted of orthodontic alignment of the dentition followed by surgical advancement of the mandible.

Main complaint:
The patient felt that his overjet was increased and his bite too deep.

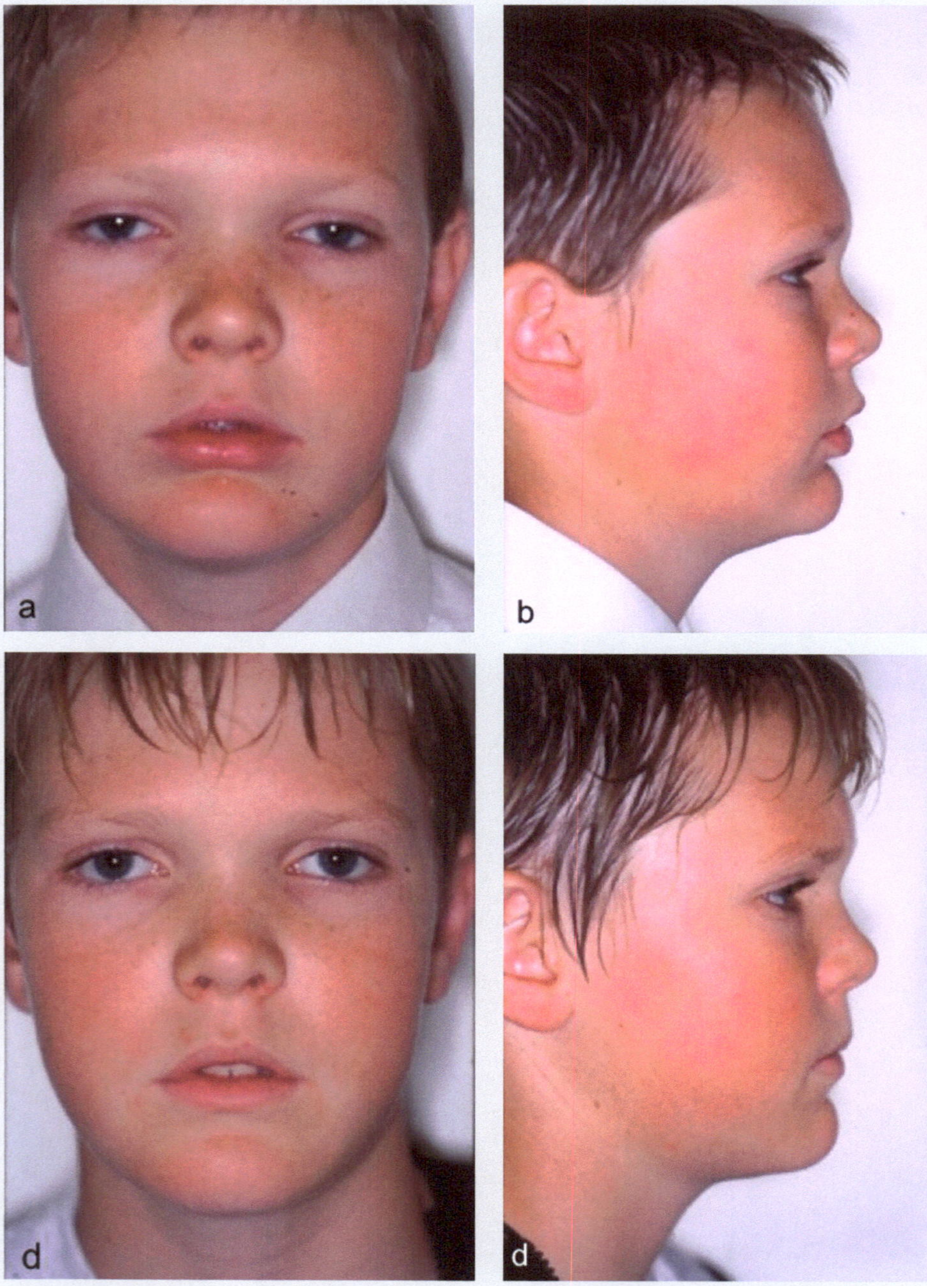

Figure 5.10 - CASE 10. *The mandibular anteroposterior deficiency of this patient is combined with macrogenia. Note the chin is also transversely deficient. Frontal (a) and profile view (b). Treatment plan consisting of mandibular advancement, reduction genioplasty and widening of the chin. Post treatment results (d).*

Diagnosis:

1. Dental: Class II dental relation.
2. Skeletal:
   - Mandibular anteroposterior deficiency.
   - Macrogenia.
   - Narrow chin.
3. Soft tissue:
   - Mandibular anteroposterior deficiency.
   - Prominent, knobby chin.
   - Deep labiomental fold.
   - Everted lower lip.
   - The chin appears narrow.

Treatment:

1. Orthodontic level and alignment of the dentition.
2. Bilateral sagittal split osteotomy, advancing the mandible.
3. Reduction genioplasty.
4. Widening the chin.

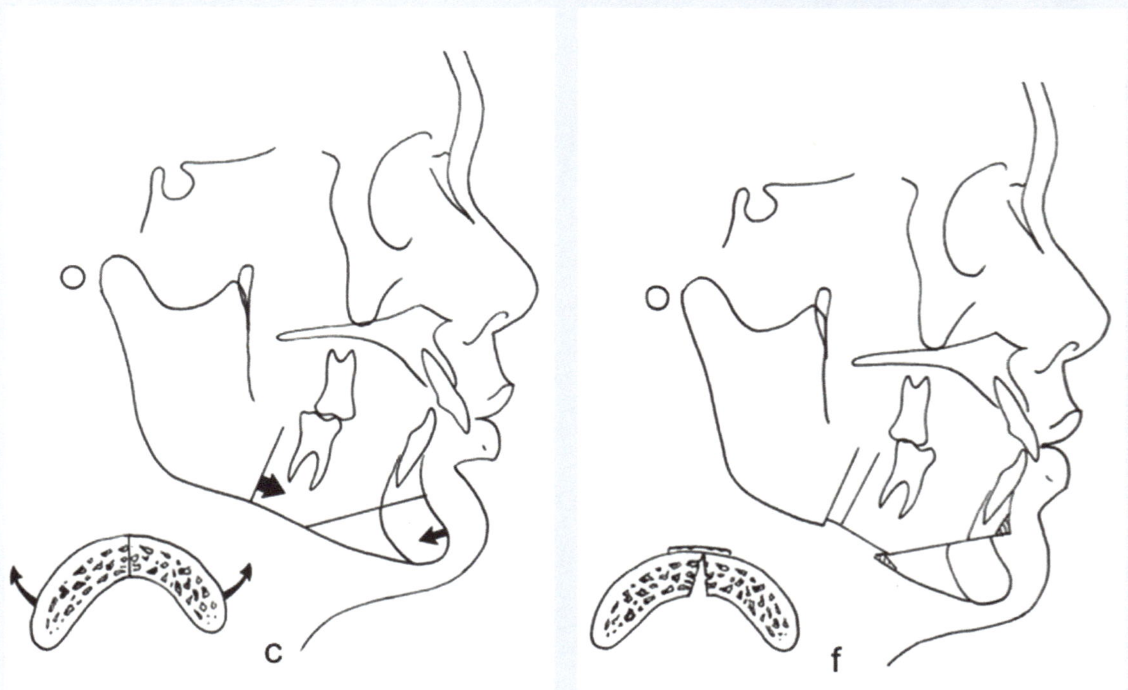

Figure 5.10 - CASE 10. *The cephalometric tracing of patient with mandibular anteroposterior deficiency combined with macrogenia. (c) Treatment plan consisting of mandibular advancement, reduction genioplasty and widening of the chin (f).*

Anteroposterior Chin Reduction Combined with a Vertical Increase of Anterior Mandibular Height

Case 11: This 30-year-old female consulted the surgeon regarding a reduction of her prominent chin.

Main complaint:
Her chin appeared too prominent.

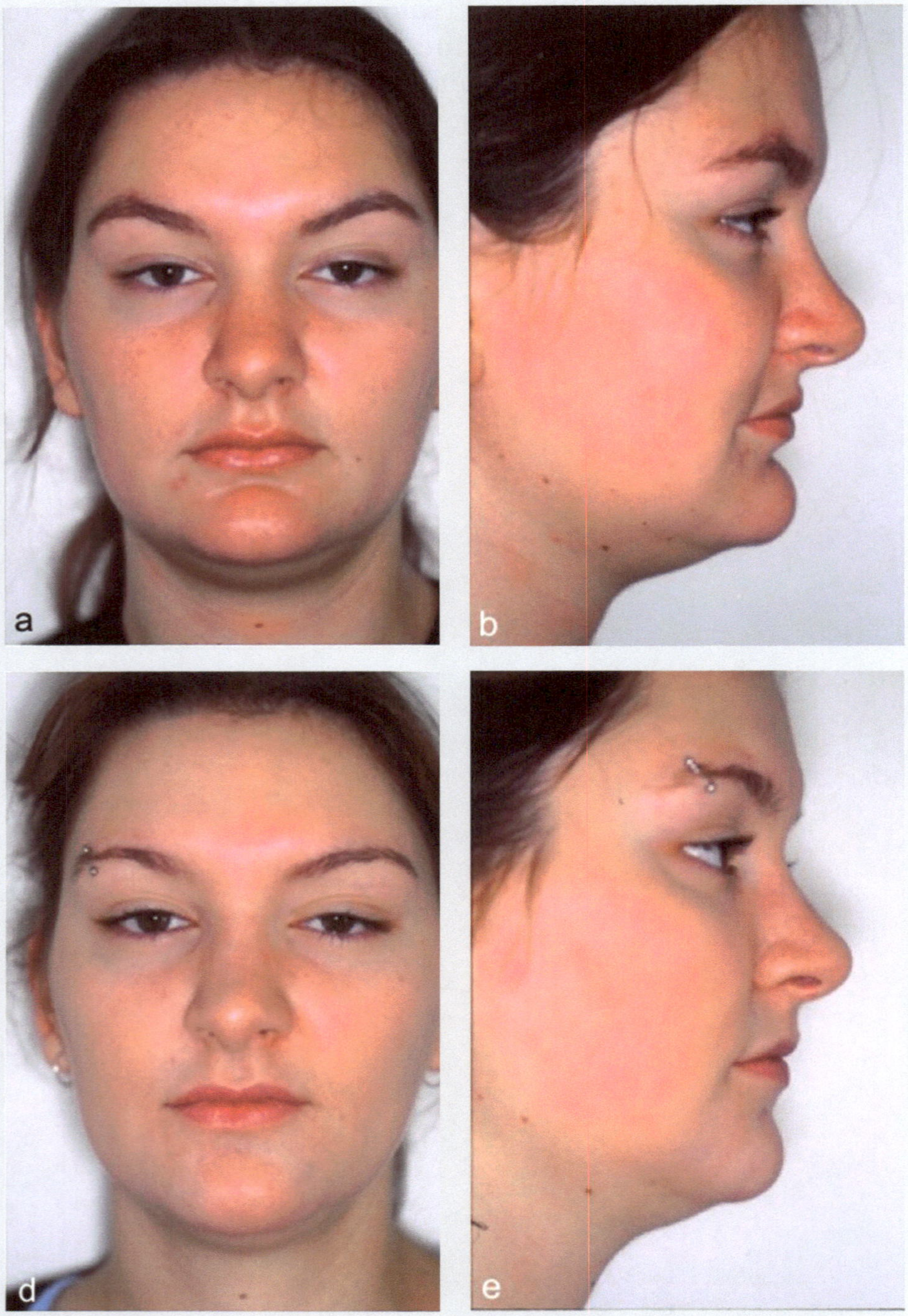

Figure 5.11 - CASE 11. *The anteroposterior excess of the chin is combined with slight vertical deficiency in the frontal (a) and profile view (b). The osteotomy is angled to allow the chin to slide backward and downward. The post treatment results in the frontal (d) and profile view (e).*

Diagnosis:

1. Dental: Class I occlusion.
2. Skeletal:
   - Macrogenia.
   - A tendency to a reduced anterior mandibular height.
3. Soft tissue:
   - Prominent chin.
   - Deep labiomental fold.

Treatment:

1. Reduction genioplasty. The osteotomy was angled to increase the height of the chin as it is moved posteriorly.

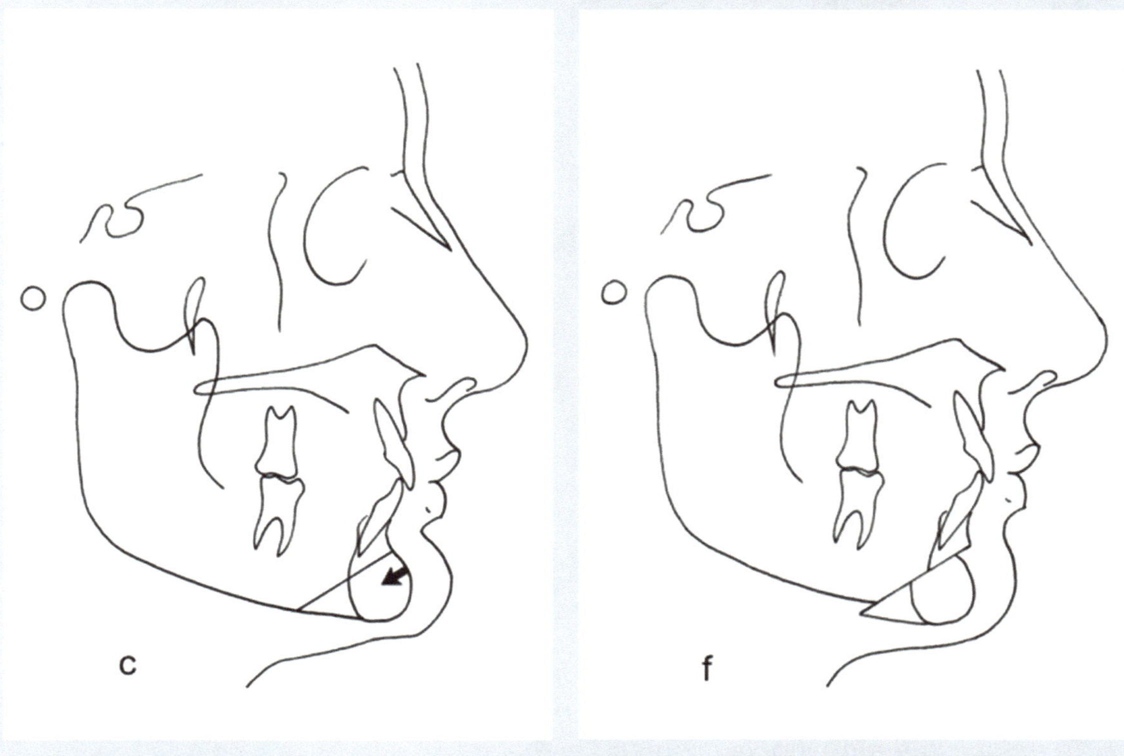

Figure 5.11 - CASE 11. *The anteroposterior excess of the chin is combined with slight vertical deficiency. The osteotomy is angled to allow the chin to slide backward and downward (c). The post treatment results (f).*

Rotation of Maxillomandibular Complex Combined with Reduction Genioplasty

Case 12: A patient with a severe Class II deep bite malocclusion.

Main complaint:
His very prominent chin

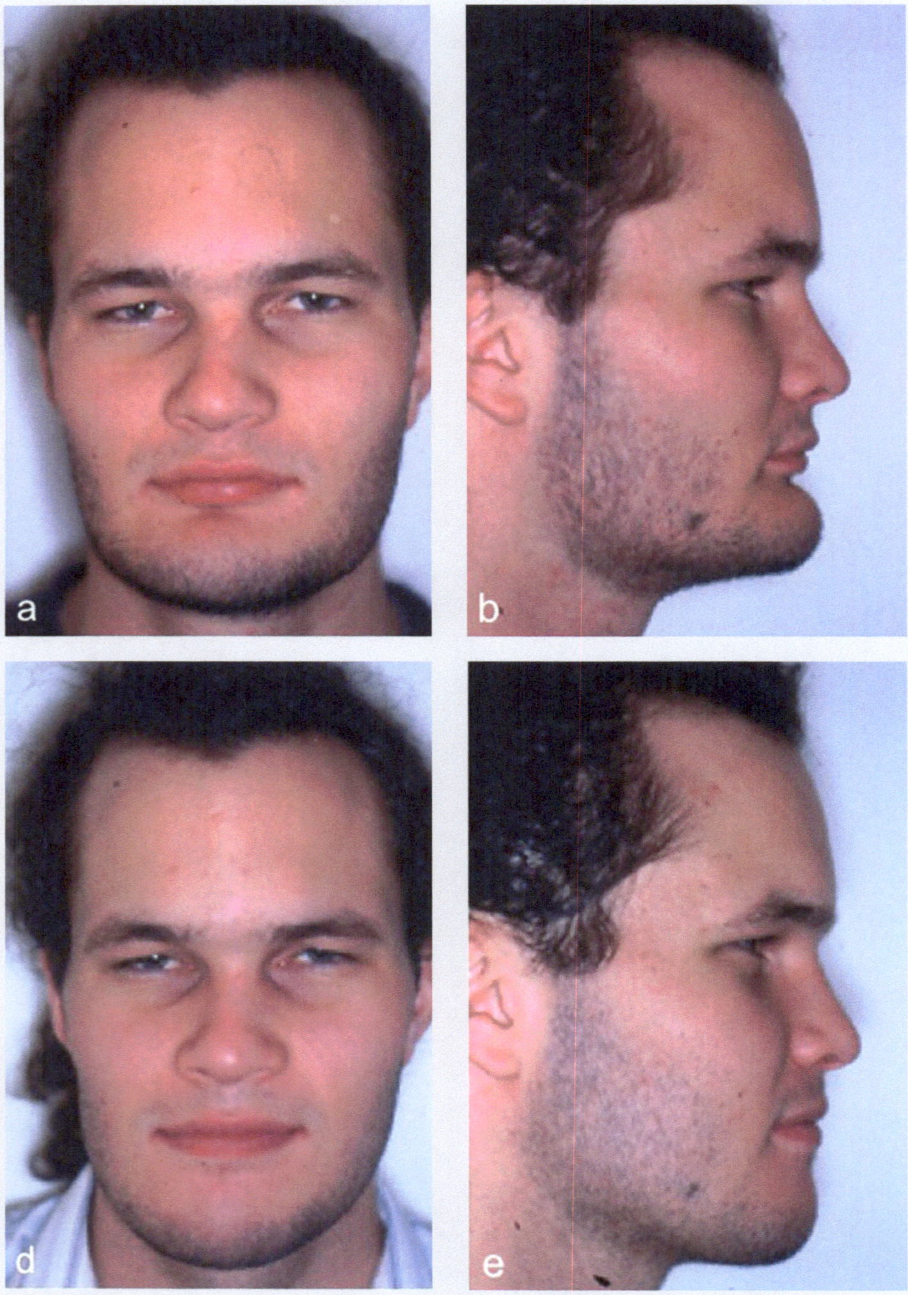

Figure 5. 12 - CASE 12. *24-year old patient with a severe low angle Class II deep bite malocclusion. Pre-surgical frontal (a) and profile view (b). To establish the best occlusion and esthetic result the maxillomandibular complex was rotated clockwise and the chin reduced by a posterior sliding genioplasty. The post-surgical frontal (d) and profile view (e).*

Diagnosis:

1. Dental: Malocclusion.
2. Skeletal:
   - Low mandibular plane angle.
   - Low occlusal plane.
3. Soft tissue:
   - Prominent chin.
   - Deep labiomental fold.

Treatment:

1. Clockwise rotation of his maxillomandibular complex.
2. Reduction genioplasty.

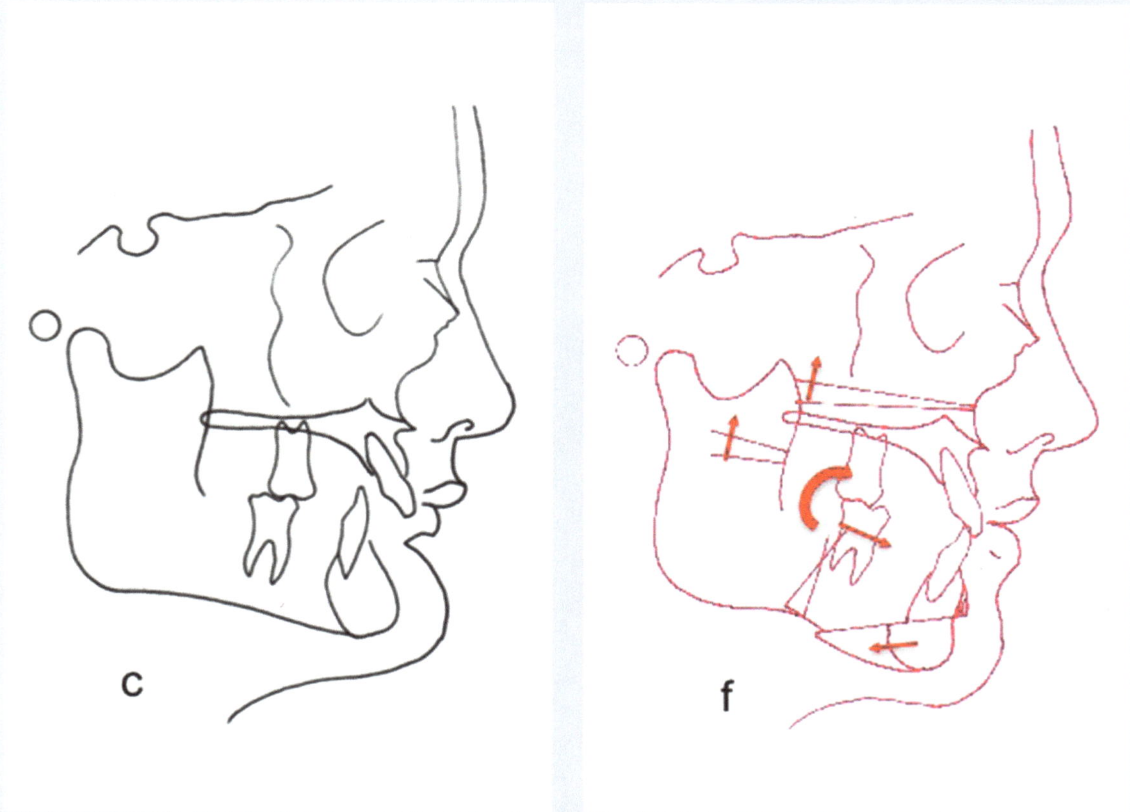

Figure 5. 12 - CASE 12. *Patient with a severe low angle Class II deep bite malocclusion. Pre-surgical cephalometric tracing (c). To establish the best occlusion and esthetic result the maxillomandibular complex was rotated clockwise and the chin reduced by a posterior sliding genioplasty. The post-surgical visual treatment objective (f).*

Posterior Sliding Genioplasty

Case 9: A 28-year-old patient presented with a main complaint of a prominent chin. She had a Class I occlusion.

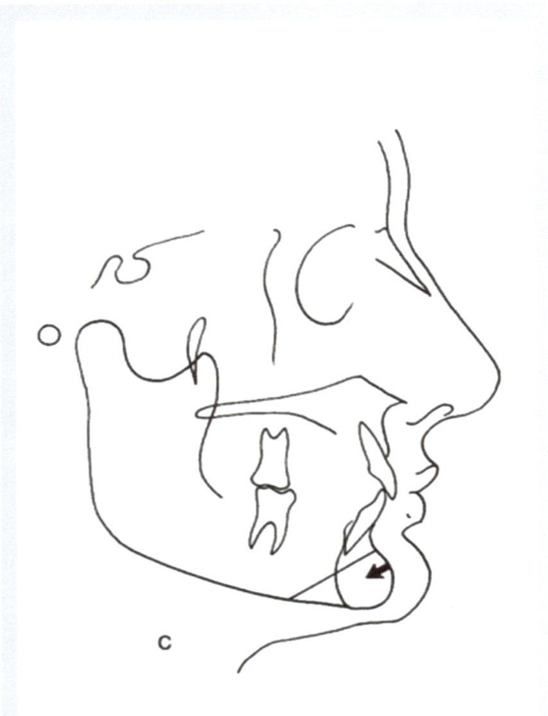

Main complaint:
Prominent chin.

Diagnosis:
1. Dental: Class I occlusion.
2. Skeletal:
   - Mandibular anteroposterior deficiency.
   - Macrogenia.
   - Narrow chin.
3. Soft tissue:
   - Prominent, knobby chin.
   - Deep labiomental fold.

Treatment:
1. Posterior sliding genioplasty, taking care not to excessively reduce the labiomental fold.

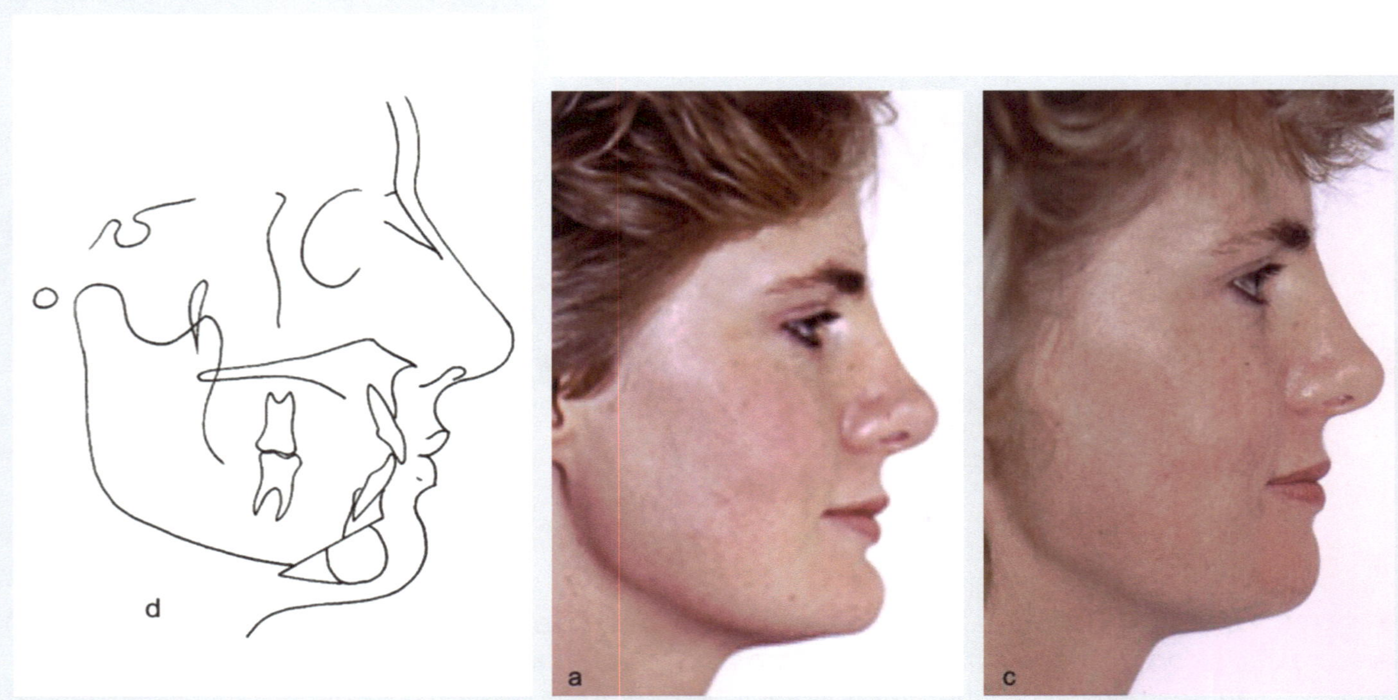

Figure 5.9 - CASE 9. *The esthetic changes to the chin is well demonstrated following a posterior sliding genioplasty. Note the importance of maintaining a pleasing labio-mental contour (arrow).*

Vertical Chin Excess

Vertical reduction genioplasty is indicated when the lower facial height is increased due to vertical excess of the anterior mandible.[14] When the lower facial height is increased, the clinician should differentiate between vertical maxillary excess and vertical mandibular excess. In cases where the maxilla is vertically excessive, the interlabial gap is increased, incisor tooth exposure is increased, and patients often have a gummy smile. When the height of the chin is excessive, the lower third of the lower facial third exceeds the normal ratio of 1:2 = Sn-Stm^{i}:Stm^{i}-Me, while the lower half of the lower facial third is excessive (Sn-Li < Li-Me).

Typical Clinical Characteristics of Vertical Chin Excess

Frontal view:

- Increased lower facial third (G'-Sn<Sn-Me').
- Increased lower half of the lower facial height (Sn-Li<Li-Me).
- Increased lower third of the lower facial third (Sn-Stm^{i}<Stm^{i}-Me').
- Flat labiomental fold.

Profile view:

- Flattened labiomental fold.
- Chin often anteroposteriorly excessive.
- Increased lower facial height with ratios discussed in the frontal view.

Treatment

The height of the chin is reduced by ostectomy of the anterior mandible, which is also called vertical reduction genioplasty.[14]

Esthetic Objectives

Careful preoperative clinical and cephalometric assessment is essential to plan the correct amount of vertical reduction. Here again, apart from the vertical deformity, the anteroposterior and transverse dimension should be considered.

- **Chin Shape.** By changing the shape of the bone to be removed from the anterior mandible, the shape of the chin may be influenced. *(See Chapter 4, Surgical Techniques.)*
- **Control the depth and height of the labiomental fold.** Establishing an esthetic labiomental fold should be one of the primary goals. It is often necessary to advance the chin after vertical reduction to create an esthetically pleasing labiomental fold. Bear in mind that after vertical skeletal reduction, some soft tissue bunching will take place, pushing the soft tissue of the chin slightly forward.
- **Vertical chin assessment.** Cephalometric parameters for vertical balance in combination with the available knowledge of soft tissue change in relation to skeletal repositioning should be utilized to calculate the ideal magnitude of vertical reduction.
- **Manage the lower border of the mandible.** The continuity of the inferior mandibular borderline should be maintained to ensure a smooth esthetic line of the lower border.

Vertical Chin Reduction Combined with Maxillary Superior Repositioning and Mandibular Setback

Case 13: A 19-year-old male was referred to the orthodontist for correction of a Class III anterior open bite malocclusion.

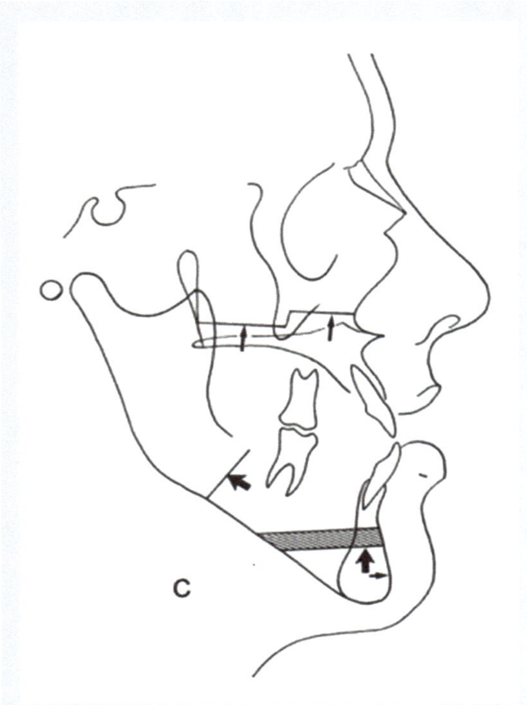

Main complaint:
The inability to bite through food with incisors.

Diagnosis:

1. Dental: Class III anterior open bite.
2. Skeletal:
   - Vertical maxillary excess.
   - Mandibular anteroposterior excess.
   - Vertical excess of the chin.
3. Soft tissue:
   - Increased height of the lower facial third.
   - Increased height of the anterior mandible.
   - Increased interlabial gap.
   - Flattened labiomental fold.
   - The chin appears large and ill defined.
   - Shortened chin–neck length.

Treatment:

1. Orthodontic alignment of both dental arches.
2. Le Fort I maxillary osteotomy superior repositioning of the maxilla.
3. Bilateral sagittal split ramus osteotomy, setting the mandible back.
4. Vertical reduction genioplasty combined by slight advancement, maintaining the chin–neck length and enhancing the labiomental fold.

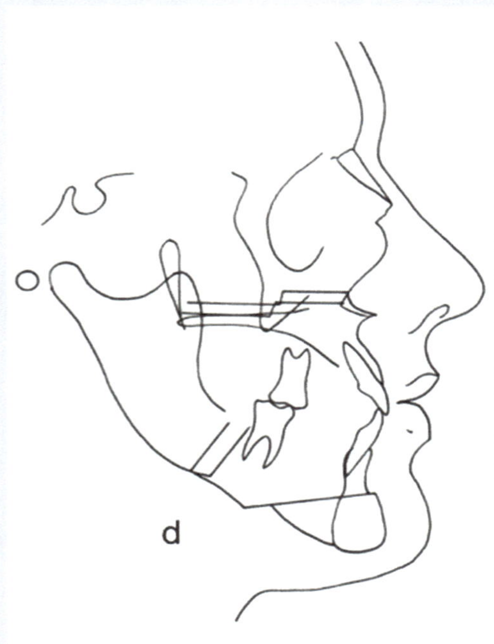

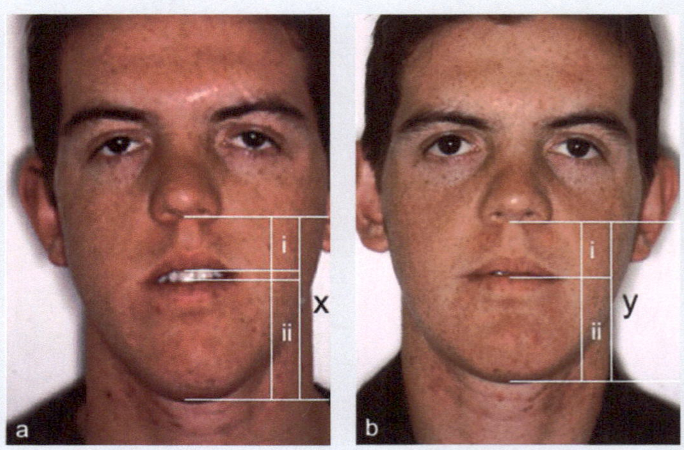

Figure 5.13 - CASE 13. *Patient with a Class III anterior open bite malocclusion, severely increased height of lower facial third, due to posterior vertical maxillary and anterior vertical mandibular excess, frontal view (a). The post treatment results (b) and (d). Note the reduction in the height of the lower facial third due to superior repositioning of the maxilla and vertical reduction of the chin (X & Y). The chin contour is maintained by slight advancement of the chin.*

Vertical Chin Reduction with Maxillary Advancement, Mandibular Setback & Dental Alignment

Case 14: This 18-year-old female was referred by her dentist for the orthognathic correction of her severe Class III malocclusion.
Main complaint: The patient was unable to chew her food properly, however, her facial appearance was the main source of her unhappiness.

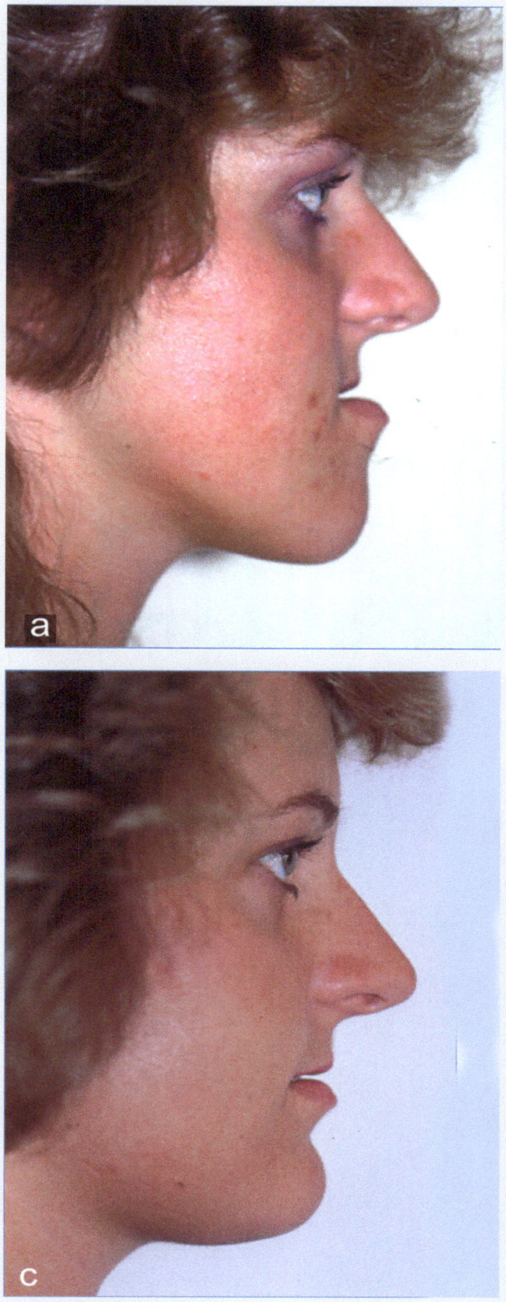

Diagnosis:

1. Dental: Class III occlusion.
2. Skeletal:
   - Maxillary anteroposterior & vertical deficiency.
   - Mandibular anteroposterior excess & asymmetry.
   - Vertical excess of the chin.
3. Soft tissue:
   - Vertical excess of the lower facial third.
   - Flattened paranasal areas.
   - Obtuse labiomental angle.
   - Acute lip–chin–submental angle.
   - Excessive chin–neck length.
   - Poor lip competence.

Treatment:

1. Preoperative orthodontic alignment of the dental arches.
2. Maxillary advancement and downgraft.
3. Mandibular setback.
4. Vertical reduction of the chin with slight advancement to enhance the labiomental fold.

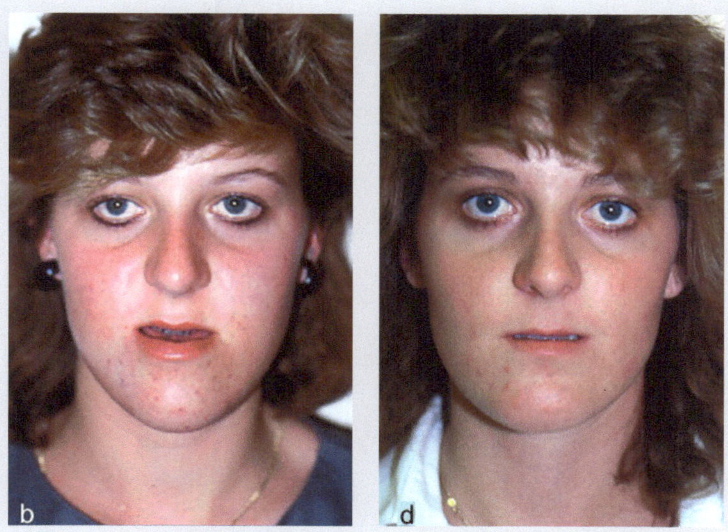

Figure 5.14 - CASE 14. *The diagnosis of maxillary anteroposterior and vertical deficiency, mandibular anteroposterior excess and vertical excess of her chin was made and is illustrated in (a) and (b). The treatment results (c) and (d). Note the reduction in chin height.*

Vertical Chin Deficiency

Vertical deficiency of the anterior mandible will lead to a decrease in the lower facial height relative to the midface height.[16,17] However, vertical chin deficiency should be differentiated from vertical maxillary deficiency and deep bite cases. All three of these dentofacial deformities will clinically and cephalometrically manifest as a diminutive or "squashed" lower facial third, which is vertically shorter than the middle third (N-Sn > Sn-Me).To aid in the specific diagnosis, additional evaluation of the lower third of the face is essential. The anterior dental height of the mandible, from lower incisor tip to menton, should be 42±2 mm. The soft tissue relation of subnasale to upper lip stomion and stomion to menton is a 1:2 ratio ($Sn\text{-}Stm^i : Stm^s\text{-}Me = 1:2$), whereas the distance between Sn and Me is halved by the lower lip vermillion border (Sn-Li : Li-Me = 1:1).

Typical Clinical Characteristics of Vertical Chin Deficiency

Frontal view:
- Decreased lower facial third.
- Decreased lower half of the lower facial third.
- Short, broad lower face.
- Deep labiomental fold.

Profile view:
- The chin appears short and "knobby."
- Deep labiomental fold.
- The chin often appears round and prominent.
- The vertical proportions are the same as observed from the frontal view.
- The lower border of the mandible often has a bowing, rounded curve.

Treatment

Vertical increase of the chin by downgrafting the chin segment. In selected cases, the height of the anterior mandible can be increased when concomitant anteroposterior excess exists.

Esthetic Objectives

Accurate preoperative planning using the surgical cephalometric treatment objective to ascertain the correct amount of vertical increase is essential:

- **Planning by cephalometric visual treatment objective.** Vertical and anteroposterior parameters, as discussed in the cephalometric analysis section, serves as a guide for three-dimensional correction.
- **Manage the lower border.** Care should be taken to maintain the smooth, continuous, and well-defined border of the mandible.
- **Manage the lower border cant.** In cases where the height is increased by downgrafting the chin segment, care should be taken to maintain a symmetric cant of the lower border.
- **Pay attention to any anteroposterior changes.** By changing the shape of the bone graft, the three-dimensional structure of the chin may be altered. *(See Chapter 4, Surgical Technique.)*

Vertical and Anteroposterior Augmentation of the Chin Combined with Mandibular Advancement

CASE 15: This 17-year-old female patient was referred to the surgeon by her orthodontist for surgical correction of her deficient mandible and Class II malocclusion.

Main complaint:
Her deep labiomental fold and the "weak" appearance of her chin were her main concerns.

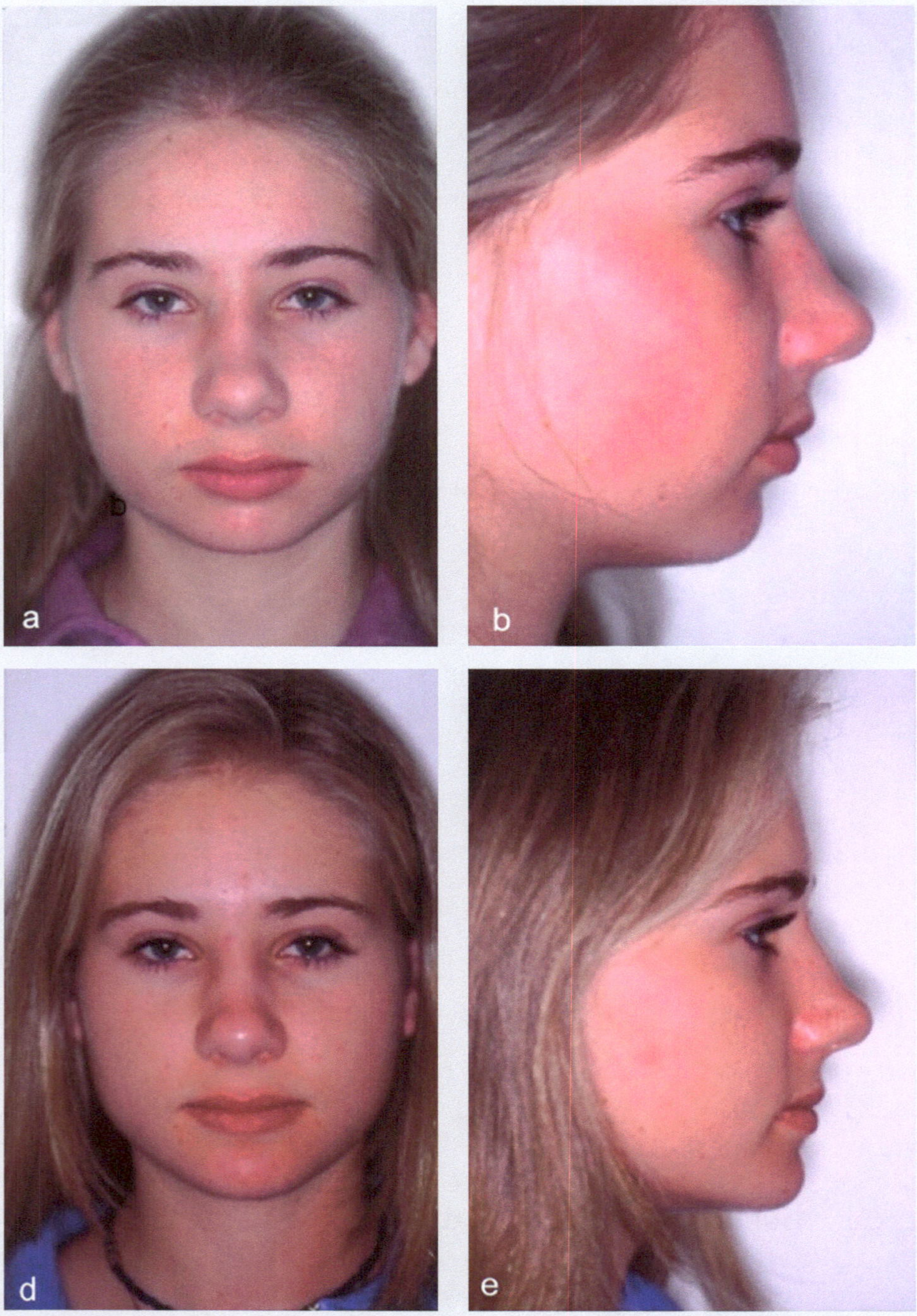

Figure 5.15 - CASE 15. *The patient's mandible is anteroposteriorly deficient and she has a Class II malocclusion. The chin is anteroposteriorly and vertically deficient as seen in frontal (a) and profile view (b). Mandibular advancement combined with a sliding genioplasty advancing the chin and downgrafting the chin segment to increase chin height resulted in (d) and (e).*

Diagnosis:

1. Dental: Class II anterior open bite following orthodontic treatment.
2. Skeletal:
   - Microgenia.
   - Vertical deficiency of the chin.
3. Soft tissue:
   - Convex profile.
   - Decreased height of lower facial third.
   - Deep labiomental fold.
   - Everted lower lip.
   - Increased lip–chin–submental angle.

Treatment:

1. Orthodontic leveling and alignment of the dental arches.
2. Surgical advancement of the mandible and genioplasty, advancing the chin with anterior downgrafting of the segment.

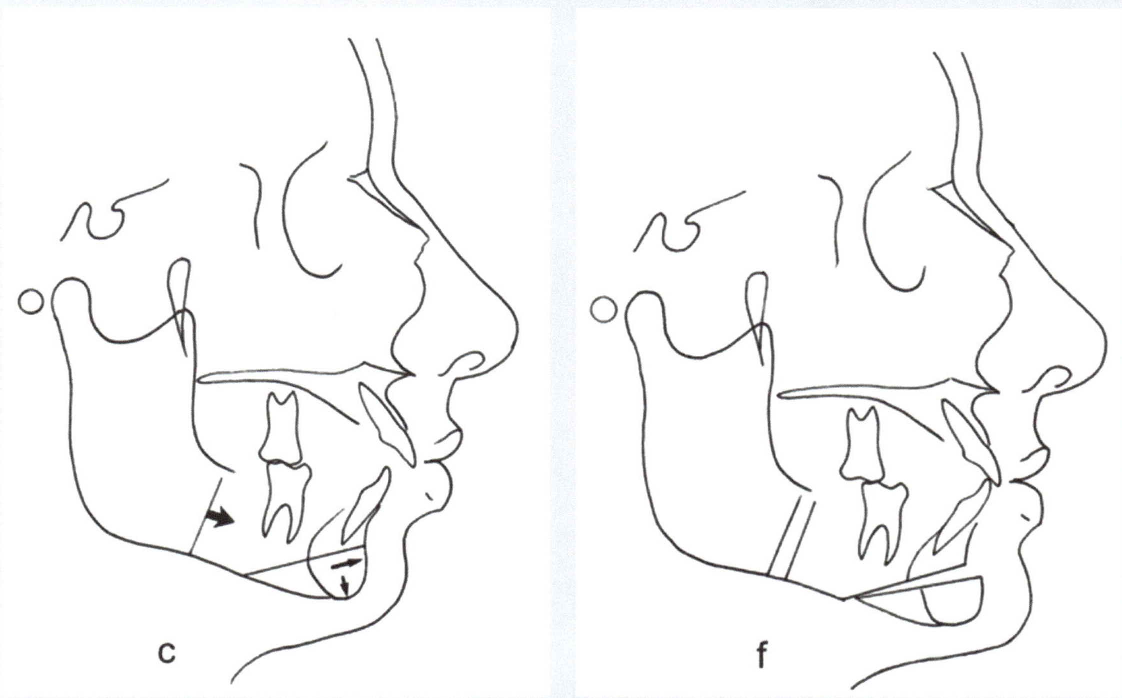

Figure 5.15 - CASE 15. *The patient's mandible is anteroposteriorly deficient and she has a Class II malocclusion. The chin is anteroposteriorly and vertically deficient. The treatment plan: mandibular advancement combined with a sliding genioplasty advancing the chin. The height of the chin is increased by downgrafting the chin segment as shown in the cephalometric tracing (c). The post-surgical visual treatment objective is shown in (f).*

Vertical and Anteroposterior Augmentation of the Chin Combined with Mandibular Advancement

CASE 16: After seeking help from a new dentist, this 36-year-old male was referred to an orthodontist for treatment of his severe Class II deep bite malocclusion.

Main complaint:
The patient's main concern was the fact that he chronically injured his palatal mucosa with his mandibular incisors.

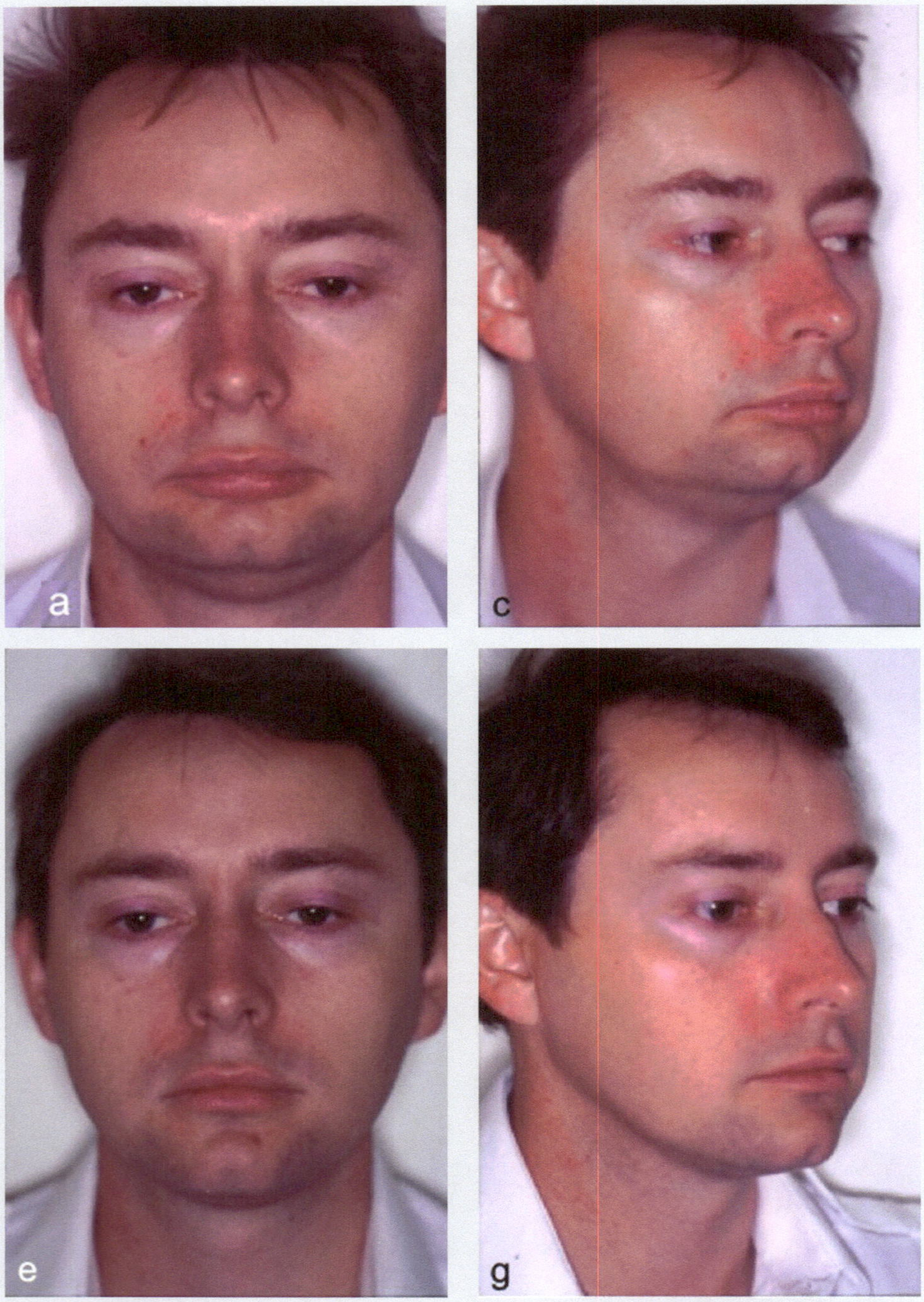

Figure 5.16 - CASE 16. *The preoperative frontal (a) and three-quarter view (c) show Class II deep bite malocclusion, mandibular anteroposterior deficiency, vertically and anteroposteriorly deficient chin. A bilateral sagittal split osteotomy advancing the mandible and a sliding genioplasty advancing and downgrafting the chin at the same time. Post treatment results (e) & (g).*

Diagnosis:

1. Dental: Class II deep bite occlusion.
2. Skeletal:
   - Mandibular anteroposterior deficiency.
   - Reduced height of the anterior mandible.
3. Soft tissue:
   - Convex profile.
   - Reduced lower facial height.
   - Deep labiomental fold.
   - Everted lower lip.
   - Short chin-neck length.

Treatment:

1. Orthodontic alignment of the dental arches. No attempt was made to open the deep bite or level the curve of Spee preoperatively. This would enhance the height of the mandible as it is advanced.
2. Bilateral sagittal split ramus osteotomy advancing the mandible.
3. Genioplasty advancement and downgrafting of the chin. (Note the shape of the graft in Figure 5.16h.)

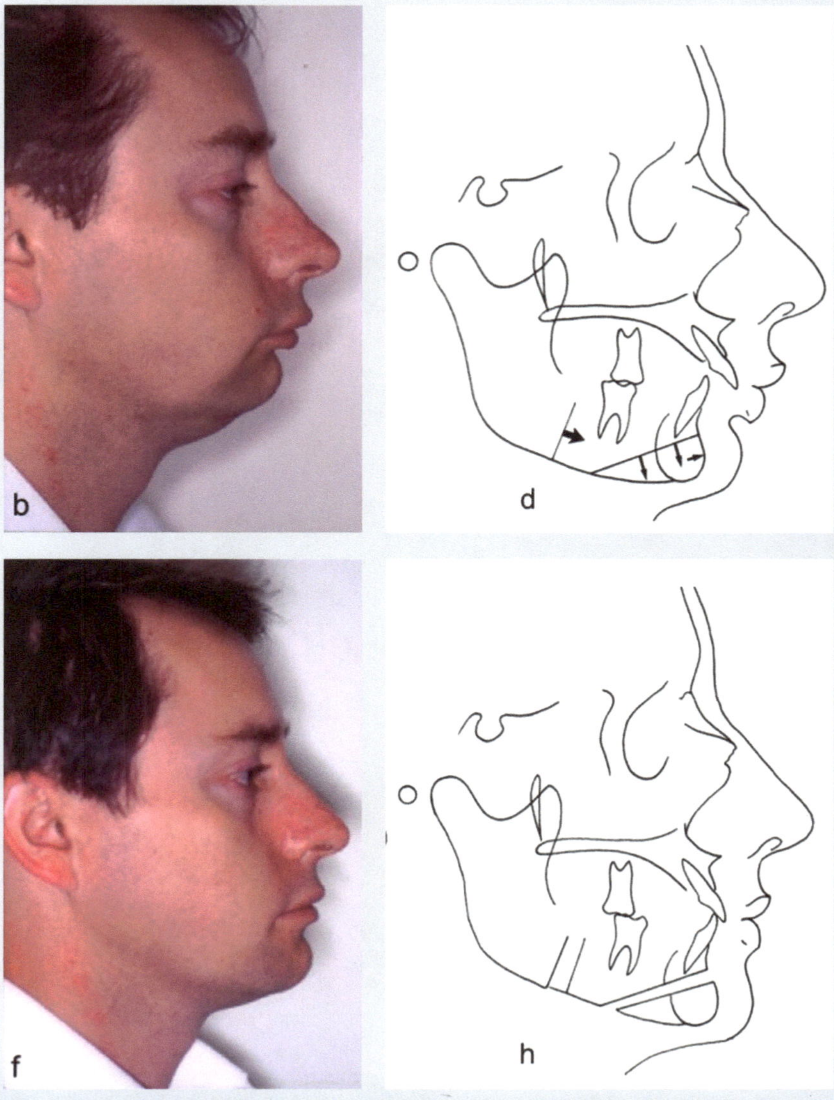

Figure 5.16 - CASE 16. *The preoperative profile view (b) shows a Class II deep bite malocclusion, mandibular anteroposterior deficiency, vertically and anteroposteriorly deficient chin. This is also illustrated by the cephalometric tracing (d). The surgical treatment plan: a bilateral sagittal split osteotomy advancing the mandible and a sliding genioplasty advancing the chin. The chin is downgrafted at the same time. Note the shape of the graft: the anterior and posterior part of the chin segment is downgrafted the same amount. The post-surgical visual treatment objective is shown in (h) and further illustrated by the patient profile photo (f).*

Vertical Augmentation and Anteroposterior Reduction Combined with Mandibular Advancement

CASE 17: The orthodontist referred this 37-year-old female patient for surgical correction of a Class II deep bite malocclusion.

Main complaint:
The patient's main complaints were her "knobby" chin and deep labiomental fold.

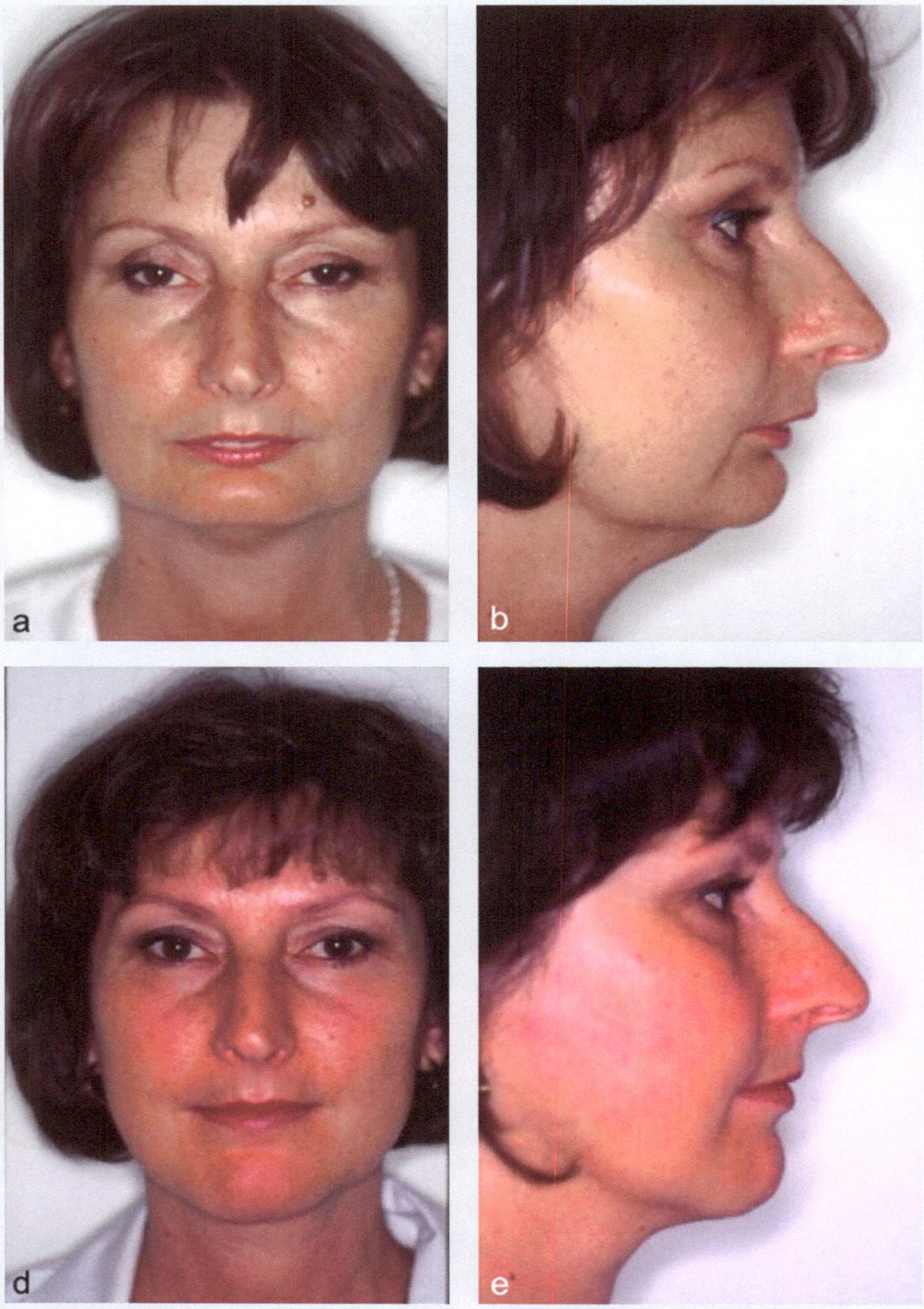

Figure 5.17 - CASE 17. *The preoperative frontal (a) and profile view (b). The mandible is anteroposteriorly deficient and a Class II deep bite mal-occlusion is present. The chin is anteroposteriorly excessive, but vertically deficient. The nose appears relatively large. Mandibular advancement, reduction genioplasty and vertical augmentation of the chin results in (d) and (e).*

Diagnosis:

1. Dental: Class II deep bite.
2. Skeletal:
   - Mandibular anteroposterior deficiency.
   - Anteroposterior chin excess.
   - Vertical deficiency of the chin.
3. Soft tissue:
   - A knobby short chin.
   - Deep labiomental fold.
   - Double chin.
   - Increased submental–neck angle.
   - Decreased lower facial height.
   - Relatively prominent nose.

Treatment:

1. Orthodontic alignment of the dental arches.
2. Bilateral sagittal split ramus osteotomy advancing the mandible.
3. Genioplasty:
   - Downgrafting the chin segment.
   - Contouring the bone superior to the chin segment as well as the posterior edges of the segment.

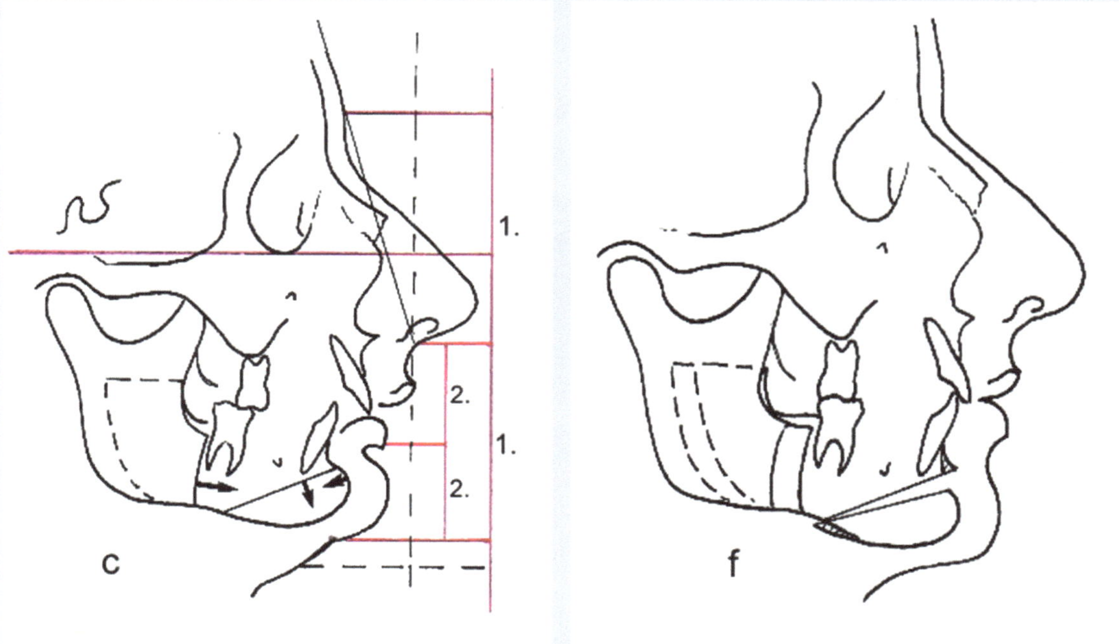

Figure 5.17 - CASE 17. *The preoperative cephalometric tracing illustrates the mandible is anteroposteriorly deficient and a Class II deep bite mal-occlusion is present (c). The chin is anteroposteriorly excessive, but vertically deficient. The nose appears relatively large. The treatment plan: mandibular advancement, reduction genioplasty and vertical augmentation of the chin, resulted in the post-surgical visual treatment objective tracing (f).*

Transverse Chin Deformities

There are relatively few guidelines to aid the clinician in evaluating the width of the chin. The transverse dimension of the chin should be related to the patient's bizygomatic and bigonial widths. The general shape of the head (brachidephalic or dolicocephalic) and face (euryprosopic or leptoprosopic) should be taken into account. The face may be described as round, oval, square, narrow, tapering or a combination of the above shapes, and the chin outline should be in harmony with the facial shape. The outline of each third should be in balance and it may be necessary to transversely reduce a square chin to establish harmony with an oval-shaped face, for example. Equally important is to establish a smooth, continuous line in the lower mandibular border connecting the chin to the rest of the face.

Typical Clinical Characteristics of Transverse Chin Deficiency

Frontal view:

- The lower face is tapered toward the narrow chin.
- The chin appears "pointy."
- Poor relationship between the anterior and posterior facial width.
- Often vertically and anteroposteriorly deficient.

Profile view:

- The chin is often vertically deficient as well as anteroposteriorly deficient.
- The lower border of the mandible does not follow a smooth line.

Treatment

The chin segment can be widened in the anterior area by grafting between the chin segments, the posterior area by rotating the posterior aspects of the segmemnts, or both areas by combining the above.

Transverse Deficiency

The chin may be widened in the posterior area by sectioning the chin segment in the midline, after placement of a rigid fixation boneplate on the outer surface of the chin, and rotating the posterior ends outward. The chin is often widened in combination with correction of anteroposterior chin deficiency or excess. When the chin is advanced, especially where the horizontal osteotomy is extended posteriorly to the molar region, the posterior ends of the segment will provide lateral augmentation. *(See Chapter 4, Surgical Technique.)* In cases where the soft tissue chin is pointy and narrow with parasymphyseal indentations, the chin should be widened in addition to the advance.

Advancing a narrow, pointed chin without lateral augmentation (widening) of the posterior area may cause "marionette grooves." Although the profiles of these individuals may be improved, from the front, the result will be an accentuation of the pointed chin, which is cosmetically disappointing.

Widening the posterior aspect of the chin segment may be indicated after anteroposterior reduction. Posterior widening of the segment will prevent the creation of an irregular step on the inferior border of the mandible after posterior repositioning of the chin.

Certain individuals require a transverse increase in the anterior part of the chin giving it a square appearance. Enhancing the anterior width of the chin is often indicated in male patients and can be achieved by sectioning the mobilized segment in the middle and placing a bone graft between the segments. The size of the graft can be varied according to the esthetic requirements. *(See Chapter 4, Surgical Techniques.)*

Widening the Chin in Combination with Maxillary Superior Repositioning and Mandibular Advancement

CASE 18: The dentist referred this 32-year old female patient to an orthodontist for treatment of her severe bimaxillary protrusion.

Main complaint:
The prominence of her teeth and inability to keep her lips together when relaxed.

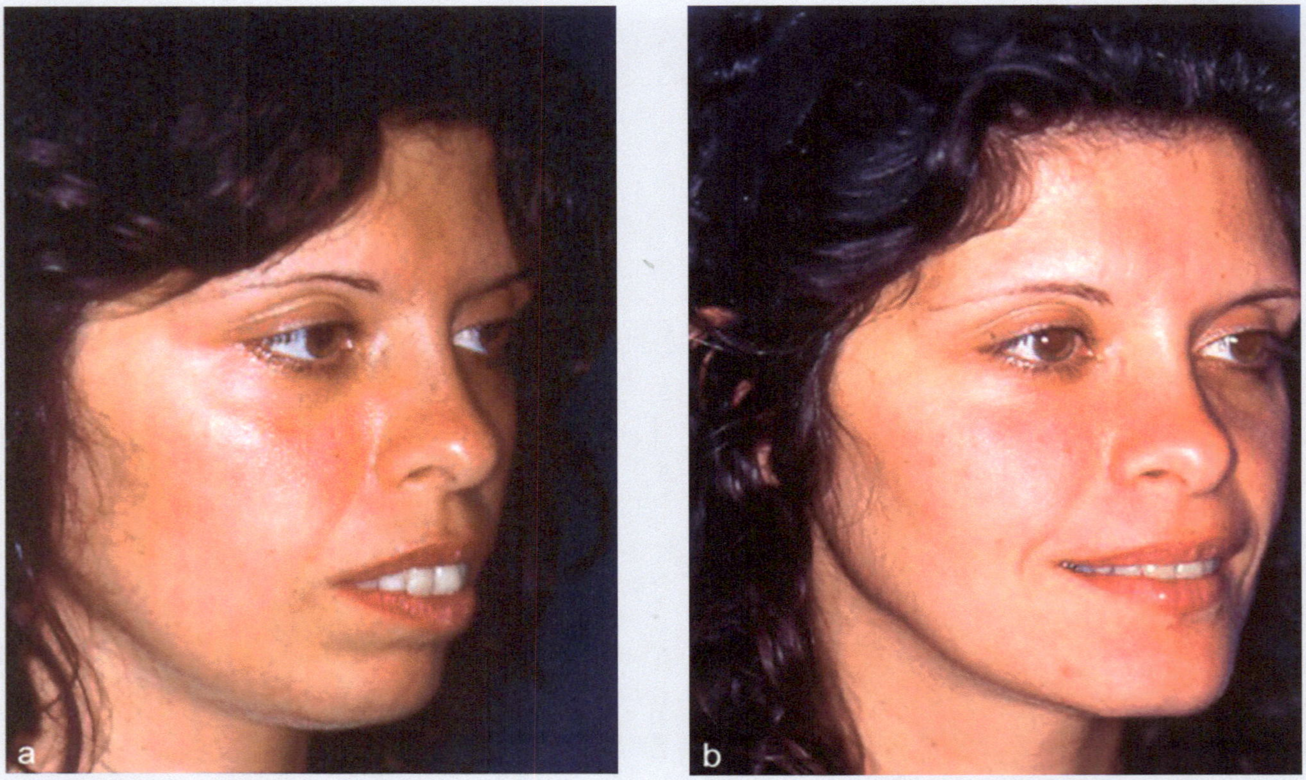

Figure 5.18 - CASE 18. *The preoperative three-quarter view (a) of a patient with microgenia and transverse deficiency of her chin. She also has bimaxillary protrusion, vertical maxillary excess and mandibular anteroposterior deficiency. The treatment plan consisted of: an advancement genioplasty and at the same time widening of the chin. Her occlusion was corrected by means of a le Fort I maxillary osteotomy and a bilateral sagittal split mandibular osteotomy. The improved chin contour is illustrated in (b).*

Diagnosis:

1. Dental: Class II occlusion with severe bimaxillary protrusion.
2. Skeletal:
   - Vertical maxillary excess.
   - Mandibular anteroposterior deficiency.
   - Microgenia.
   - Maxillary transverse deficiency.
3. Soft tissue:
   - Convex profile.
   - Prominent and incompetent lips.
   - Increased interlabial gap.
   - Hyperactive mentalis muscle.
   - Everted lower lip.
   - An acute labiomental fold.
   - Increased lip-chin-submental angle.
   - Narrow chin.

Treatment:

1. Orthodontic alignment of both dental arches in preparation for orthognathic surgery.
2. 3-piece le Fort I maxillary osteotomy:
   - Superiorly repositioning the maxilla.
   - Expanding the posterior segments of the maxilla.
   - Slight setback of the anterior maxillary segment.
3. Bilateral sagittal split ramus osteotomy advancing the mandible.
4. Genioplasty:
   - Advancing the chin.
   - Widening the chin by means of a midline osteotomy.

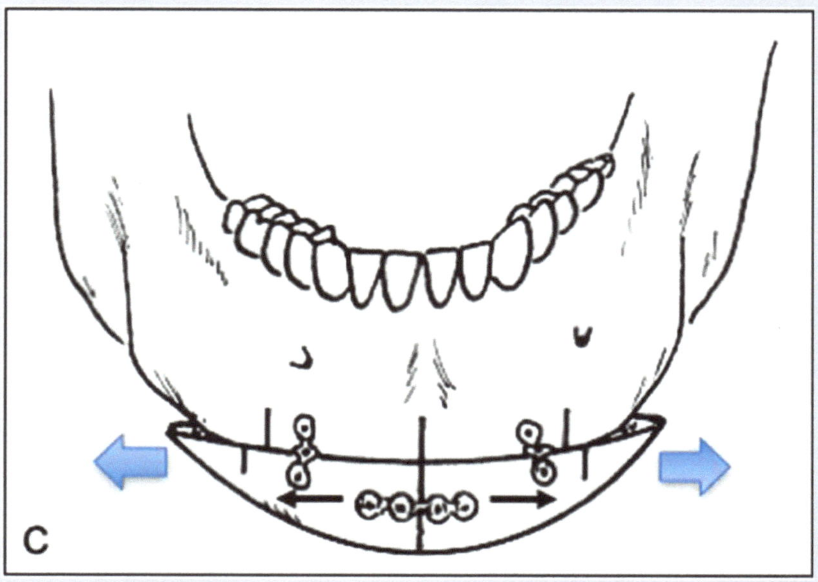

Figure 5.18 - CASE 18. *The treatment plan consisted of: an advancement genioplasty and at the same time widening of the chin as illustrated above. Her occlusion was corrected by means of a le Fort I maxillary osteotomy and a bilateral sagittal split mandibular osteotomy.*

Vertical Reduction & Widening of Chin with Maxillary Advancement & Mandibular Setback

Case 19: The severe vertical increase of the lower facial third is due to vertical chin excess. The patient also suffered of a Class III anterior open bite malocclusion that was treated by a le Fort I maxillary osteotomy and a bilateral sagittal split mandibular osteotomy.
The chin deformity was managed by vertical reduction and widening the chin.
Main complaint: The patient was unhappy with his appearance and found it difficult to bite food with his incisor teeth.

Diagnosis:

1. Dental: Class III anterior open bite malocclusion.
2. Skeletal:
   - Maxillary anteroposterior deficiency
   - Mandibular anteroposterior excess and asymmetry.
   - Vertical excess of the chin.
3. Soft tissue:
   - Vertical excess of the lower facial third.
   - Flattened paranasal areas.
   - Obtuse labiomental angle.
   - Acute lip–chin–submental angle.

Treatment:

1. Le Fort I maxillary osteotomy (advance).
2. Bilateral sagittal split mandibular osteotomy (setback).
3. Genioplasty with vertical reduction and widening of the chin

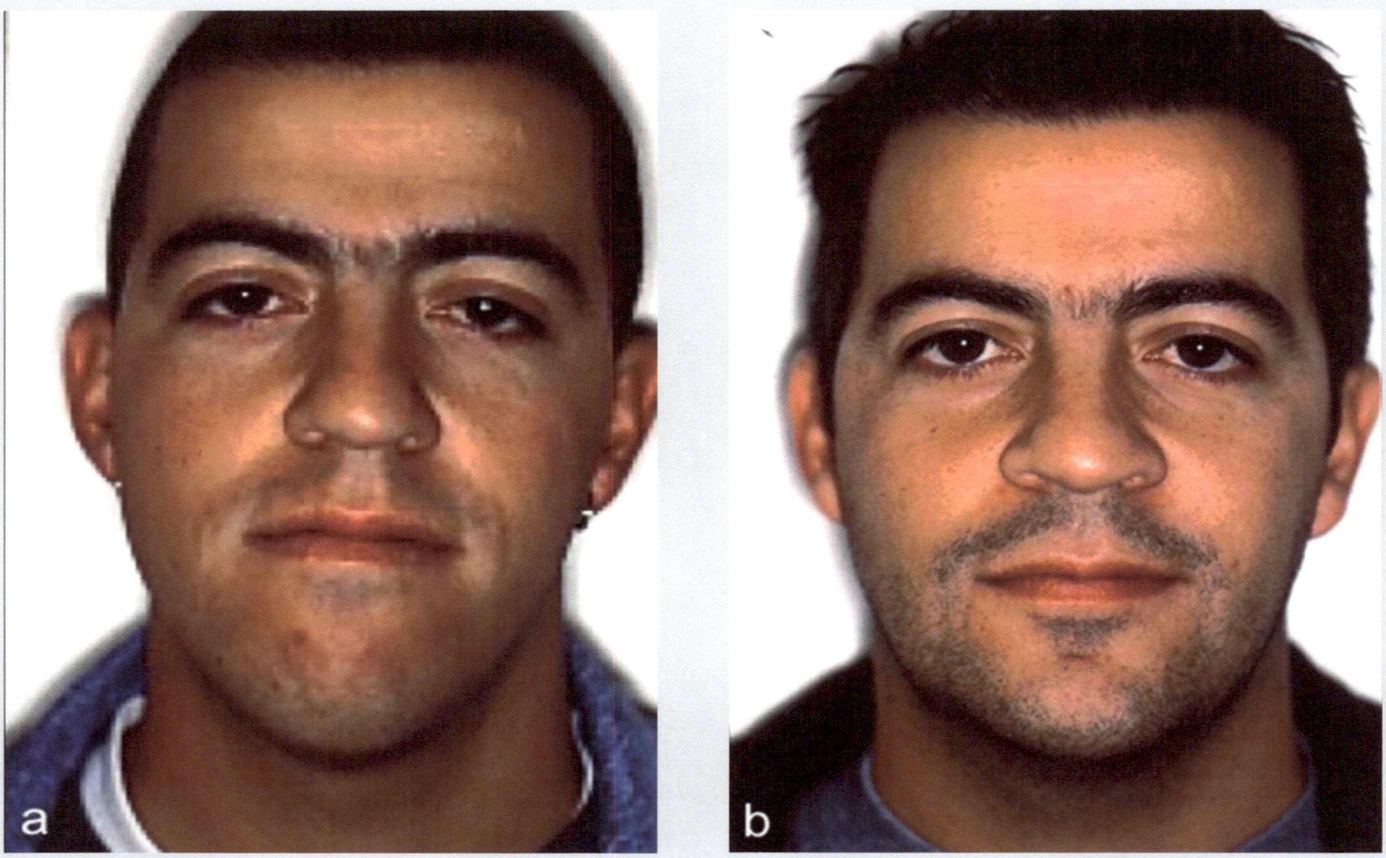

Figure 5.19 - CASE 19. *Vertical reduction and widening of the chin is demonstrated in pre-operative frontal view (a) and post-operative frontal view (b).*

Transverse Excess

The chin may be narrowed or tapered by sectioning the chin segment in the middle and removing a triangular section of bone from the lingual aspect. The boneplate placed on the anterior surface of the segment before mobilization will allow the segments to be "bent" narrower. (See Chapter 4, Surgical Techniques.) Individuals requiring large transverse posterior chin reductions may need additional contouring of the lateral surface of the mandible. When performing this contouring, special attention should be given to protect the mental nerve.

A very square, broad chin may be narrowed by removing a rectangular section of bone in the middle of the chin segment, which will reduce the width of the anterior aspect of the chin. (See Chapter 4, Surgical Techniques.) In severely broad chins the outer surface of the proximal mandible, superior to the chin segment may be contoured. When contouring this part of the mandible the mental nerve should be protected.

Narrowing of the Chin Combined with Mandibular Setback

CASE 20: This 28-year-old female patient was referred to the surgeon for surgical correction of her mandibular prognathism.

Main complaint:
Her strong lower jaw was the patient's main concern.

Diagnosis:
1. Dental: Class III malocclusion.
2. Skeletal:
   - Maxillary anteroposterior deficiency.
   - Mandibular anteroposterior excess.
   - Broad chin.
3. Soft tissue:
   - Short upper lip.
   - Flattened paranasal areas.
   - Prominent, broad lower jaw.
   - Increased chin–neck length.

Treatment:
1. Orthodontic decompensation, leveling and alignment of the dental arches.
2. Rotation of the maxillomandibular complex:
   - Advancement of the maxilla and superior repositioning of the posterior maxilla.
   - Setback and rotation of the mandibular occlusal plane.
   - Genioplasty narrowing the chin by means of a midline osteotomy.

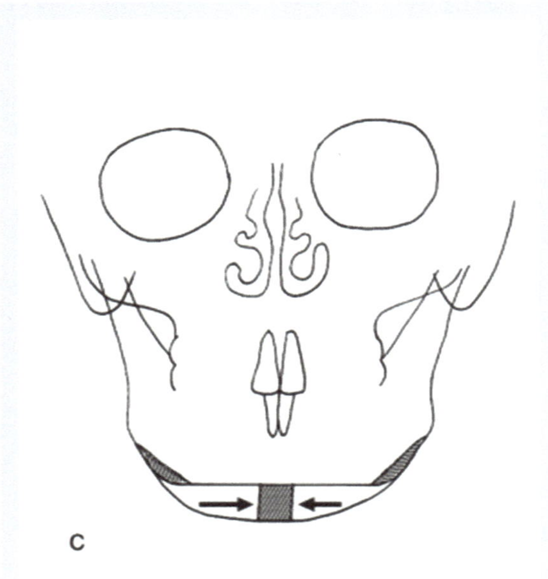

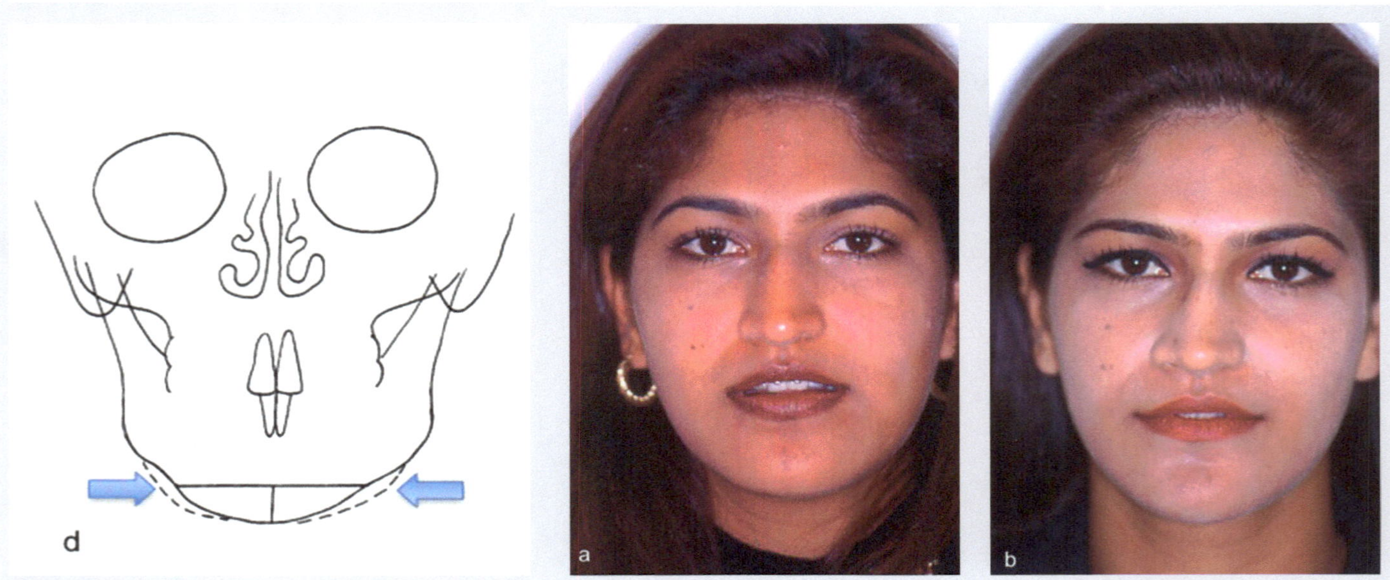

Figure 5.20 - CASE 20. *The broad chin is demonstrated in the frontal view (a). The treatment plan: narrowing the anterior part of the chin by means of a midline ostectomy (c). The post-surgical visual treatment objective is illustrated in (d) and post treatment result is illustrated in frontal view (b).*

Narrowing & Advance of the Chin with Lateral Contouring of Mandibular Body & Augmentation with Implants

CASE 21: Patient's mandibular contour was improved by the placement of bilateral angle implants, combined with a genioplasty advancement and narrowing of his chin

Main complaint:
The patient felt that his lower jaw appeared weak.

Diagnosis:
1. Dental: Class I occlusion.
2. Skeletal:
   - Broad, rounded chin.
3. Soft tissue:
   - Poorly defined mandibular lower border
- Broad lower jaw with poorly defined angles.

Treatment:
1. Genioplasty narrowing the chin by a midline osteotomy.
2. Augmentation of the mandibular angles by subperiosteal implants.

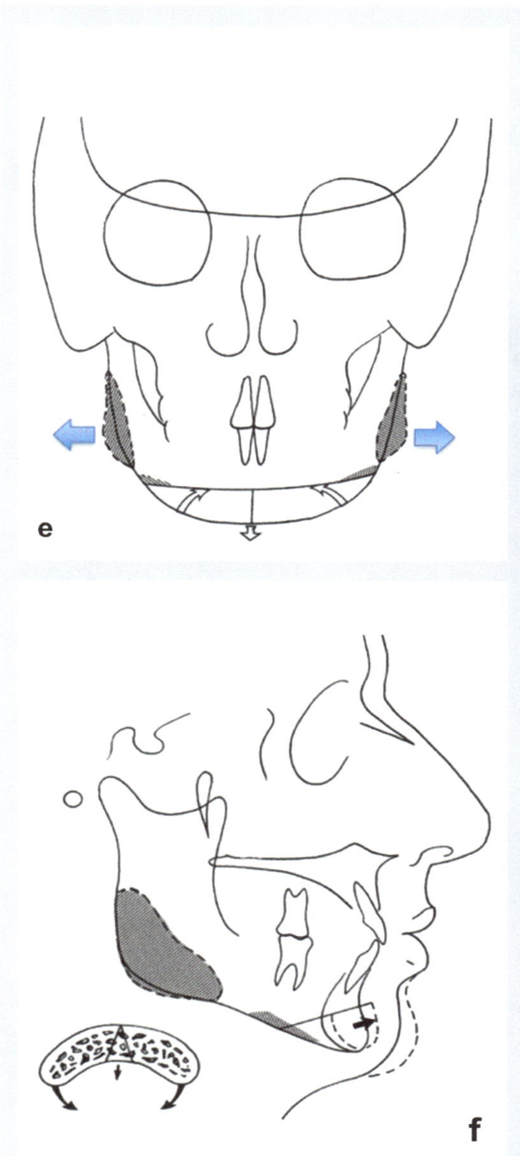

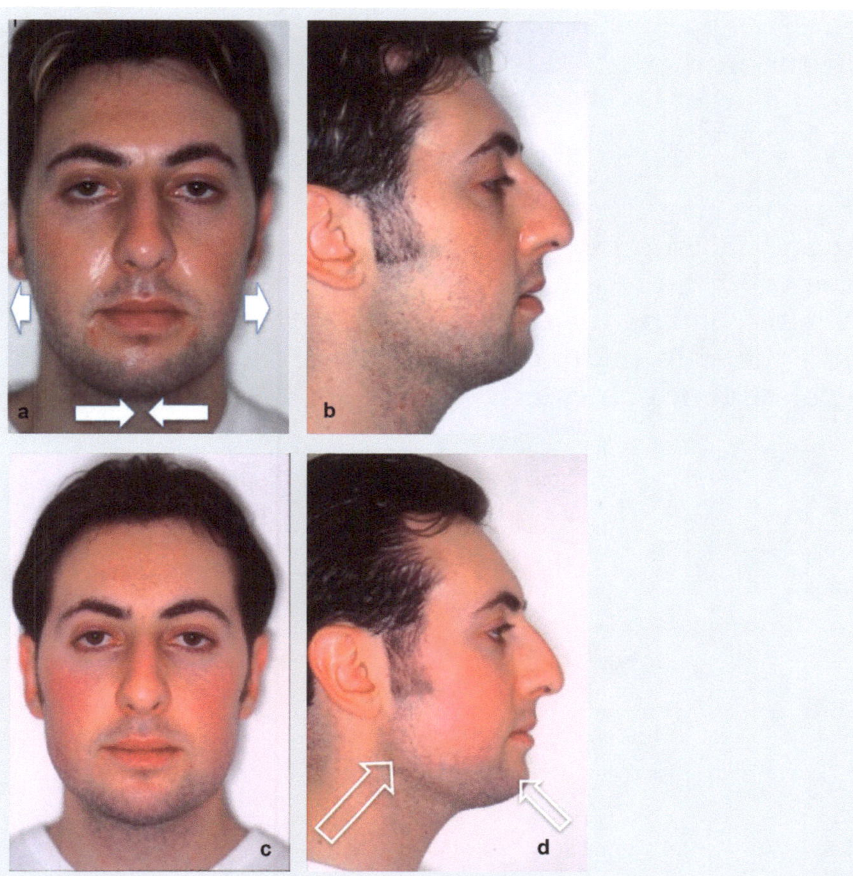

Figure 5.21 - CASE 21. *The broad, rounded chin and poorly defined mandibular angles are evident (a & b). The mandibular angles were emphasized by onlay grafts, while the chin was narrowed by means of a two piece genioplasty. Treatment plan tracing (e & f) Post treatment results (c & d).*

Correction of Chin Asymmetry

Asymmetry of the chin is rarely an isolated entity and is most often part of mandibular asymmetry. Facial asymmetry is the most chanllenging deformity to assess and correct, as the deformity is often three-dimensional.

Surgical correction usually involves:

- Correction to match skeletal, soft tissue and dental midlines to the facial midline.
- Leveling of the occlusal planes.
- Leveling of mandibular inferior borders. Leveling chin cants.
- Ensuring parasymphyseal symmetry.
- Establishing anteroposterior balance by augmentation and/or reduction.

For the purpose of this text, it is assumed that all other facial structures are symmetric or corrected to be symmetric.

The chin may be asymmetric to the dental and facial midlines. Correction in this case will require a horizontal osteotomy of the chin, sliding the chin to the left or right until the chin midline, dental midline and facial midline coincides.

The cant of the lower border of the chin may differ from the cant of the occlusal or interpupillary plane. Correction of the lower border cant will be influenced by the relative height of the chin and may involve unilateral vertical reduction, augmentation or a combination of the above performed on the left and right sides. *(See Chapter 4, Surgical Techniques.)*

Anteroposterior parasymphyseal asymmetry may be present requiring rotational repositioning of the chin to balance the left and right side fullness of the chin. *(See Chapter 4, Surgical Techniques.)*

It is possible, in fact, it is often the case that chin asymmetry will involve all three dimensions of space, requiring a combination of the above corrective procedures. Only by meticulous and critical clinical examination, lateral cephalometric and P.A. cephalometric radiograph analysis and/or three-dimensional computer scan, can the various aspects of the deformity be appreciated and an accurate treatment plan formulated.

Bilateral Sagittal Split Osteotomy and Sliding Genioplasty and Advancement

CASE 22: This 18-year-old female consulted the surgeon regarding correction of her facial asymmetry. She was referred to the orthodontist for alignment of both dental arches in preparation for the surgical correction of her mandibular asymmetry.

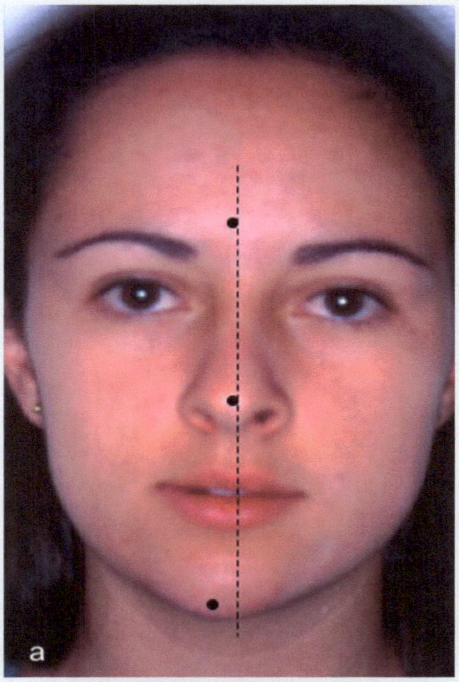

Main complaint: Her facial asymmetry.

Diagnosis:

1. Dental:
   - Class II occlusion right and Class I occlusion left.
   - Maxillary dental midline coincided with GM, while mandibular midline was 3mm to the right.
2. Skeletal:
   - Mandibular asymmetry towards the right.
   - Chin midline is 6mm to the right of the facial GM
   - Microgenia.
3. Soft tissue:
   - Mandibular asymmetry.
   - Anteroposterior chin deficiency.

Treatment:

1. Orthodontic decompensation of incisors and posterior teeth, level and alignment of the dental arches.
2. Bilateral sagittal split ramus osteotomy correcting the mandibular asymmetry and dental midlines.
3. Genioplasty – sliding chin to the left, correcting the chin symmetry and advancing the chin segment.

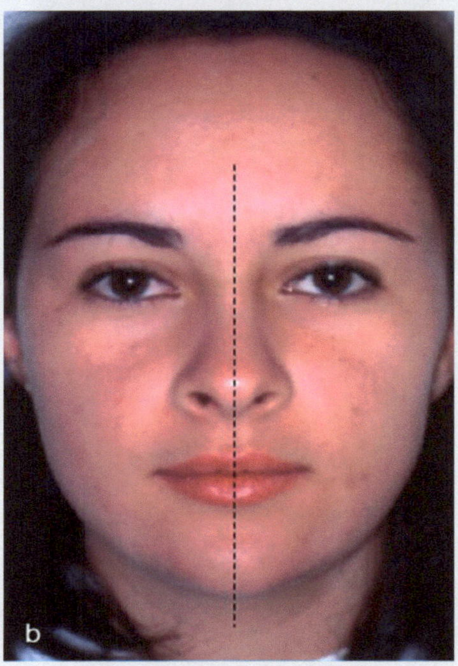

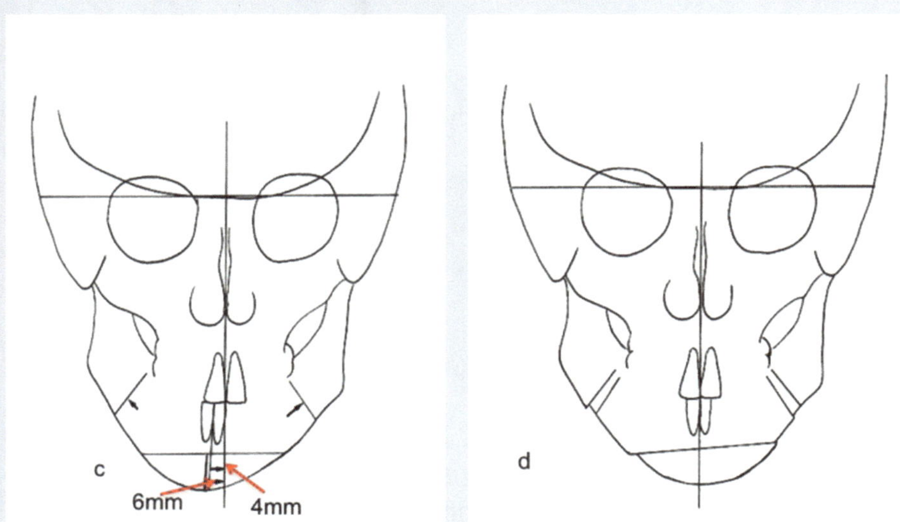

Figure 5.22 - CASE 22. *The mandibular asymmetry is evident in the frontal view (a). The lower dental midline is 4mm, and the midpoint of chin is 6mm to the right of facial midline (c). Surgical repositioning of the mandible to correct the dental midlines and occlusion. The chin is advanced and moved left (c) and (d). The treatment results are illustrated in (b).*

Le Fort I Osteotomy, Bilateral Sagital Split Osteotomy, and Propellor Genioplasty

CASE 23: Severe cants of the lower border of the chin is often present in patients suffering from unilateral condylar hyperplasia.

Main complaint: Her facial asymmetry.

Diagnosis:

1. Dental: Maxillary occlusal cant.
   - Maxillary dental midline to the left.
   - Posterior open bite on the right.
2. Skeletal: Hyperplastic right mandibular condyle.
   - Bowing of the right mandibular body.
   - Cant of the lower border of the chin.
3. Soft tissue: Facial asymmetry to the left.
   - Right facial height increased.

Treatment:

1. Le Fort I osteotomy, correcting the dental midline symmetry and occlusal cant.
2. Bilateral sagittal split mandibular osteotomy correcting the occlusal cant.
3. Ostectomy of the right mandibular body and use the bone as a graft to the leftside lower border.
4. A propellor genioplasty, correcting the asymmetry and lower border cant.

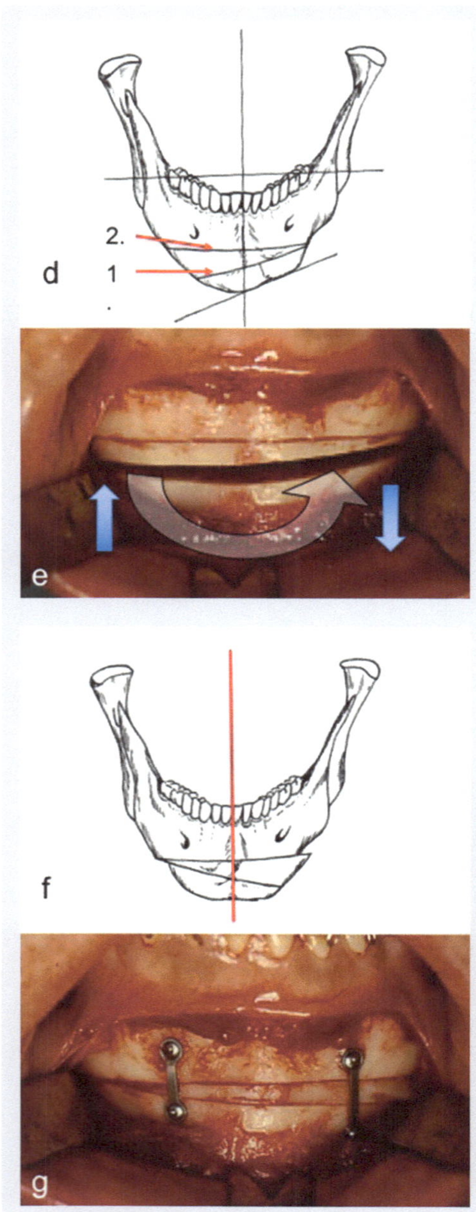

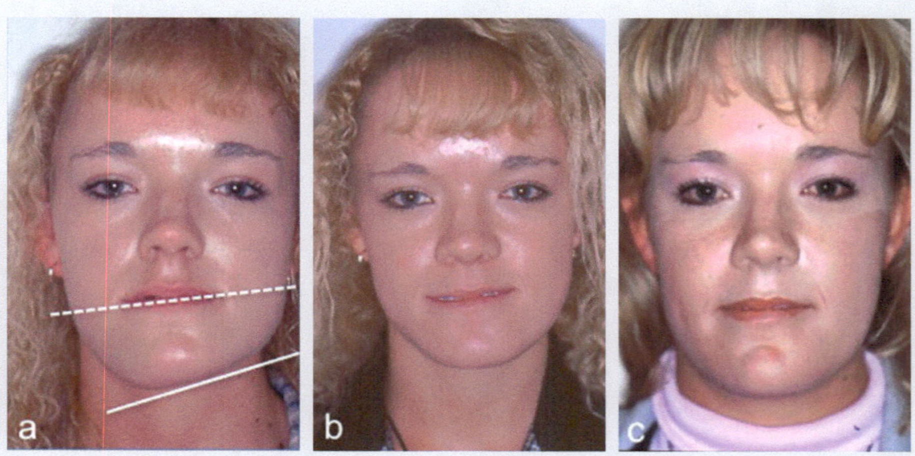

Figure 5.23 - CASE 23. *Patient with unilateral condylar hyperplasia. The facial asymmetry and bowing of the right mandibular lower border is evident in the frontal view. Also note the severe cant of the lower border of the chin. The dotted line demonstrates the extent of the transverse cant of the occlusal plane (a). The post-operative frontal view (b) and the improved symmetry 9 years following surgery (c). The severe cant of the lower border of the chin was corrected by means of a propeller osteotomy.The first osteotomy is performed parallel to the lower border of the chin (d, arrow 1). The next osteotomy is performed parallel to the inter pupillary line (d, arrow 2) The intermediate bone segment is rotated by 180° and fixated aligning the bone marks (f and g).*

Adjunct Surgical Procedures

There are various surgical procedures that augment the soft tissues and enhance the esthetic results of chin surgery.[18-20] These procedures influence the structures around the chin and are usually used as parameters for relative esthetic evaluation. These structures include the lips, submental area, soft tissue thickness over the chin and the width of the mandibular angles.

Lips. Much of the soft tissue analyses used during evaluation of chin projection employ the upper and lower lip position as relative references, e.g., the E-line and S-line. In some cases, however, the lips excessively protrude. This may lead the clinician to believe that the chin is deficient or more deficient than it actually is. Incorrect diagnosis, inaccurate treatment planning, and, poor post-treatment esthetics may result.[18-19]

It is therefore essential that more than one diagnostic analysis is used during evaluation, and that all other structures used as a reference in the analysis also be evaluated for any possible deformity.

Vermillionectomy of Upper and Lower Lips in Combination with Mandibular and Chin Advancement

CASE 24: Patient with excesssively everted lips and excessive vermillion exposure. The lips in this case should not be used as a parameter against which to evaluate the chin.

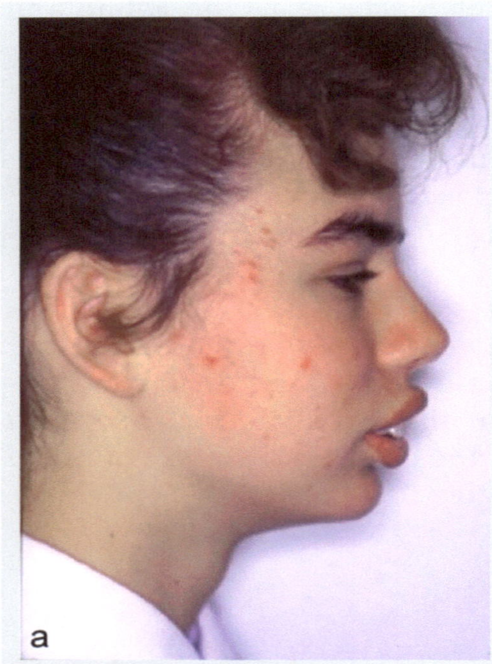

Main complaint: Inability to close lips.

Diagnosis:

1. Dental:
    - Class II division 1.

Skeletal:

- Maxillary anteroposterior deficiency.
- Mandibular anteroposterior defiency.

3. Soft tissue:
    - Anteroposterior chin deficiency.
    - Excessive vermillion exposure.
    - Protrusive lips.
    - Everted upper and lower lips.

Treatment:

1. Mandibular advancement.
2. Genioplasty, advancing the chin.
3. Upper and lower lip vermillionectomies.

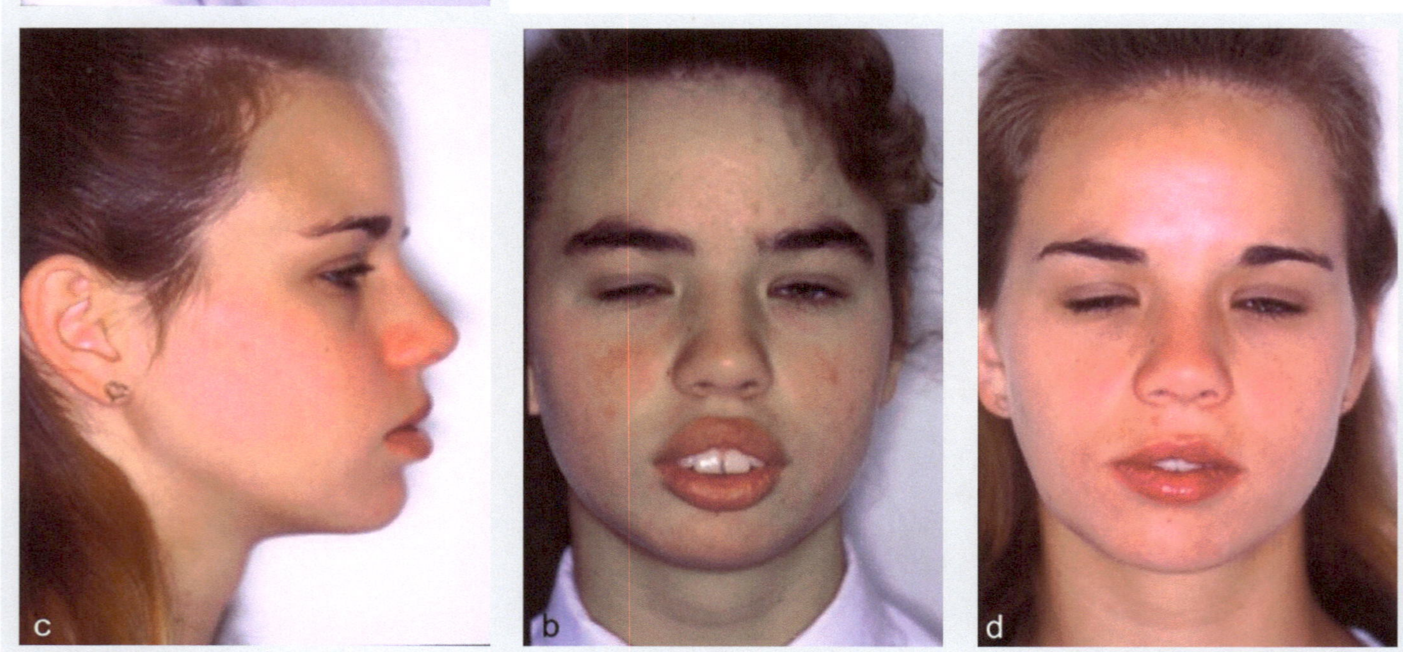

Figure 5.24 - CASE 24. *The pre-treatment frontal (b) and profile view (a) illustrating the excessive vermillion exposure and protrusive lips. The mandible and chin is anteroposteriorly deficient. The frontal view (d) and profile view (c) following upper and lower lip vermilionectomy and mandibular and chin advancement. Note: 1) The improvement in facial contour, 2) the more defined contour of the mandibular lower border, 3) increase in chin-neck length and 4) decreased lip protrusion and vermillion exposure.*

Submental Area

CASE 25: The patient illustrates the improved esthetics after mandibular advancement, advancement genioplasty, and submental liposuction.

The submental area plays an important role in the overall evaluation of chin esthetics, e.g., the lip–chin–submental angle, submental–neck angle, chin–neck length, etc.[21] Excessive submental fat adds to poor chin esthetics and submental liposuction or lipectomy should be considered as an adjunct procedure to enhance chin esthetics.[22]

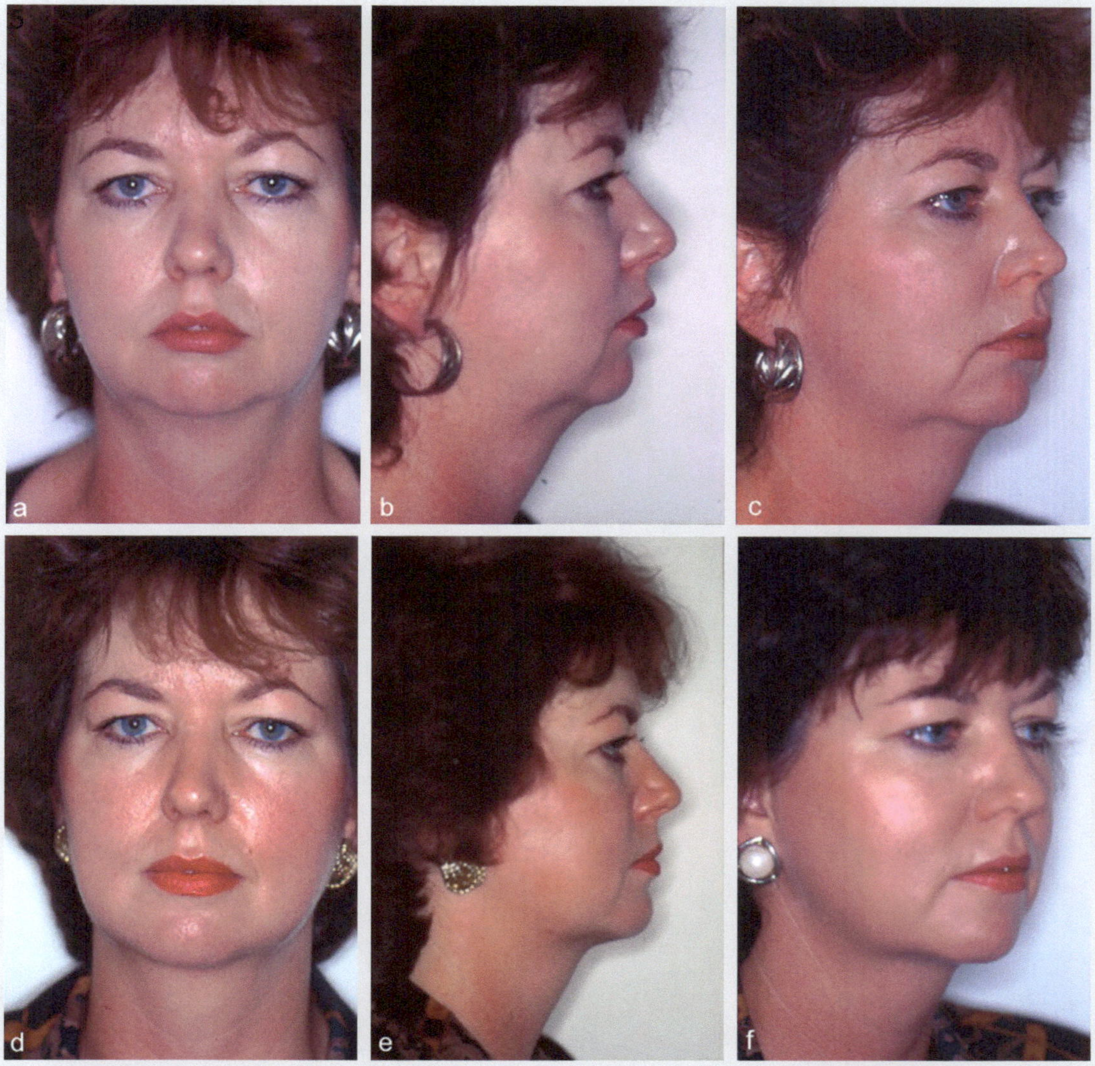

CASE 25 - CASE 25. *Patient had surgical advancement of her mandible for correction of a skeletal Class II malocclusion. The mandibular surgery (bilateral sagittal split osteotomy and genioplasty) was combined with submental liposuction. The pre-surgical frontal, profile and three-quarter views are demonstrated in (a, b and c) and the postoperative results in (d, e and f).*

Augmentation of the Mandibular Angles

In cases where the mandibular angles are poorly defined, the transverse dimension in this area may be augmented by sub-masseteric implants.[25] The esthetic change in a patient after increasing the mandibular width and definition, combined with narrowing and advance the chin, is demonstrated in Figure 5.21.

Submental Liposuction. Some individuals may have excessive neck fat and therefore poor definition of the lower border of the mandible and an unaesthetic chin–neck length with a tendency toward having a double chin. The above features often occur in patients with a skeletal Class II malocclusion. Esthetic improvement of the neck–cervicofacial region, with or without adjunctive platysma muscle plication, should be considered. Submental liposuction in combination with mandibular advancement and genioplasty advancement will enhance the submental esthetics. Note the improvement in the chin–throat length, lip–chin–submental angle and the lower border definition in Case 25, Figure 5.25.

Improving the Submental Facial Contour

CASE 26: This patient's severely obtuse lip–chin-–submental angle and short chin–throat length required submental liposuction, plication of the platysma muscles, and removal of a limited amount of skin to improve the cervicofacial contour.

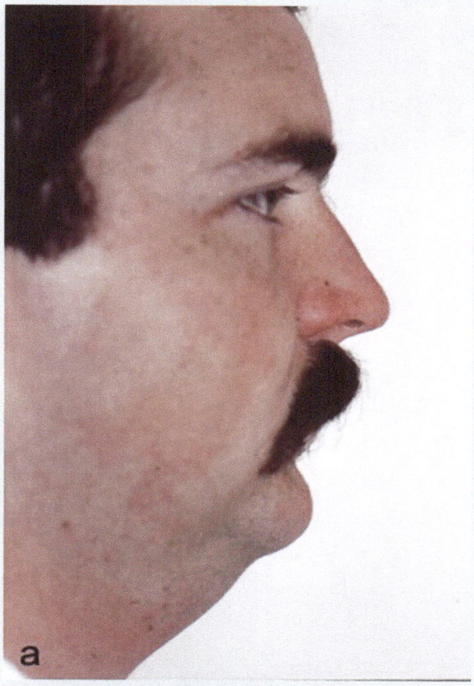

Main complaint: The patient was self-conscious about his severely deficient chin and grew a moustache to hide it.

Diagnosis:

1. Dental: A Class II anterior open bite malocclusion.
2. Skeletal:
   - Mandibular anteroposterior defficiency.
   - Anterior vertical maxillary deficiency.
   - Posterior vertical maxillary excess.
   - Microgenia.
3. Soft Tissue:
   - Excesive submental fat deposits.

Treatment:

1. Mulipiece le Fort I maxillary osteotomy (superior repositioning the posterior segments and improving the upper incisor-lip relationship).
2. Mandibular advancement by means of bilateral sagittal split osteotomy.
3. Augmentation genioplasty.
4. Submental liposuction and placation of the pla tysma muscles.

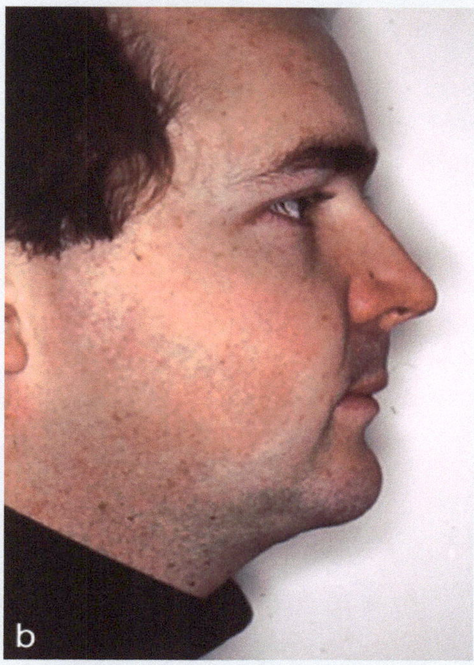

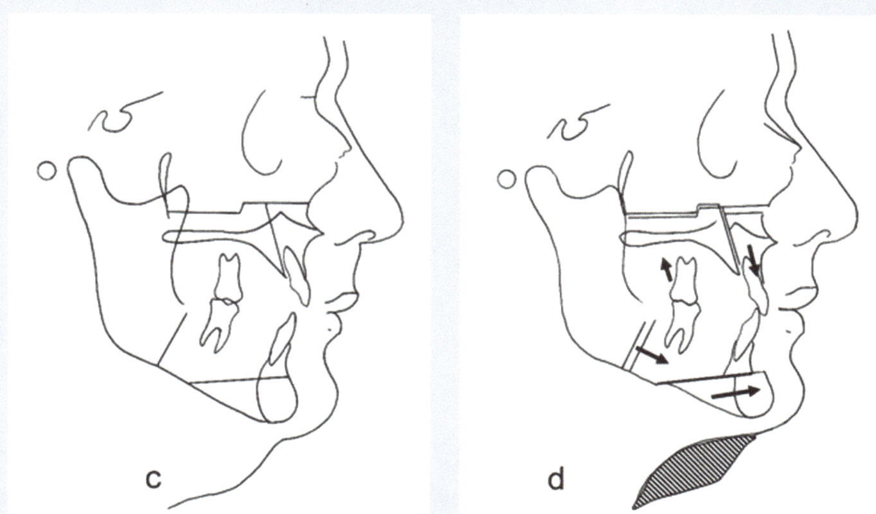

Figure 5.26 - CASE 26. *Plication of the platysma muscles, liposuction and removal of excess skin improved the cervico-facial esthetics substantially. Pre-surgical profile (a) and cephalometric tracing (c). The treatment plan is outlined in tracing (d). The final result (b).*

Masseter Reduction

CASE 27: The patient's dolicoprosopic square facial form was adressed by reducing the posterior broadness of her mandible and increasing her anterior mandidular height.

The interzygomatic, bigonial and chin width should be in balance. In patients with bilateral masseter muscle hypertrophy, this balance is disturbed and will render esthetic chin surgery difficult. Reduction of the bigonial width should be considered in these cases.[23,24] In Case 27, the mandibular angles were reduced and chin contour improved, combined with submental liposuction. *(Fig 27)*

The transverse dimension at the angles of the mandible can be reduced by reduction of the masseter muscle, which is often combined with reduction of the laterally everted mandibular angles.

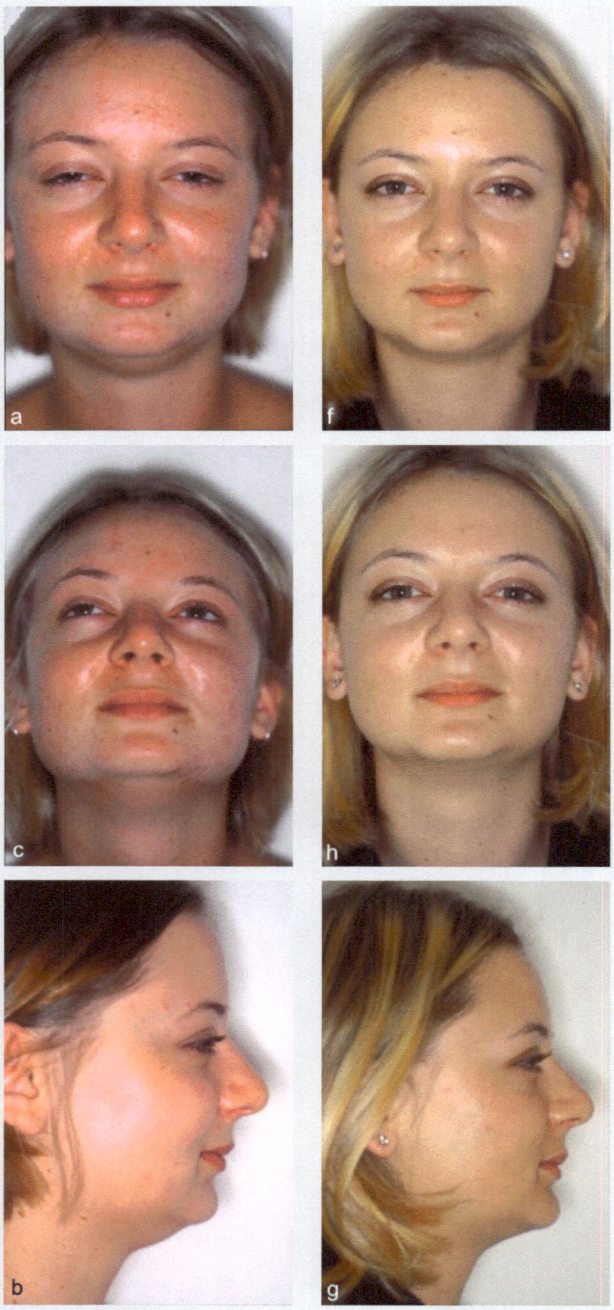

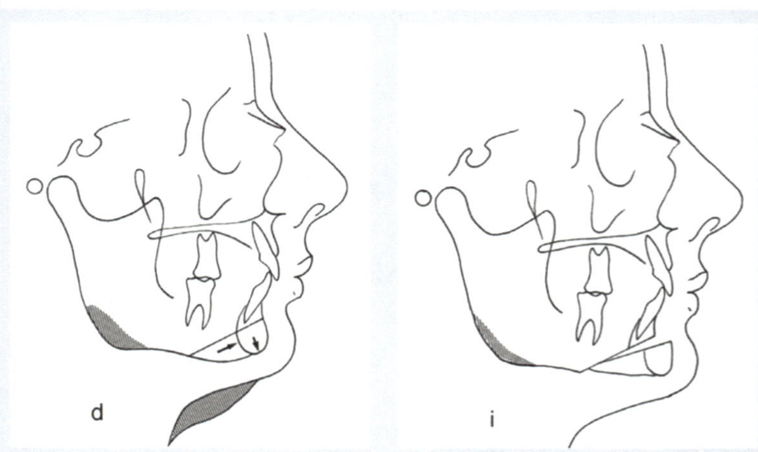

Figure 5.27 - CASE 27. *Pretreatment frontal (a), profile (b) and frontal 3/4 view (c) of patient with anteroposterior chin deficiency, square face and tendency to double chin due to fat deposit. Treatment plan tracings (d) and result after anterior sliding genioplasty and down graft of the chin, mandibular angle reduction and submental liposuction (f, g, h & i). Note: 1) increase in chin-neck length, 2) improvement in mandibular lower border definition, 3) improvement in facial contour angle and 4) improvement in parasymphyseal depressions.*

Soft Tissue Thickness

CASE 28: A patient with excessive lipid tissue in her mandibular symphyses. Apart from excessive fat in the submental area, excessive fat may be found in the chin area, increasing the soft tissue thickness over the chin. This excessive fat is often unattractive and makes correction by bone repositioning impossible. Extra-oral removal of the excessive fat and skin is indicated in these cases.

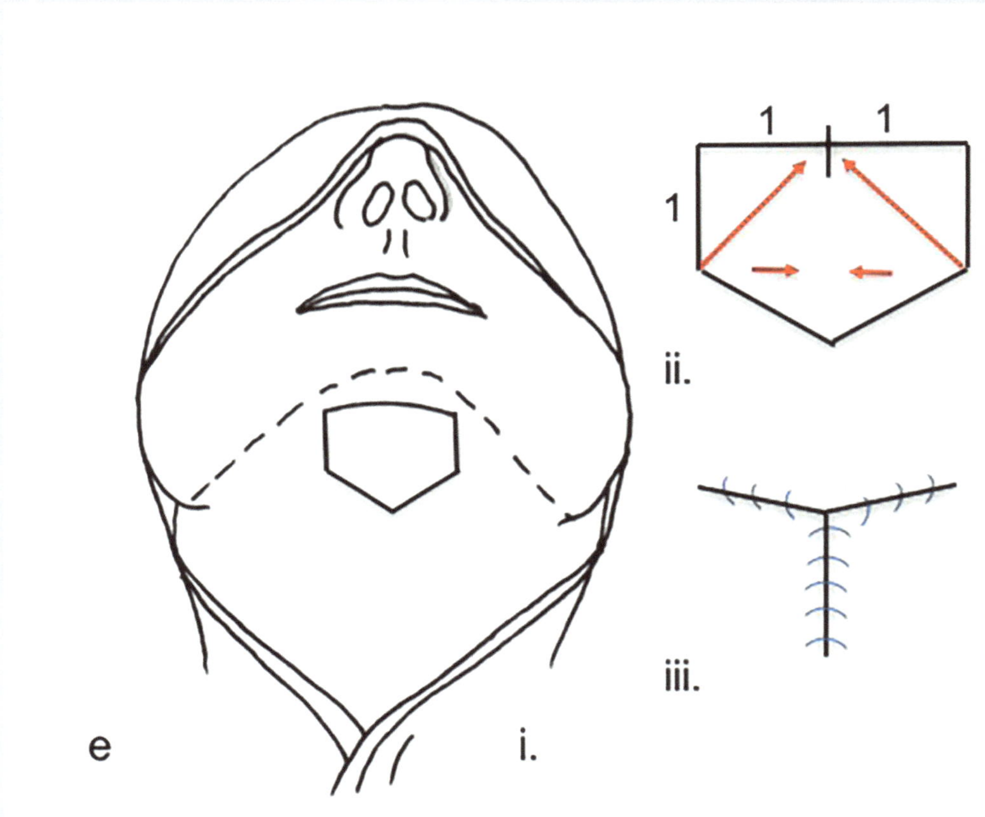

Figure 5.28 - CASE 28 *The female patient demonstrates excessive chin projection, due to increased fat in the chin area. Removal of the fat through an extra-oral approach and V-Y skin closure after excision of a triangular area of skin. The design of the skin incision is demonstrated in (i) and (ii) (Fig 5.28e).*

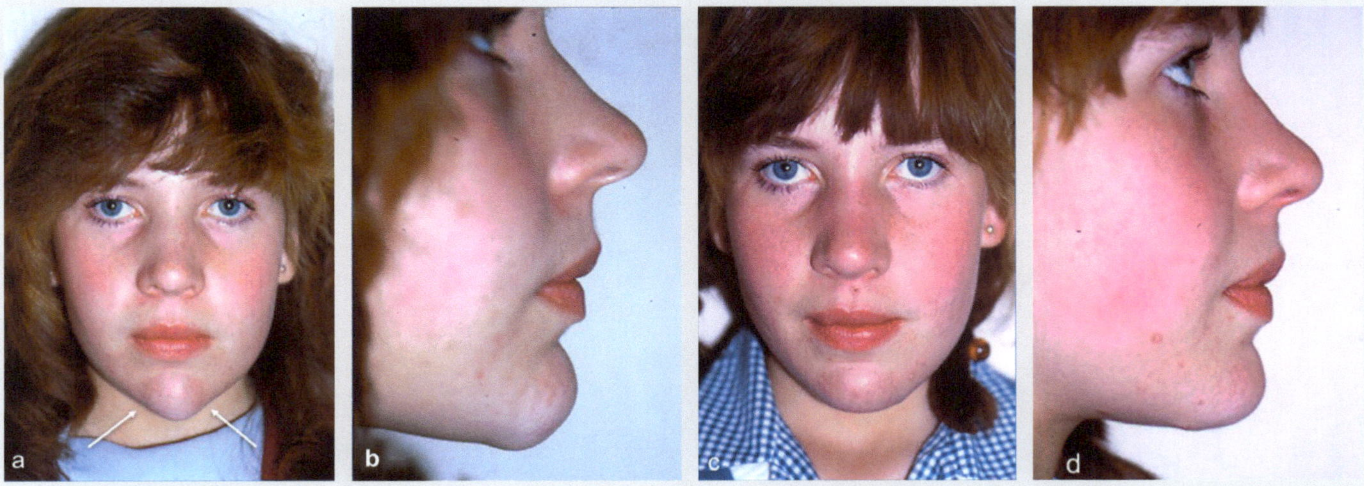

Figure 5.28 - CASE 28 *The pre-treatment frontal (a) and profile view (b) of a patient with excessive lipid tissue in her mandibular symphyses. The outcome is illustrated in (c) and (d).*

Chapter 6 - Complications of Sliding Genioplasty

Although relatively uncommon, complications do occur following the sliding genioplasty. Unexpected sequelae usually occur due to inadequate planning, failure to follow a meticulous stepwise surgical technique and performing surgery without respect for hard and soft tissue structures. Complications may occur intraoperatively or postoperatively and may involve the hard or soft tissue structures of the chin.[1,2]

Soft Tissue Complications

Neurologic complications. Postoperative parasthesia of the mental nerves occurs to some degree in most cases and all patients should be warned about this possible complication. In the vast majority of cases, paresthesia is transient and resolves within a short period of time, usually a few weeks.[3,4]

Prolonged parasthesia is usually caused by excessive traction, inadequate exposure, and poor protection of the mental nerve when performing the horizontal osteotomy inferior and/or posterior to the mental foraminae.

Other orthognathic procedures performed during the same operation may be responsible for loss of sensation in the mental nerve distribution due to neuropraxia of the inferior alveolar nerve (mandibular), e.g., bilateral sagittal split osteotomy.

Permanent anesthesia, however, may be caused when the nerve or some of its small terminal branches are transected. This may occur at two locations:

1. By performing the osteotomy less than 5mm below the mental foramen, the nerve may be transected in the inferior alveolar canal before its exit from the fo-

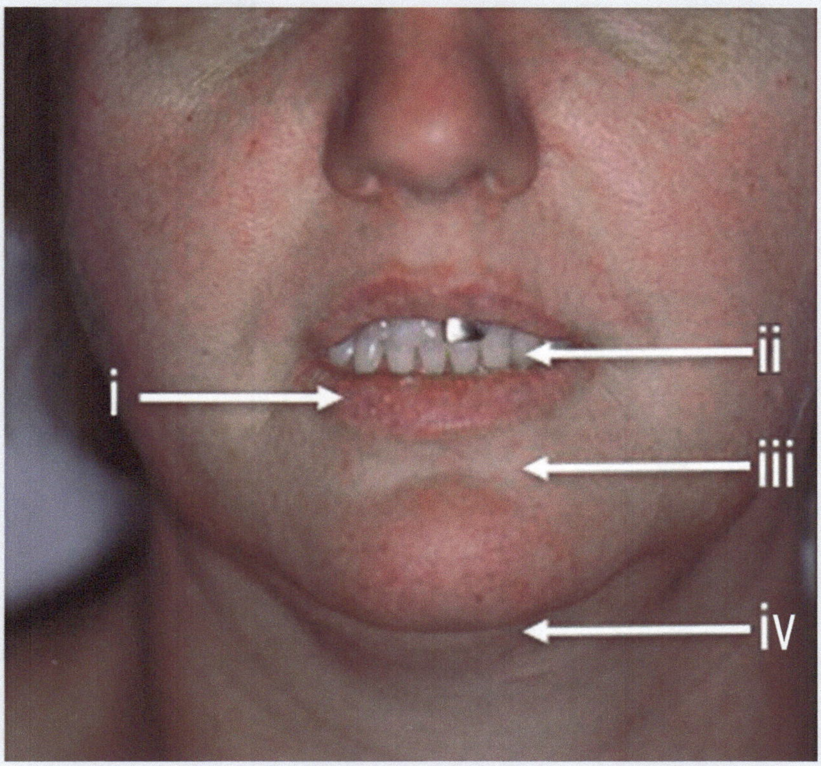

Figure 6.1 - CASE 1. *Inaccurate re-approximation of the mentalis muscle and mucosa may lead to asymmetry of the lower lip (i), exposure of the lower incisors (ii), flattening of the labiomental fold (iii) and unevenness of the chin contour (iv).*

ramen. Keep in mind that the nerve exits from the foramen from below and backwards.

2. When the soft tissue incision is placed too far labially or laterally, some of the terminal branches of the mental nerve may be transected. *(Refer to Chapter 4, Surgical Technique Step 3.)*

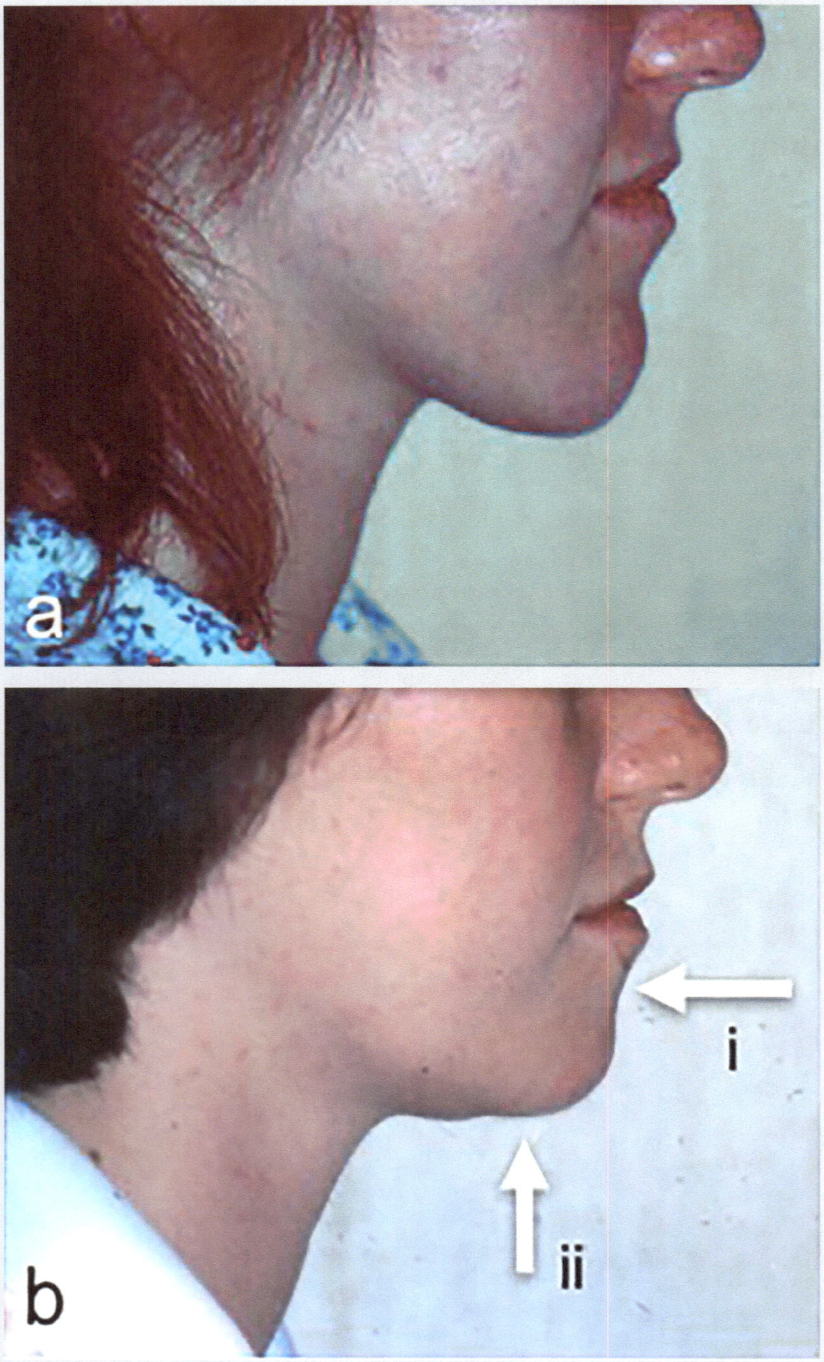

Figure 6.2 - CASE 2. *Vertical reduction of the chin is shown both (a) preoperative and (b) postoperative. In this case, the chin height was reduced without any anteroposterior augmentation leading to flattening of the labiomental fold (i) and poor submental contour (ii).*

Vascular Complications. While performing a surgical procedure, the patient's blood pressure should be lowered by the anesthesiologist. When the mean blood pressure is maintained below 90mm of mercury, capillary oozing and bleeding are minimized. Local anesthetic with a vasoconstrictor should be infiltrated into the labial sulcus about 10 minutes before surgery. Blood loss with this procedure may occur as persistent oozing from transected vessels in the genioglossus, geniohyoid, mylohyoid or digastic muscles. Significant bleeding may occur due to perforation of the submental artery (a small terminal branch of the facial artery). Intramedullary vessels may also be a source of hemorrhage and should be controlled prior to bone fixation.

It is vital that intraoperative hemorrhage be controlled promptly by burnishing medullary bleeders, cauterizing soft tissue bleeders and where necessary, placing a suture to secure homeostasis.

A postoperative sublingual hematoma may develop once the patient becomes normotensive following anesthesia. A sublingual hematoma will push the tongue and floor of the mouth upwards with black discoloration of the submucosa. This may distress the patient and make normal speech difficult.

Airway compromise is fortunately rare and treatment with a pressure dressing, ice and hot packs usually leads to quick recovery. Placement of the pressure dressing will also prevent subperiosteal hematoma formation on the anterior mandibular surface.[5]

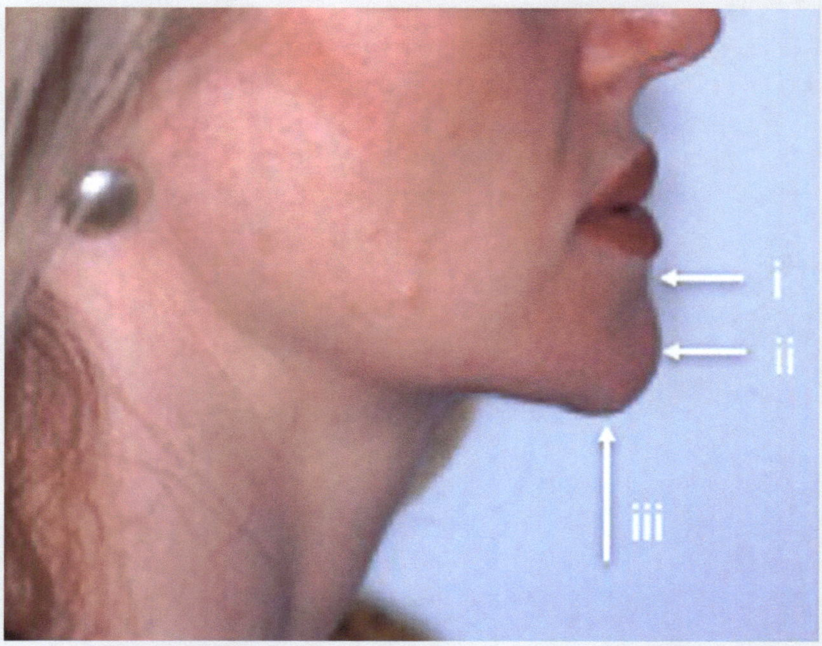

Figure 6.3 - CASE 3. *A patient with a Class III dental relationship with compensated incisors was treated by anteroposterior and vertical "shaving" of the chin. In an attempt to correct the poor esthetic result achieved, after the first surgery, a silastic implant was placed in a second procedure. Note in the profile view of the patient: The flattening of the labio-mental fold (i), the poor chin contour arrow (ii) and the drooping chin (iii).*

Muscle Displacement. Extensive reflection of the periosteum over the anterior and lower border of the chin (degloving) should be avoided. The only muscle that will be incised with the labial surgical approach is the mentalis muscle. Care should be taken to suture the incision in a double layer fashion, and to accurately re-approximate the muscle during closure.[6] Poor technique regarding the above aspects may lead to: chin ptosis (witch's chin), flattening of the labiomental fold, lip incompetence, excessive lower incisor teeth exposure, and/or poor submental esthetics.[7,8]

Total degloving of the anterior mandible and stripping of the lingual muscle attachments from the mobilized chin segment will increase the risk of extensive bone resorption leading to unpredictable and disappointing soft tissue results. This complication often occurs when a double sliding genioplasty is performed and it is one of the reasons why this procedure is not recommended.

Mucosal Complications. Final closure of the mucosa following muscle and submucosal layer closure should be done meticulously. Closure of the last layer can be considered the surgeon's signature on his/her work and is often a reflection of the surgery performed.

Incorrect approximation of the midlines of the incision will lead to an asymmetric lower lip, which may often be very obvious to the patient, causing disappointment with the result.

Suturing should be done with 4/0 resorbable suture, taking thin, even bites with symmetric approximation. Failure to adhere to the above will result in an asymmetric and uneven lower lip. Deep sutures with large bites will tend to shorten the lower lip and may cause muco-gingival damage.[9]

Periodontal Complications. The mucosal incision for the surgical approach to the bony chin should be placed at least 5mm labially to the keratinized epithelial border. This will not only facilitate easy suturing but also prevent muco-gingival stripping.

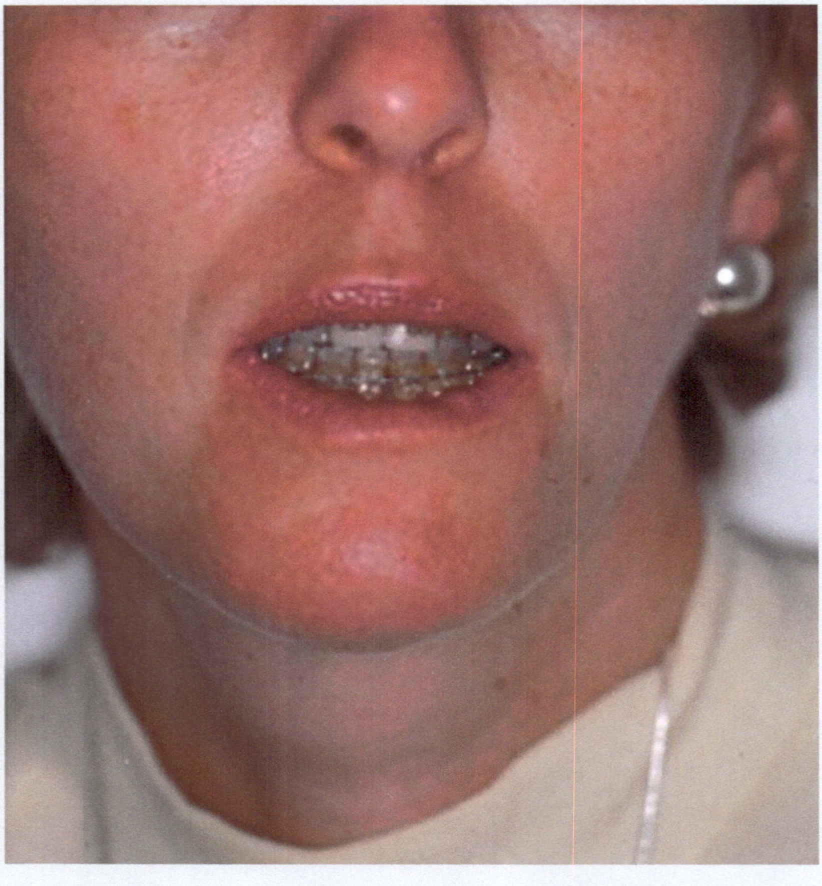

Figure 6.4 - CASE 4. *Inaccurate re-approximation of the mentalis muscle resulted in lower lip shortening and asymmetry with excessive lower incisor exposure.*

A thin zone of attached gingiva, existing periodontal disease, and high attachment of the mentalis muscles should be noted preoperatively and complications avoided by placing the soft tissue incision further labially. *(Refer to Chapter 4, Surgical Technique, Step 21-22.)*

Soft Tissue Esthetic Complications. Poor esthetic results are mostly the consequence of inaccurate diagnosis, poor treatment planning and inadequate, incorrect, sloppy surgical technique.[9-11]

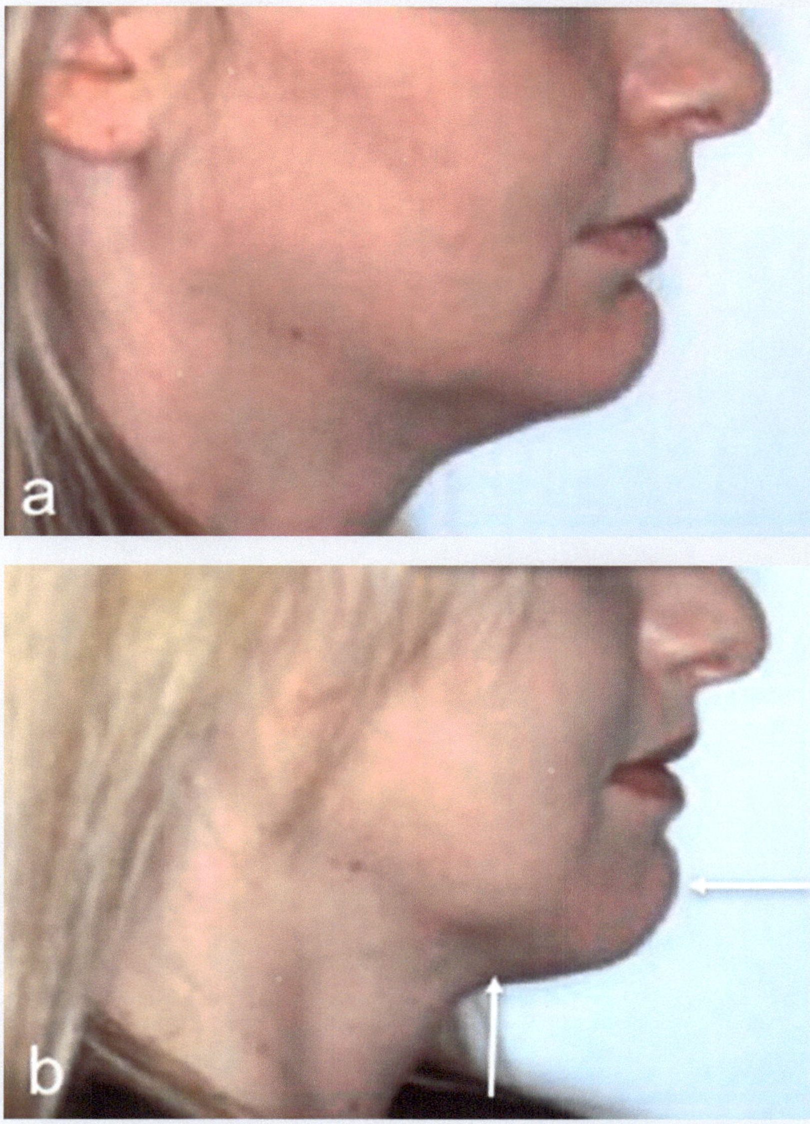

Figure 6.5 - CASE 5. *Poor definition of the mandibular lower border resulted after a large chin setback procedure without contouring the posterior edges of the chin segment. Pre-surgical (a) and post-surgical (b).*

Some of the Most Common Aesthetic Complications

Soft Tissue Complications.

1. Shortening of the lower lip *(Fig 6.1)*.
2. Obliteration of the labiomental fold *(Fig 6.2)*.
3. Development of chin ptosis and submental unevenness *(Fig 6.3)*.
4. Lower lip shortening and asymmetry *(Fig 6.4)*.
5. Poor lower border definition after setback procedures *(Fig 6.5)*.

Prevention of the above complications have been noted in the text accompanying Figure

Hard Tissue Complications.

1. Poor chin contour, lip shortening and mentalis strain, and postoperative chin and lip asymmetry *(Fig 6.6)*.
2. Genioplasty performed for incorrect indication.
    - Accentuation of anteroposterior chin augmentation when mandibular advancement is indicated *(Fig 6.7)*.
    - Vertical and anteroposterior chin reduction when mandibular setback is indicated *(Fig 6.8)*.
    - Performing an anteroposterior chin augmentation when a mandibular advancement is indicated *(Fig 6.9)*.

Prevention of the above complications have been discussed in Chapter 4, Surgical Techniques.

Hard Tissue Complications

Incomplete Osteotomy. By not completing the horizontal osteotomy through the lower border of the mandible, downfracture of the chin segment will lead to a fracture of the lower border posteriorly. Failure to remove the bone specule from the segment will lead to inaccurate bone approximation. *(Refer to Chapter 4, Surgical Technique, Step 7.)*

Inadequate Fixation. Fixation of the repositioned segment may be performed by bicortical screws, boneplates or interosseous wires. Inadequate fixation may lead to postoperative loosening of the segment requiring reoperation. *(Refer to Chapter 4, Surgical Technique, Step 13.)*

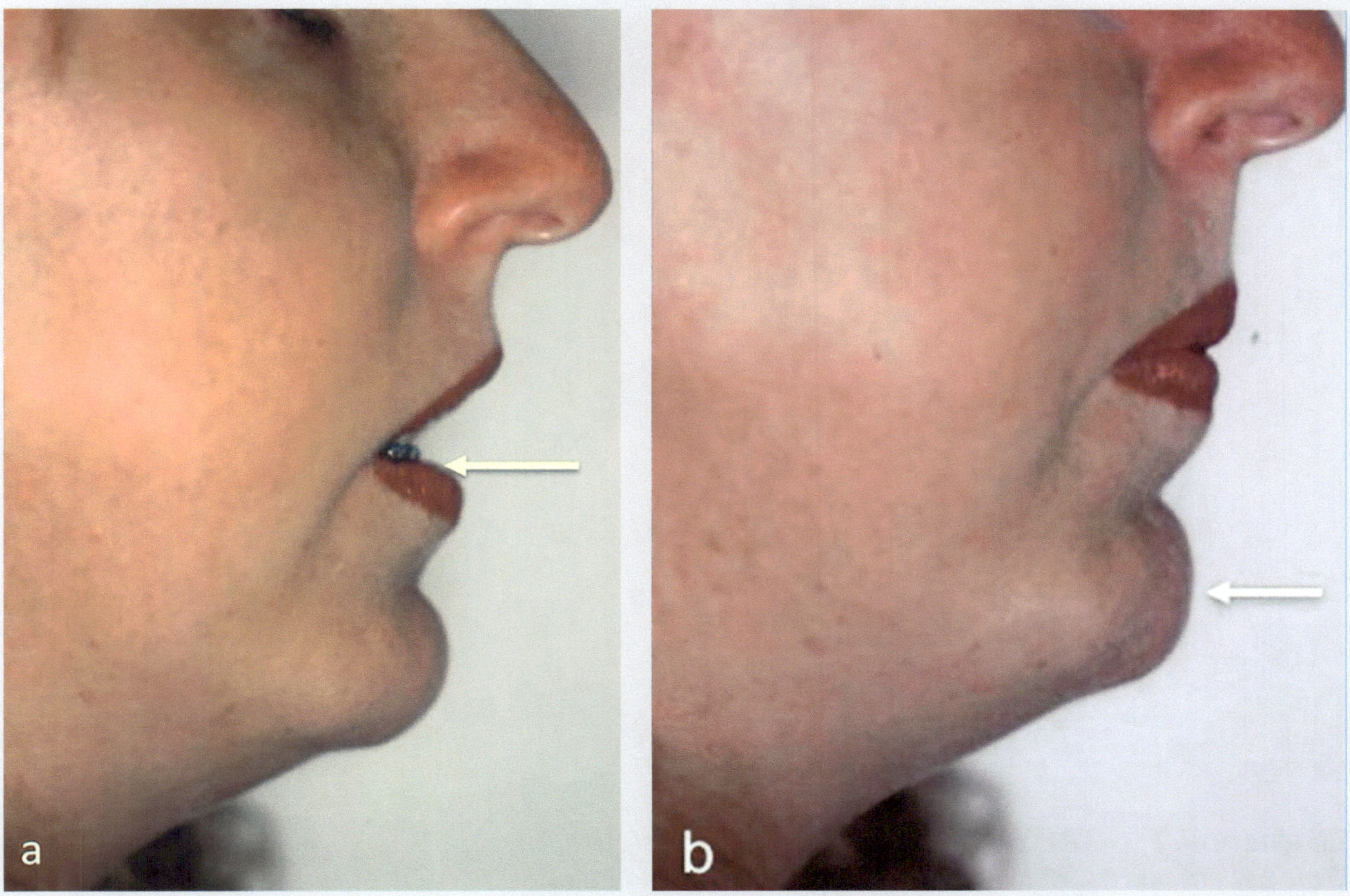

Figure 6.6 - CASE 6. *Inaccurate suturing of the submucosal tissues and mucosa resulted in lip shortening, poor chin contour and severe soft tissue soft tissue strain when the lips are forced together. Lips relaxed (a) and the lips forced together (b).*

Inaccurate Bone Repositioning. Orientation marks should be placed on the outer cortex of the chin before performing the horizontal osteotomy. The preoperative surgical plan will be a guide for placement of reference marks and accurate repositioning of the chin. *(Refer to Chapter 4, Surgical Technique, Step 5.)*

Devitalization of Teeth. The horizontal osteotomy should be performed at least 5mm below the apices of the teeth. The lower incisors and canine teeth are involved. The preoperative panoramic radiograph should be used as a guide to estimate root length and location for the safe placement of the horizontal osteotomy.

An osteotomy placed too high may devitalize the teeth, or compromise the pulpal blood flow. Long-term loss of vitality, the presence of pain or periapical changes may necessitate endodontic intervention. *(Refer to Chapter 4, Surgical Technique, Step 6.)*

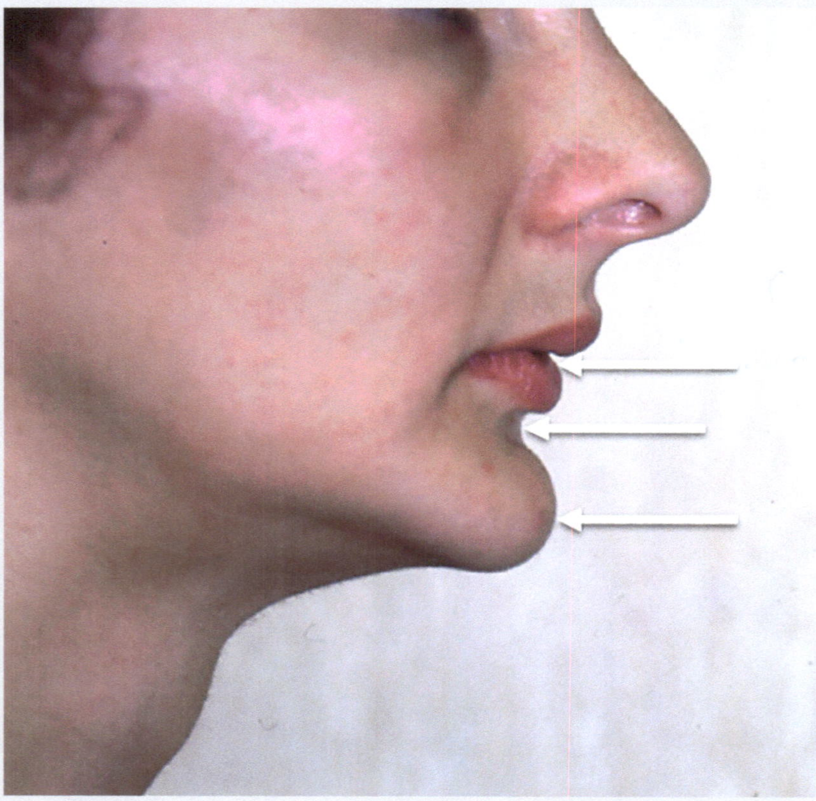

Figure 6.7 - CASE 7. Top *Inappropriate surgery. This patient has a Class II dental occlusion and mandibular anteroposterior deficiency requiring mandibular advancement. The compromised treatment by means of a "double sliding genioplasty" resulted in an everted lower lip (i), deep labiomental fold (ii) and a "knobby" chin (iii).*

Infection. Prophylactic antibiotics are used routinely to prevent infection. Postoperative infection seldom occurs after genioplasty. Soft tissue infection usually follows wound dehiscence with pain and swelling of the chin. The surgical wound should be irrigated daily through the wound margins using an antibiotic solution. Healing usually takes place within 10 days with granulation tissue and re-epithelization.

Infection of the pedicled bone segment is rare and should be treated as above.

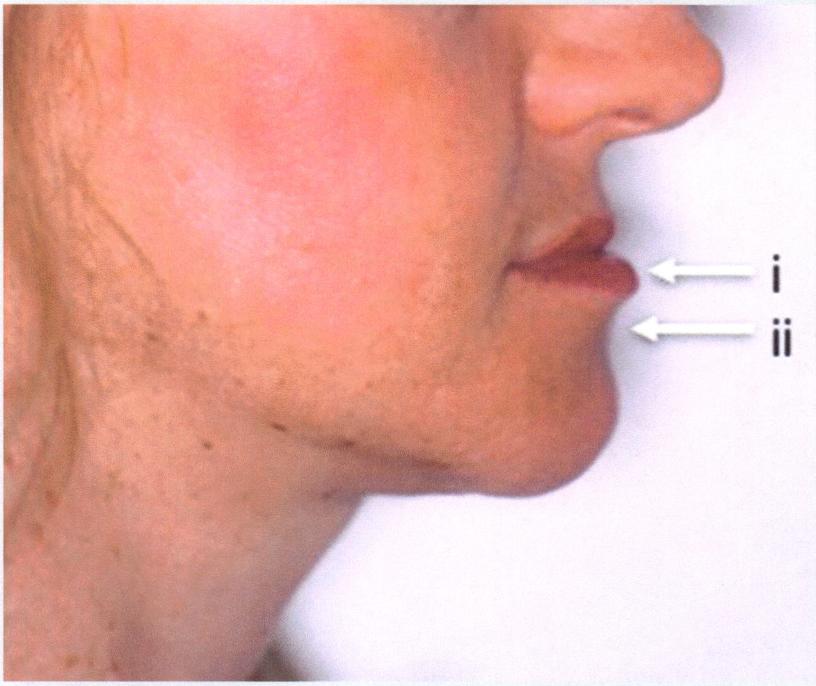

Figure 6.8 - CASE 8. Bottom *The patient's "prominent chin" was treated by shaving the chin button. Note the still existing the prominent lower lip and mandible (i) and the obtuse labio-mental fold (ii).*

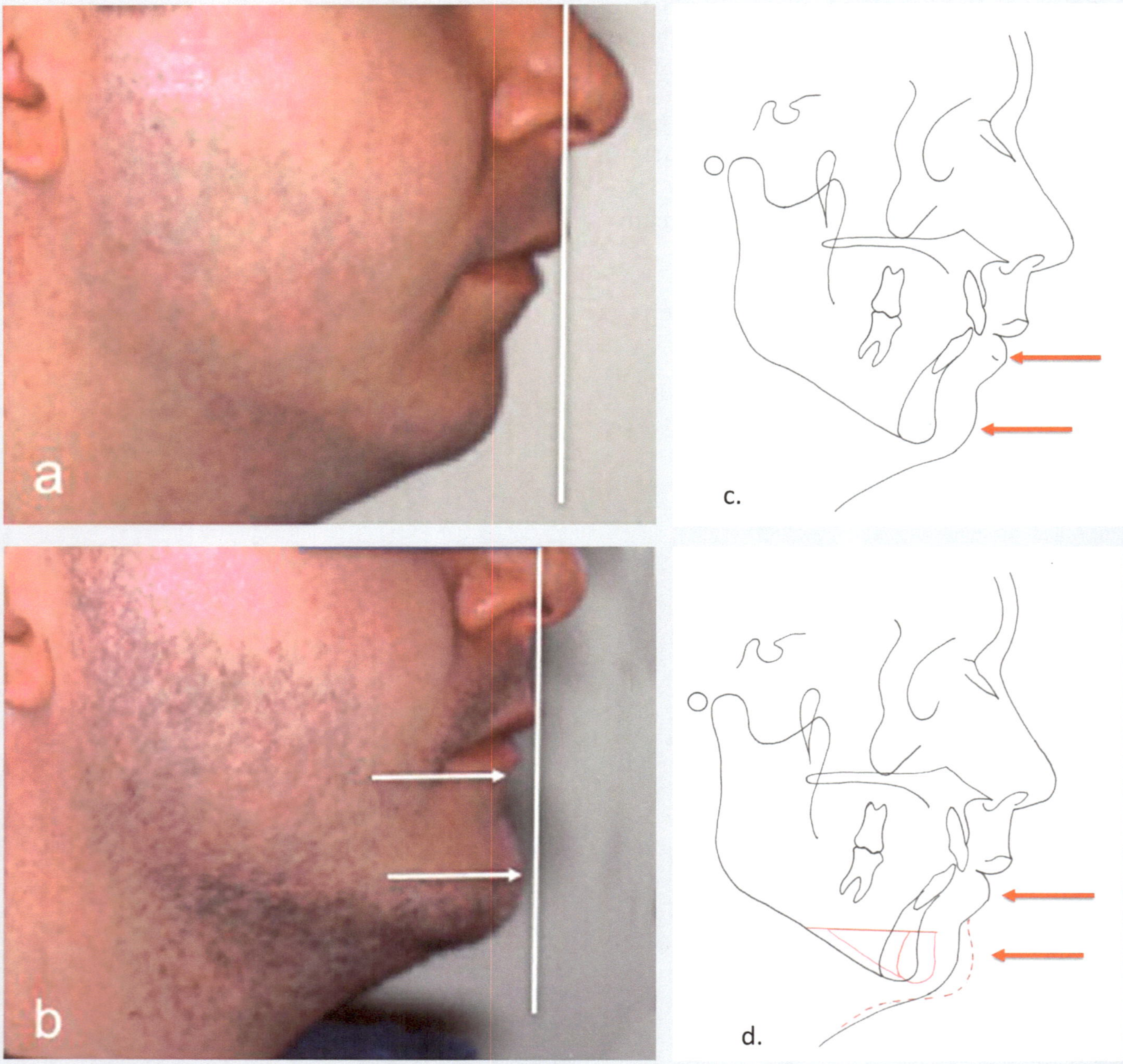

Figure 6.9 - CASE 9. *Genioplasty is not a substitute for mandibular surgery. The patient required mandibular surgery for the correction of a Class II occlusion (a). As a compromise, a genioplasty was performed. Note the improved chin prominence however the lower lip remains deficient (arrows)(b). A cepalometric tracing of Case 9. The dentition is compromised, lower incisors are protruded and upper incisors retrocined (arrows) (c). The poor chin shape is predicted in the surgical visual treatment plan after advancement genioplasty (arrows) (d).*

SCIENCE and art

Medicine consists of science and art
in a certain relationship to each other, yet wholly distinct.
Science can be learned by anyone, even the mediocre.
Art, however, is a gift from heaven.
So you cannot count yourselves among the great doctors
by simply acquiring knowledge.

The scientist continually and receptively gathers
a vast amount of material,
while the artist creates new roads of thought.
Knowledge suffocates the scientist,
whereas it gives the artist fresh inspiration.
Therefore, gentlemen, learn as much as you can ~
but your learning must be the basis
for your art, not an end in itself.
A little less science and a little more art, Messieurs!

Armand Trousseau
(to his students)

References

Chapter 1

1. Leakey R, Lewin R. Origins reconsidered. In: Search of What Makes Us Human. London, Abacus Publishers, 1992, pp. 205-209.
2. Ibid, pp. 137-152.
3. Johanson D, Edgar B. From Lucy to Language. New York, Simon & Schuster, 1996.
4. Parker S. Evolution: The Whole Story. Thames and Hudson, London, 2015.
5. Goose DH, Appelton J. Growth of the mandible. In: Human Dentofacial Growth. Oxford, Pergamon Press, 1982, pp. 77-78.
6. Cicero. De Oratore, Vol. III, 55 BC.
7. Bates B, Cleese J. The Human Face. London, Dorling Kindersley Publishers, 2001.
8. Converse JM, Wood-Smith D. Horizontal osteotomy of the mandible. Plast Reconstr Surg 1964;34:464-471.
9. Guyuron B. Genioplasty. Boston, Little, Brown and Company, 1990.
10. Precious AD, Armstrong JE, Morais D. Anatomic placement of fixation devices in genioplasty. Oral Surg Oral Med Oral Oral Pathol 1992;73:2-8.
11. Blomquist DS, Lee JJ. Mandibular orthognathic surgery. In: Peterson's Principles of Oral and Maxillofacial Surgery, Vol 2, Miloro M, Ghali GE, Larsen P, Waite P, eds. Bejing, People's Medical Publishing House, 2012, pp. 1350-1359.
12. Enlow HD. Introductory concepts of the growth process. In: Facial Growth, 2nd ed. Philadelphia, WB Saunders, 1990, pp. 25-49.
13. Enlow DH, Harris DB. A study of the postnatal growth of the human mandible. Am J Orthodont Dentofac Orthoped 1964;50:25-50.
14. Moss ML. Functional analysis of human mandibular growth. J Prosth Dent 1960;10:1149-1159.
15. Enlow DH. The facial growth process. In: Facial Growth, 2nd ed. Philadelphia, WB Saunders, 1990, pp. 83-97.
16. Björk A. Prediction of mandibular growth rotation. Am J Orthodont Dentofac Orthoped 1969;55:585-599.

Chapter 2

1. Enlow HD. Faces. In: Facial Growth, 3rd Ed. Philadelphia, WB Saunders, 1990, pp 2-9.
2. Epker BN. The chin: genioplasty. In: Esthetic Maxillofacial Surgery. Philadelphia, Lea & Febiger, 1994, pp. 2-4.
3. Legan HL, Burstone CJ. Soft tissue cephalometric analysis for orthognathic surgery. J Oral Surg 1980;38:744-751.
4. Schendel SA, Eisenfeld J, Bell WH, Epker BN, Mishelevich DJ. The long face syndrome: vertical maxillary excess. Am J Orthod 1976;70:398-408.
5. Arnett GW, Bergman RT. Facial keys to orthodontic diagnosis and treatment planning - Part II. Am J Orthod Dentofac Orthoped 1993;5:395-411.
6. Cineros GJ, Kaban LB. Computerized skeletal scintigraphy for assessment of mandibular asymmetry. J Oral Maxillofac Surg 1984;42:513.
7. Reyneke JP. Systematic Patient Evaluation in Essential in Orthognathic Surgery, 2nd ed. Quintessence, Chicago, 2014.
8. Burstone CJ. Lip posture and its significance in treatment planning. Am J Orthod 1967;53:262-284.
9. Epker BN, Wolford LM. Reduction cheiloplasty: its role in the correction of dentofacial deformities. J Maxillofac Surg 1977;5:134.
10. Rosen HM. Aesthetic refinements in genioplasty: the role of the labiomental fold. Plast Reconst Surg 1990;88:760.
11. Epker BN, Stella JP. Systematic aesthetic evaluation of the neck for cosmetic surgery. Oral Maxillofac Surg Clin North Am 1990;2:217.
12. Elam MV, Berkowitz F. Submental and submandibular lipectomy by liposuction surgery. Am J Cosmet Surg 1988;2:3.
13. Vinas JC, et al. Surgical correction of the double chin. Plast Reconstr Surg 1972;50:119-122.
14. Marino H, Galeano EA. Plastic correction of double chin-importance of the hyoid bone. Plast Reconstr Surg 1963;31:45-50.
15. Costa LE, et al. Orthognatic surgical alteration of the cervicomental angle. Birmingham, 1987 University of Alabama School of Dentistry, unpublished.
16. Sommerville JM, Sperry TP, Be Gole EA. Morphology of the submental and neck area. Int J Adult Orthod 1988;3:97-106.
17. Hayes RJ, Sarver DM, Jacobson AJ. Quantification of cervicomental angle changes with mandibular advancement. Am J Orthod Dentofacial Orthop1994;4:105.
18. Burstone CJ. Lip posture and its significance in treatment planning. Am J Orthod 1967;53:262-284.
19. Legan HL, Burstone CJ. Soft tissue cephalometric analysis for orthognathic surgery. J Oral Surg 1980;38:747-751.
20. Bell WH, Jacobs JD, Quajada JG. Simultaneous repositioning of the maxilla, mandible, and chin. Am J Orthod 1986;89:28-50.
21. Ricketts RM. Esthetics, environment of the law of lip relation. Am J Orthod 196854:272.
22. Scheideman GB, Bell WH, Legan HL, et al. Cephalometric analysis of dentofacial normal. Am J Orthod 1980;74:404-420.
23. Solow B, Tallgren A. Head posture and craniofacial morphology. Am J Phys Anthropol 1976;44:417-436.
24. Steiner CC. The use of cephalometrics as an aid to planning and assessing orthodontic treatment. Am J Orth 1960;46;721.
25. Merrifield LL. The profile line as an aid in critically evaluating facial esthetics. Am J Orthod 1966;52:804-822.
26. Wolford LM, Hilliard FW, Dugan DJ. Surgical Treatment Objective: A Systematic Approach to the Prediction Tracing. St. Louis, Mosby 1985.

27. Ricketts RM. Cephalometric analysis and synthesis. Angle Orthod 1961;31:141-156.
28. Jacobson A. Radiographic Cephalometry. From Basics to Video Imaging. Chicago, Quintessence, 1995, pp. 243-253.
29. Steiner CC. Cephalometrics as a clinical tool. In: Vistas in Orthodontics, Kraus BS, Riedel RA, eds. Philadelphia, Lea and Febiger, 962.
30. Downs WB. Analysis of the dentofacial profile. Angle Orthod 1956;26:191-211.
31. Holdaway RA. A soft tissue cephalometric analysis and its use in orthodontic treatment planning: Part I. Am J Orthod 1983;84:1-28.
32. Holdaway RA. A soft tissue cephalometric analysis and its use in orthodontic treatment planning: Part II. Am J Orthod 1984;85:279-293.
33. Zide BM, McCarthy J. The mentalis muscle: an essential component of chin and lower lip position. Plast Reconstr Surg 1989;83:413.
34. Jacobson A. Radiograpic Cephalometry. From Basics to Video Imaging. Chicago, Quintessence, 1995, pp. 69-71.
35. Bütow KW, van der Walt PJ. The "Stellenbosch" – triangle analysis of postero-anterior and basilar cephalograms. J Dent Assoc South Afr 1981;36:461.
36. Bütow KW, van der Walt PJ. The use of the triangle analysis for cephalometric analysis in three dimensions. J Maxillofac Surg 1984;12:54-62.
37. Reyneke JP. Surgical technique, Chapter 5. In: Essentials in Orthognathic Surgery, 2nd ed. Chicago, Quintessence, 2014.

Chapter 3

1. McNeil RW, Profitt WR, White RW. Cephalometric prediction for orthognathic Surgery. Angle Orthod 1972;42:154-164.
2. Wolford LM, Hilliard FW, Dugan DJ. Surgical Treatment Objective: A Systematic Approach to the Prediction Tracing. St. Louis, CV Mosby, 1985.
3. Epker BN, Stella JP, Fish LC. Dentofacial Deformities – Integrated Orthodontic and Surgical Correction, 2nd ed. St. Louis, CV Mosby, 1995.
4. Proffit WR, Epker BN. Treatment planning for dentofacial deformities. In: Surgical Correction of Dentofacial Deformities, Bell WH, Proffit WR, White RP, eds. Philadelphia, WB Saunders, 1980, pp. 183-197.
5. Ricketts RM. Planning treatment on the basis of the facial pattern and an estimate of its growth. Angle Orthod 1957;27:14.
6. Legan HL, Burstone CJ. Soft tissue cephalometric analysis for orthognathic surgery. J Oral Surg 1980;38:744-751.
7. Bell WH, Dann JJ. Correction of dentofacial deformities by surgery in the anterior part of the jaws: a study of stability and soft tissue changes. Am J Orthod 1973;64:162.
8. McDonnell JP, McNeil RW, West RA. Advancement genioplasty: a retrospective cephalometric analysis of osseous and soft tissue changes. J Oral Surg 1981;39:505.
9. Bell WH. Correction of mandibular prognathism by mandibular setback and advancement genioplasty. Int J Oral Surg 1981;10:221.
10. Scheideman GB, Legan HL, Bell WH. Soft tissue changes with combined mandibular setback and advancement genioplasty. J Oral Surg 1981;39:505.
11. Bell WH, Galaghar DM. The versatility of genioplasty using a broad pedicle. J Oral Maxillofac Surg 1983;41:763.
12. Galaghar DM, Bell WH, Storum KA. Soft tissue changes associated with advancement genioplasty performed concomitantly with superior repositioning of the maxilla. J Oral Maxillofac Surg 1984;42:238.
13. Epker BN, Fish LC. Definitive immediate presurgical planning. In: Epker BN, Fish LC, eds. Dentofacial Deformities – Intergrated Orthodontic and Surgical Correction, Vol 1. St. Louis, Mosby, 1986, pp. 103-127.
14. Park HS, Ellis E, Fonseca RS, et al. A retrospective study of advancement genioplasty. Oral Surg Oral Med Oral Pathol 1989;67:481-489.
15. Reyneke JP, Van Eeden SP. Skeletal and soft tissue changes following advancement genioplasty. J Dent Assoc S Africa 1993;48:627-630.
16. Hohl TH, Epker BN. Macrogenia, a study of treatment results, with surgical recommendations. J Oral Surg 1976;41:545-552.
17. Wessberg GA, Wolford LM, Epker BN. Interpositional genioplasty for the short face. J Oral Surg 1980;38:584.

Chapter 4

1. Bell WH, Proffit WR, White RP. Surgical Correction of Dentofacial Deformities. Philadelphia, Saunders, 1980, pp. 1210-1280.
2. Epker BN. Esthetic Maxillofacial Surgery. Philadelphia, Lea and Febiger, 1994, pp. 4-19.
3. Sullivan SM. Genial procedures. In: Oral and Maxillofacial Surgery. Fonseca RJ, ed. Philadelphia, WB Saunders, 1999, pp. 7-10.
4. Epker BN, Stella JP, Fish LC. Dentofacial deformities. Integrated Orthodontic and Surgical Correction, Vol I, 2nd ed. St. Louis, Mosby, 1994.
5. Reyneke JP, Johnson T, van der Linden WJ. Screw osteosynthesis compared with wire osteosynthesis in advancement genioplasty: a retrospective study of skeletal stability. Br J Maxillofac Surg 1997;35:352-356.
6. Bell WH, Brammer JA, McBride KL, et al. Reduction genioplasty: surgical techniques and soft tissue changes. Oral Surg Oral Med Oral Pathol 1981;51:471.
7. Hinds EL, Kent JN. Genioplasty. The versatility of

horizontal osteotomy. J Oral Surg 1969;27:690-700.
8. Totonchi A, Molavi S, Guyuron B. Osseous genioplasty. In: Orthognathic Surgery – Principles, Planning and Practice, Naini FB, Daljit SG, eds. London, Wiley Blaskwell, 2016.
9. Precious DS, Armstrong JE, Morais D. Anatomical placement of fixation devices in genioplasty. Oral Surg Oral Med Oral Pathol 1992; 73:2-8.
10. Reyneke JP, Sullivan SM. A simplified technique of genioplasty with simultaneous widening or narrowing of the chin. J Oral Maxillofac Surg, 2001;59:1244-1245.

Chapter 5

1. Park HS, Ellis E, Fonseca RS, Reynolds ST, Mayo KH. A retrospective study of advancement genioplasty. Oral Surg Oral Med Oral Pathol 1989;67:481-489.
2. Converse JM, Wood-Smith D. Horizontal osteotomy of the mandible. Plast reconstr Surg 1964;34:464-471.
3. Davis WH, Davis CL, Daly BW, Taylor C. Long-term bony and soft tissue stability following advancement genioplasty. J Oral Maxillofac Surg 1988;46:731.
4. Kawamoto H, Foster CA, Tolleth H, Wolfe SA. Panel discussion. Finesse in genioplasty. Aesth Surg J 1999;19:141-147.
5. Cohen SR, Mardach OL, Kawawata HK. Chin disfigurement following removal of alloplastic chin implants. Plast Reconstr Surg 1991;88:62-67.
6. Guyyron B, Raszewski RL. A critical comparison of osteoplastic and alloplastic augmentation genioplasty. Aesthetic Plast Surg 14:1990.
7. Peled IJ, Wexler MR, Ticher S, et al. Mandibular resorbtion from silicone chin implants in children. J Oral Maxillofac Surg 1986;44:346.
8. Robinson M, Shuken R. Bone resorbtion under plastic chin implants. J Oral Surg 1969;27:116.
9. Friedland JA, Coccano PJ, Converse JM. Retrospective cephalometric analysis of mandibular bone absorbtion under silicone rubber chin implants. Plast Reconstr Surg 1976;57:144.
10. Bell WH, Brammer JA, McBride KL, Finn RA. Reduction genioplasty: surgical techniques and soft tissue changes. Oral Surg, Oral Med, Oral Pathol 1981;52:471.
11. Putman JM, Donovan MG. Modified reduction genioplasty. J Oral Maxillofac Surg 1989;47:200.
12. Hohl T, Epker BN. Macrogenia: a study of tissue changes with surgical recommendations. Oral Surg 1976;41:545-67.
13. Precious DS, Delaire J. Correction of anterior mandibular vertical excess: the functional genioplasty. Oral Surg Oral Med Oral Pathol 1988;59:229.
14. Epker BN. Esthetic Maxillofacial Surgery. Philadelphia, Lea & Febiger 1994, pp. 58-67.
15. Wessberg GA, Wolford LM, Epker BN. Interpositional genioplasty for the short face syndrome. J Oral Surg 1980;38:584.
16. Rosen HM. Surgical correction of the vertical deficient chin. Plast Reconstr Surg 1988;81:247.
17. Calhoun KH. Aesthetic Lip Surgery: Surgery of the Lip. New York, Theime Medical Publishers, 1992, pp. 74-83.
18. Stucker FJ Jr. Reduction cheiloplasty. An adjunctive procedure in the black rhinoplasty patient. Arch Otolaryngol Head Neck Surg 1988;114:779.
19. Turvey TA, Epker BN. Soft tissue procedures adjunctive to orthognathic surgery for improvement of facial balance. J Oral Surg 1974;32:572.
20. Epker BN, Stella JP. Systematic aesthetic evaluation of the neck for cosmetic surgery. In: Cosmetic Oral and Maxillofacial Surgery. Oral and Maxillofacial Surgery Clinics of North America. Philadelphia, WB Saunders, 1990.
21. Elan MV, Berkowitz F. Submental and submandibular lipectomy by liposuction surgery. Am J Cosmet Surg 1988;2:3.
22. Chee LF, Fei YJ. Surgical correction of masseter muscle approach. J Oral Maxillofac Surg 1989;48:883.
23. Roncevic R. Masseter muscle hypertrophy. Aetiology and therapy. J Maxillofac Surg 1986;14:344.
24. Romano JJ, Wellizz T, Manson PN, Hiff NT. Experience with porous high density polyethylene implants in 97 patients with facial fractures. Intl Symp Plast Surg 1990;1-7.

Chapter 6

1. Sullivan SM. Genial procedures. In: Oral and Maxillofacial Surgery, Fonseca RJ, ed. Philadelphia, WB Saunders 1999, pp. 112-114.
2. Posnick JC. Avoiding pitfalls during chin surgery. In: Orthognathic Surgery Principles and Practice, Vol 2, Posnick JC, ed. New York, Elsevier, 2014.
3. Lindquist CC, Obeid G. Complications of genioplasty done alone or in combination with sagittal split ramus osteotomy. Oral Surg Oral Med Oral Pathol 1988;66:13-16.
4. Zide BM, McCarhy J. The mentalis muscle: an essential component of chin and lower lip position. Plast Reconstr Surg 1989;83:413.
5. Schendel SA, Delaire J. Facial muscles: form, function, and reconstruction in dentofacial deformities. In: Surgical Correction of Dentofacial Deformities, Bell WH, Proffit WR, White RP, eds. Philadelphia, WB Saunders, 1980, pp. 259-280.
6. Mercuri L, Laskin DM. Avascular necrosis after anterior horizontal augmentation genioplasty. J Oral Surg 1977;35:413.
7. Trauner RT, Obwegeser H. The surgical correction of mandibular prognathism and retrognathia with consideration of genioplasty. Part I: surgical procedures to correct mandibular prognathism and reshaping of the chin. Oral Surg Oral Med Oral Pathol 1957;10:677.
8. Reyneke JP. Genioplasty. In: Essentials in Orthognathic Surgery. Chicago, Quintessence, 2014.

www.ingramcontent.com/pod-product-compliance
Lightning Source LLC
Chambersburg PA
CBHW041324210926
51847CB00003B/38
9781948083133